Nursing Care
of Adolescents

Nursing Care
of Adolescents

Jeanne Howe, R.N., Ph.D.

Associate Professor
School of Nursing and Health Sciences
Western Carolina University

McGraw-Hill Book Company

New York St. Louis San Francisco Auckland Bogotá Düsseldorf
Johannesburg London Madrid Mexico Montreal New Delhi
Panama Paris São Paulo Singapore Sydney Tokyo Toronto

NOTICE

Medicine is an ever-changing science. As new research and clinical experience broaden our knowledge, changes in treatment and drug therapy are required. The editors and the publisher of this work have made every effort to ensure that the drug dosage schedules herein are accurate and in accord with the standards accepted at the time of publication. Readers are advised, however, to check the product information sheet included in the package of each drug they plan to administer to be certain that changes have not been made in the recommended dose or in the contraindications for administration. This recommendation is of particular importance in regard to new or infrequently used drugs.

NURSING CARE OF ADOLESCENTS

1 2 3 4 5 6 7 8 9 0 D O D O 7 8 3 2 1 0 9

Library of Congress Cataloging in Publication Data

Main entry under title:

Nursing care of adolescents.

    Bibliography: p.
    Includes index.
    1. Youth—Diseases—Nursing. 2. Youth—Health and hygiene. I. Howe, Jeanne.
RJ550.N87   610.73   79-13413
ISBN 0-07-030585-4

This book was set in Times Roman by Offset Composition Services, Inc.
The editor was David P. Carroll and the production supervisor was Nancy Parisotti.
The cover was designed by John Hite.
R. R. Donnelley & Sons Company was printer and binder.

To Marie Josberger,
who, during the preparation
of this book,
made a silk-purse friendship
out of sow's-ear adversity

Contents

List of Contributors

ANNE ALTSHULER, R.N., M.S.
Clinical Nurse Specialist
University of Wisconsin Hospitals;
Associate Clinical Professor
University of Wisconsin
Madison, Wisconsin

MARY ANN ANGLIM, R.N.,
  M.Ed.
Assistant Professor
Formerly Research Associate, Home
  Care for the Child with Cancer
School of Nursing
University of Minnesota
Minneapolis, Minnesota

PHYLLIS J. BALDWIN, R.N.,
  M.S.N.
Clinical Director of Psychiatric
  Nursing
University of Michigan Hospital
Ann Arbor, Michigan

SUSAN ANN CLEMEN, R.N.,
  M.P.H.
Associate Professor
Community Health Nursing Graduate
  Program
School of Nursing
University of Michigan
Ann Arbor, Michigan

CAROL J. DASHIFF, R.N., C.S.,
  Ph.D.
Associate Professor
School of Nursing
University of Alabama in Birmingham
Birmingham, Alabama;
Formerly Clinical Nurse Specialist
Private Practice in Psychiatric-Mental
  Health Nursing
Tallahassee, Florida

ELIZABETH FITZPATRICK, R.N.,
  S.N.P.
Formerly Medical Services
  Coordinator
Office of Youth Services
Department of Corrections
State of Colorado
Denver, Colorado

DOROTHY P. GEIS, R.N., M.Ed.
Formerly Research Associate and
  Project Director in Charge of
  Service, Home Care for the Child
  with Cancer
School of Nursing
University of Minnesota
Minneapolis, Minnesota

EVANGELINE C. GRONSETH,
  R.N., Ph.D.
Assistant Professor and Research
  Associate, Home Care for the Child
  with Cancer
School of Nursing
University of Minnesota
Minneapolis, Minnesota

LEONA J. HAVERKAMP, R.N.,
  P.H.N., S.N.P.
Staff Nurse
Cedar Rapids Community Schools
Cedar Rapids, Iowa;
President, Iowa School Nurse
  Organization;
Director, National Association of
  School Nurses

SUSAN HILDEBRAND, R.N., M.S.
Clinical Nurse Specialist, Private
  Practice
Parent-Child Consultation
Bonner Springs, Kansas

JEANNE HOWE, R.N., Ph.D.
Associate Professor
School of Nursing and Health
  Sciences
Western Carolina University
Cullowhee, North Carolina

JUDITH B. IGOE, R.N., M.S.
Associate Professor and Program
  Director, School Nurse Practitioner
  Program
Schools of Nursing and Medicine
University of Colorado
Denver, Colorado

SALLY A. JULIEN, R.N.
Washtenaw County Community
  Mental Health Center
Ann Arbor, Michigan

ROSEMARIE B. KING, R.N., M.S.
Assistant Director of Nursing
Rehabilitation Institute of Chicago
Chicago, Illinois

RITA BAYER LEYN, R.N.,
  M.N.Ed.
Formerly Nurse Consultant
Community Human Services
Pittsburgh, Pennsylvania

IDA M. MARTINSON, R.N., Ph.D.,
  F.A.A.N.
Professor and
  Director of Research
Principal Investigator, Home Care for
  the Child with Cancer
School of Nursing
University of Minnesota
Minneapolis, Minnesota

PEGGIE J. MOYER, R.N., M.S.
Director of Nursing
Children's Hospital
Santa Rosa Medical Center
San Antonio, Texas;
Formerly Assistant Director
University Health Service
University of Georgia
Athens, Georgia

SALLY WINN NICHOLSON, R.N.,
   Ph.D.
Professor and Assistant to
   the Dean
College of Nursing
University of North Carolina at
   Charlotte
Charlotte, North Carolina

JUDI ODIORNE, R.N., M.S.N.
Director of Nursing
Department of Child Psychiatry
Mount Carmel Mercy Hospital and
   Medical Center;
Associate Professor
Department of Child and Adolescent
   Mental Health Nursing
Wayne State University
Detroit, Michigan

ANN WIZINSKY PATTULLO,
   R.N., M.N.
Program Director for Nursing
Institute for the Study of Mental
   Retardation and Related
   Disabilities;
Associate Professor
School of Nursing
University of Michigan
Ann Arbor, Michigan

ELIZABETH RANDALL-DAVID,
   R.N., M.A.
Formerly Executive Director
Gainesville Women's Health Center
Gainesville, Florida

RAE SEDGWICK, R.N., Ph.D.
Private Clinical Practice
Individual-Family Therapy
Bonner Springs, Kansas

SUSAN M. STRAWN, R.N., B.S.N.
Head Nurse, Pediatric Unit
Rehabilitation Institute of Chicago
Chicago, Illinois

CAROL TENEROWICZ, R.N.,
   M.S.N.
Assistant Professor
Department of Psychiatric Mental
   Health Nursing
Wayne State University
Detroit, Michigan

JANE WENTWORTH, Ph.D.
Assistant Professor
Community and Public Health
   Nutrition
Department of Human Nutrition and
   Food
Virginia Polytechnic Institute and
   State University
Blacksburg, Virginia

DEE WILLIAMS, R.N., C.S., M.N.
Clinical Specialist
Community Alcohol Program
North Central Florida Community
   Mental Health Center
Gainesville, Florida

PATRICIA S. YAROS, R.N., M.N.
Doctoral Student
College of Nursing
Wayne State University
Detroit, Michigan

Preface

It is past time for adolescence to come into its own as a health care specialty. I hope this book will give impetus to that development.

I do not intend by those statements to minimize the facts that there are nurses, physicians, and practitioners of other health disciplines who already specialize quite competently in the care of adolescents and that some have done so for a long time. Many of the authors of this book are just such specialists, in fact, and their chapters reveal a well-developed framework for practice and carry the ring of authenticity that comes only from extensive, effective clinical experience. But there are about 48 million people between the ages of 10 and 21 in the United States alone—between a fourth and a fifth of the population—and if health services are going to be adapted on a suitably large scale to serve this age group, the health professions' *education programs* are going to have to acknowledge adolescence as a specialty and teach about it. Some schools of nursing do offer either undergraduate or graduate courses in the care of adolescents, and some nurse practitioner programs also teach about adolescents as a special group of nursing care clients. Faculty and students in such courses generally have had to manage without the assistance a textbook can provide, and I believe still other nurse educators have been discouraged from allotting adolescence a place of its own in their curricula because there has not been an adequate text to support the teaching and learning of nursing care of young people. It is my hope that this book will meet that need and encourage the proliferation of educational offerings in the clinical care of adolescents.

A second purpose of the book is to assist students and practicing nurses who wish to improve the quality of their nursing care for young people. This objective is undertaken in two ways, with two rather different types of chapters. The first 11 chapters describe adolescents themselves. Each chapter deals with one substantive topic related to adolescent health: growth and development, the nurse-adolescent relationship, health assessment, responses to illness and disability, nutrition, drugs, mental retardation, sexuality, crisis, death and dying, and health teaching and counseling. These chapters help the student or practitioner understand adolescent behavior and both physical and psychosocial development, particularly as they pertain to health and health care. The last 10 chapters describe health care delivery: programs, services, physical facilities, personnel, interface with the community, and issues such as the ethics of treating minors. These chapters discuss a broad range of settings in which adolescents receive health care: general hospital, rehabilitation center, free "street" clinic, school, college health service, drug detoxification and rehabilitation centers, women's health clinic, mental health counseling service, juvenile detention facility, and psychiatric inpatient setting. The health needs and other characteristics of the subgroups of adolescents who seek services in each setting are presented, as are effective ways of organizing and operating the facilities to optimize health care for young people.

The book has been influenced by a number of my personal beliefs—about books as well as about adolescence and nursing. First, the people who write professional books absolutely must know what they are talking about. Knowledge has expanded so terrifically in recent years that texts on all but the narrowest topics must be collaboratively prepared. In order to collect truly excellent, up-to-date material about each of the subtopics I wanted to include in this book, I have used a multiauthor approach. The 25 other nurses and one nutritionist who have written the book were selected for their expertness as practitioners and for their ability to share their specialized knowledge and demonstrate its application by clinical examples. These women have been an exciting and gratifying group to work with, and I am very pleased to be able to provide the vehicle for making their knowledge available to a wide audience.

Second, I believe that the teaching and practice of nursing are the responsibility and prerogative of *nurses*. It follows that nursing texts should be written by nurses, except when there is a very good reason for having someone else do the writing. This book conforms to that belief.

I also believe there is little justification for producing a new book that duplicates content that is already adequately available elsewhere. Accordingly, this book includes so-called medical model information (pathology, etiology, symptomatology, pharmacology, etc.) only where that kind of material is needed, such as in the chapter that discusses physical assessment. Nor is this another book about adolescents' illnesses or the application of the nursing process in the care of young people with specific health disorders. Readers seeking those kinds of information are referred to *Comprehensive Pediatric Nursing*, by Gladys Scipien et al., and to the *McGraw-Hill Handbook of Clinical Nursing*.

I think of adolescents as people whose destiny, unless they are dying, is adulthood. A successful adolescence, then, is one that (among other things) equips a young person for a successful adult life. Mental and physical health enormously affect the quality of living for young people as well as adults. Nursing as presented throughout this book, therefore, includes helping adolescents to develop abilities and attitudes that facilitate their optimal health not only while they are teenagers but also in later life. Adolescence is the ideal time for learning to make informed decisions about matters affecting one's health and for preparing for a lifelong role as health care consumer. The book deals to a considerable extent with active nursing interventions designed to promote health-seeking behavior and help clients become able to claim and wisely use their rightful functions as decision-makers and responsible participants in their own care.

A related bias is my belief that all people, not just ill or disabled people, are candidates for nursing care. The nursing of well persons is directed at helping them stay well, and nursing care for all people includes helping them learn to maneuver to their own best advantage as consumers in the health care system. The provision of therapeutic services for the developmentally deviant, ill, injured, and handicapped is the other segment of nursing practice addressed in this book. Identification and care of the young person whose physical or mental health or development is suboptimal are examined throughout the book in a way that emphasizes who the young person *is*, and what constitutes effective nursing care and why.

Two additional explanatory remarks are in order here. One is that, somewhat to the chagrin of the photographers who asked whom they should and should not photograph and of those authors who sought my guidance about whom they should and should not write about, I have adhered to no specific age limits to define who is and who is not an adolescent. Adolescence is better delimited by physical and social phenomena than by chronological age, and its termination is even more difficult to specify than its beginning. My general objective in putting the book together has been to deal with the part of the life span that begins approximately with the physical or sociocultural onset of pubescence and gradually resolves with the establishment of an adult physique and an adult life-style (however that is defined in any particular subculture). The second comment I want to make is that the photographs used throughout the book, and particularly the statements that accompany them, are of my own selection; in no case should the chapter authors be criticized for that material.

I thank Sally Barhydt for her generous and capable counsel and enthusiasm while the book was being planned; Gladys Scipien, Martha Barnard, Marilyn Chard, and Patricia Phillips for their encouragement and suggestions; Molly Dougherty and Carolyn Stoll for their assistance in recommending authors; and my Western Carolina University colleagues for their interest in this work and for the patience and support they extended to me during the book's preparation.

Jeanne Howe

Nursing Care
of Adolescents

Chapter 1

Growth and Development

Sally Winn Nicholson

To provide effective nursing for any person, it is important to know where the person is developmentally. With no group is such knowledge more important than with adolescents. The teenage years are a period of developmental crisis. Perhaps there is no other phase of the life span in which people are called upon to adjust to so many personal changes at one time. Adolescence is a period of great physical growth accompanied by hormonal changes that alter not only physical structure but also thoughts, desires, and emotions. Following the relatively quiescent period of late childhood, when the world seemed under control, these changes inevitably disrupt the young person's self-concept—the sense of who and what kind of person he or she is. However longed for the signs of physical maturity are, they signal not only the beginning of desired maturity but also the end of the comfortable period of childhood. The attractiveness of the Peter Pan fable is not surprising.

All of the changes that characterize adolescence—physical, social, psychological, and cognitive—interact and compound one another. Despite this, it is necessary to look at each before the interacting whole can

1

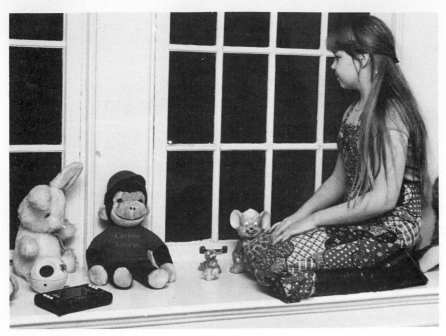

The onset of adolescence brings both welcome and anxiety-producing new opportunities and capabilities. It also forces the child and significant others to relinquish many established patterns of behavior. (*Copyright © 1980 by Patricia Yaros.*)

be understood. Consequently, this chapter will deal with the following subparts of adolescent development: the rhythm and timing of the beginning of the growth spurt, physical changes that take place, psychosocial development, changing self-concept, role in the peer group, cognitive development, and relationships with adults.

Some definitions are in order. There is rather general agreement that *puberty* is the point in life at which a person becomes physically capable of reproduction, i.e., the time at which mature sex cells begin to be produced. The period that precedes puberty, during which rapid growth occurs and the secondary sex characteristics begin to appear, is called *pubescence*.

On the meaning of *adolescence* there is less agreement. In his classical work on adolescent psychology, G. Stanley Hall in 1904 described adolescence as "a period of storm and stress beginning with puberty and ending when full adult status is reached."[1] A problem with this definition is that the period is described as beginning with a physiologic event and ending with a psychologic or sociologic one. The end point of adolescence, as defined by Hall, is more difficult to identify than the beginning. Does "full adult status" refer to achievement of emotional and financial independence or to legal maturity? If the former, should a 25-year-old graduate student being supported by parents be considered an adolescent? If the latter, should 18-year-olds, legally of age in the United States, be excluded?

Dorothy Rogers describes adolescence as "a process rather than a period, a process of achieving the attitudes and beliefs needed for effective participation in [adult] society."[2] She points out that definitions of adolescence are of several kinds. Adolescence is variously defined as a period of physical development, an age span, a discrete developmental stage, a sociocultural phenomenon, and a way of life or state of mind.[3] The picture is further clouded because some young people who have not reached puberty nevertheless assume the behavioral characteristics of adolescence exhibited by their physically more advanced peers. Also, as has been noted, full adult status is not always attained by the time legal emancipation is achieved.

Throughout this chapter, then, the attempt will be put forward to discuss the changes that constitute the process of adolescence—that is, to describe what happens to transform prepubescent children into adults. It is with some apologies that age referents will be used in many places; although age categories and cutoffs must not be taken as prescriptive for any one individual, they do help to make content more manageable.

RHYTHM AND TIMING OF THE BEGINNING OF THE GROWTH SPURT

The first signal that a child is beginning the countdown to physical maturity is a period of rapid physical growth. This growth rate increase begins approximately two years before the reproductive organs become capable of adult function. The period of maximum growth rate occurs during the year preceding puberty. There is not only an increase in height and weight but also a conspicuous change in body proportions, as the rate of growth varies among the parts of the body. For example, the extremities and neck grow faster than the head and trunk. The young person is apt during the growth spurt to find his or her body less easy to manage than before: Hands and feet seem to be in different places now.

Growth begins, on the average, about two years earlier in girls than in boys. The growth spurt in girls begins between 8.5 and 11.5 years of age and in boys between 10.5 and 14.5 years.[4] From about 11 to 14, girls are likely to be taller than the boys in their age group. After that the boys catch up and are again generally taller and bigger, as they were before the growth spurt.

The Secular Trend

Studies during the past century have revealed that, throughout the period of childhood and adolescence, youngsters have been becoming larger for their age and maturing earlier than children did several years previously.

This *secular trend* has been observed in different populations and cannot be entirely attributed to social and environmental influences. The earlier development has been demonstrated by studies of height, weight, and age at which menarche occurs.

Tanner[5] reports that for the last one hundred years there has been a trend toward earlier growth spurt and earlier menarche. At all ages, children born in the 1930s and 1950s were larger than those born between 1900 and 1910. North American, British, Swedish, Polish, and German data all show similar trends. Many observers attribute this change to better nutrition, but the range of heights for each age has not narrowed as would be expected if the effect had occurred mainly among the undernourished segment of the population.[6]

Another proposed explanation for the secular trend is increasing mobility of populations and a consequent decrease in inbreeding within groups. Tanner reports that some studies have supported this view. However, the change has occurred too quickly for natural selection to be the only explanation. Others have attributed the acceleration in growth to climatic changes, specifically to a gradual increase in world temperature. Mills (in Tanner[7]) predicted that there would be a reversal in the secular trend in the 1940s and 1950s as the increase in world temperature reached a point when the retardant effect of hot climate became dominant. This reversal has not occurred, but current evidence indicates that the secular trend has now stopped.[8]

PHYSICAL CHANGES IN ADOLESCENCE

Maturation during adolescence involves changes in all body systems. The acceleration is first noticeable in musculoskeletal growth.

Bone and Muscle Growth

As was previously mentioned, growth of the extremities and neck is more rapid than that of the head or trunk during early adolescence. This gives boys and girls of this age an awkward, long-necked, leggy look. The hands and feet grow faster than the arms and legs and consequently may seem out of proportion to the rest of the body. These changes require adjustment of the young teenager's perception of self in space as well as of body image (mental picture of one's own body).

During the period of maximum growth, girls may grow 2 to 4 inches per year and boys 4 to 5 inches per year. In the initial phase much of the height increase is due to lengthening of the legs. In middle and late adolescence, height continues to increase at a slower rate, but most of the increment is in length of the trunk. Growth grids are presented in Chapter 5, Figures 5-1 through 5-4.

Skeletal age, also called bone age, is a widely used measure of physical maturity (biologic age). Skeletal age is determined by x-ray examination, usually of the wrist and hand, to assess the maturity of epiphyseal growth. From birth onward until maturity, girls are more advanced in bone age than boys. The more advanced the skeletal age is at the beginning of the growth spurt, the less time there is left for linear growth; hence, girls grow less than boys during adolescence, stop growing earlier, and are shorter at maturity. Bone age is a more accurate method of measuring biologic age than is chronologic age. Boys' maximal rate of growth (*peak height velocity*) occurs at an average bone age of 14 years, and girls' around 12.

Muscle mass and strength begin to increase in early adolescence. In boys, muscle strength may double between the ages of 12 and 16. This increase is usually accompanied by an increase in skill in using the muscles. Girls' strength increase is less. One factor that probably contributes to this sex difference is that less emphasis is placed on young women's muscular strength and skill by society and their peer group. Physical fitness test performances of adolescent girls have shown small, steady improvement in running and jumping since the feminist movement began and fitness and athletic programs in schools have become more available to females.[9]

The growth rates of a teenager's muscle tissue and bone may be different. If so, disproportion between the length of bones and their attached muscles may result. If the muscle grows more rapidly, strength may be diminished temporarily and movements may be slow because more time is needed to contract the longer muscle. On the other hand, if bone length exceeds muscle growth and the muscle is stretched by the longer bone, movements may be tight and jerky.

Changes of Body Proportions

In girls, the pelvis widens while the thorax remains proportionally narrow. In boys the reverse is true. The extremities reach adult proportions so that by late adolescence the length of the lower extremities equals the sitting (crown-rump) height. Since maximum cranial size is reached early, the head's proportion of total body length decreases as other growth proceeds. During late adolescence the lower jaw grows larger and the lips become fuller. The disproportions of early adolescence smooth out. The nose, which has seemed too large, looks as if it fits better.

Fat Distribution and Body Weight

Just before the growth spurt, the amount of subcutaneous fat often increases in both sexes. This common, normal ''plump'' stage is sometimes misdiagnosed as hypogonadism, especially in boys. Actually these heavier boys and girls tend to be early developers, and with the beginning of the growth spurt the boys' subcutaneous fat tends to decrease. In contrast, adolescent girls are likely to add more subcutaneous fat. In late adolescence there is a second and greater increase in weight for both sexes when the relatively slender body of early adolescence assumes the more filled out proportions of the adult. This change is particularly easy to observe in young men and women who play basketball: The coltish freshman becomes the well-coordinated, powerful senior. Boys commonly double their weight between age 10 and 18, and many girls nearly do so. Figures 5-1 through 5-4 present growth norms.

Cardiovascular Changes

The heart, like the other muscles, increases in size during adolescence, more in boys than in girls. The increase is thought to be the result of enlargement in muscle cell size. During the whole period of growth from infancy to maturity, heart rate gradually decreases. The decrease in rate for boys parallels that for girls until about 11 years of age, but after that boys have slower heart rates than girls, and heart rates in adult men are, on the average, lower than those of adult women. Blood pressure rises steadily during childhood. At adolescence the rate of increase jumps, and adult ranges are rapidly reached. There is great fluctuation from day to day, but pressures in the pathological range should not be disregarded. Even one systolic reading greater than 140 mmHg may be a danger sign of future hypertension.

Both hemoglobin level and circulating blood volume increase during adolescence. The increments are greater in boys than in girls. This difference between the sexes is thought to be related to the effect of males' higher testosterone level and greater muscle mass.

Skin and Hair Changes

The skin undergoes changes to assume the greater thickness and toughness that distinguish adults' skin from children's. Both boys and girls develop additional hair on their bodies. Fine hair appears on girls' cheeks and upper lip. Boys begin to grow a beard. In both sexes the activity of sebaceous and sweat glands increases. Acne caused by plugged sebaceous glands occurs in about 85 percent of adolescents. Acne may seem a minor problem to adults, but even one blemish can seem a catastrophe to the young person on whose face it appears. Increased sweating leads to body odor, which is a source of much embarrassment among adolescents.

Changes in Special Sense Organs

The eyes participate in the adolescent growth spurt, lengthening particularly in the axial plane. Consequently, there is an increased incidence of myopia in early adolescence and a worsening of preexisting myopia in teenagers who were nearsighted as children. The rise in incidence and degree of nearsightedness shows a secular trend paralleling that of earlier maturity.[10]

Auditory acuity is on the average greater in women than in men. The standard for audiometric measurement is the hearing of the average 13-year-old girl. From that age on, hearing acuity gradually diminishes. The greater decreases noted in males are thought by some to be related to the higher noise levels in traditionally male occupations and avocations that involve machinery.

Some sex difference in sensitivity to odors seems to develop at puberty. Women's greater sensitivity to musklike fragrances may be an estrogen-induced effect.

Other Areas of Physical Growth

In both sexes the voice changes, becoming lower and more mature, partly because of growth of the larynx. This growth is of course greater in boys as evidenced by the larger Adam's apple, and boys' voice change is more pronounced. The paranasal sinuses reach adult proportions and increase the resonance of the voice. The lower jaw grows and the face lengthens and acquires a more adult appearance. Sometime in late adolescence most young people's wisdom teeth begin to erupt.

The Endocrine Changes of Adolescence

The centrality of the endocrine system to adolescent growth and sexual maturation is unquestioned. However, the precise ways in which the hormones produce these changes (and even the fundamental matter of what it is that initiates pubescence) are still quite poorly understood. The endocrinology literature reflects the historically greater focus on pathology than on the physiology of normal growth processes.

When one thinks of the hormonal changes of the adolescent period, one immediately thinks of those producing the pubertal changes, the gonadal hormones. There are, however, changes in other hormonal systems. These will be discussed first.

Growth Hormone Some investigators report that the amount of growth hormone excreted by the anterior pituitary increases during the growth spurt, but others do not.[11] In any case it is clear that growth hormone, which is a major regulator of growth in childhood, is replaced by the sex hormones as the main impetus for the pubescent growth spurt,[12,13] although growth hormone no doubt remains important.

Thyroid Hormones Thyroid hormones play a major role in metabolism and hence in growth throughout childhood and adolescence. However, the interactions among thyroid hormones and other hormones that affect growth are complex, and the exact functions and importance of the thyroid in adolescence are unknown. The thyroid gland enlarges during adolescence and may temporarily increase some parts of its hormone production.

Adrenal Hormones   The adrenal glands enlarge during the growth spurt. Their production of adrenaline and noradrenaline from the medulla shows a sharp increase around 11 years of age, but the significance of this higher output is unclear.[14]

The adrenals produce androgens and estrogens in both sexes, at low levels throughout childhood and at markedly more rapid rates throughout adolescence. The ovaries and testes, of course, are the major sources of these sex steroids, but the adrenal cortex is the main and possibly only source of estrogen in males and androgens in females.

Insulin   Insulin is obviously important in metabolism and is necessary for proper growth at all stages of childhood and in adolescence, as is demonstrated by the growth failure and delayed puberty of children with poorly controlled diabetes mellitus. Growth hormone evidently requires insulin in order to be effective. The islets of Langerhans increase in size during adolescence.

The Anterior Pituitary Gland   The anterior pituitary increases in weight about the time of puberty, particularly in females. This gland, also called the adenohypophysis, was for many years considered to be the body's "master gland" because its several hormones stimulate other endocrine glands ("target organs") to produce *their* hormones. It is now understood that the anterior pituitary actually operates under the influence of the hypothalamus (neurohypophysis). The hypothalamus and the pituitary are in turn regulated by circulating hormones produced by the target endocrine glands; i.e., cyclic feedback arcs exist to turn the hypothalamus and pituitary "up" or "down" in accordance with the blood levels of the various target organ hormones.

The mechanisms that stimulate the hypothalamus to signal the pituitary to initiate the production of gonadotropic hormones (the hormones that cause the ovaries or testes to secrete *their* hormones) are unknown. It is thought that this triggering depends on the maturation of certain centers in the central nervous system. This maturation may remove some nerve cell inhibition and result in stimulation of the anterior pituitary, possibly through the formation of a gonadotropin-releasing factor in the hypothalamus. Frisch and Revelle have hypothesized that body weight is a critical factor in the occurrence of menarche (and also in the beginning of the growth spurt) and have reported that in their research menarche occurred at essentially the same weight (about 105 pounds) regardless of the age at which girls attained that weight.[15] They speculate that achieving a certain weight produces an alteration in metabolism which in turn increases the hypothalamus's regulated level of ovarian hormones and results in menstruation.

The Gonadal Hormones   The gonads are stimulated by the two gonadotropic hormones from the anterior pituitary, follicle-stimulating hormone and luteinizing hormone. Under the influence of these substances, the ovaries secrete estrogens and progesterone, and the testes produce androgens. The result is maturation of the primary sex characteristics and appearance of the secondary sex characteristics, i.e., sexual maturity.

Primary sex characteristics are those structures directly involved in reproductive function, i.e., the internal and external genitalia. The secondary sex characteristics are the physical signs that distinguish mature members of the two sexes from children and from adults of the other sex but do not play a direct part in reproduction. Secondary sex characteristics of males include pubic and axillary hair, facial hair, and the growth of hair over much of the rest of the body; coarser skin with enlarged pores; changes in voice; increased shoulder breadth, chest depth, and neck circumference; and slight, temporary enlargement of the mammary glands. Females' secondary sex characteristics include increased width and roundness of the hips; more shapely legs and arms; menarche; thicker, coarser skin with enlarged pores; appearance of facial hair on the upper lip and cheeks; breast development; pubic hair; and changes in voice.

The sex hormones, in addition to promoting development of the sex characteristics, also have powerful effects on skeletal growth. Androgens from the adrenals in both sexes are credited with initiating much of the pubescent growth spurt. Conversely, it is the sex hormones (particularly androgens) which terminate growth in height by causing bone age maturity and hence epiphyseal closure and cessation of skeletal growth.

Sexual Maturation

The first sign of impending puberty in girls is the beginning of breast development. Initially, the nipple and surrounding areola become elevated to form what is called the breast bud. Rounding of the hips begins about the same time. Next, pubic hair appears. This hair, coarse and pigmented, is at first straight and located only along the labia. It spreads over the mons pubis and becomes progressively curly and more profuse. Axillary hair develops after pubic hair. Menarche follows, usually about two years after the breast bud appears.[16] The uterus grows and reaches adult size and proportions around age 18 to 20. The clitoris enlarges early in the growth spurt and becomes erectile, probably because of circulating adrenal androgens.[17] The labia also become larger, and vaginal secretions become acidic. Breast development is complete around 15 years of age, with a range from about 13 to 18 years. There is, of course, great normal variation in breast size among adult women; there may also be discrepancy in size between right and left breasts.

The average age of American girls at menarche is 12.9 years, according to Schonfeld,[18] but the age range among healthy girls is wide—quite commonly from about 10 to 16.5 years of age.[19] Menarche is a late event in the adolescent growth spurt, and most teenagers grow only another 2.5 to 3 inches afterward.[20] Although menarche is popularly regarded as the event that marks the beginning of puberty, the first menstrual periods are anovulatory, and reproductive capacity is not achieved for one to three years. By late adolescence the menstrual cycle is usually well regulated.

The first sign of puberty in boys is beginning enlargement of the testicles with enlargement and reddening of the scrotum. The penis grows in length and circumference. Straight, pigmented pubic hair appears and gradually becomes coarser, thicker, and curly, and assumes the adult male distribution. In boys there is no striking event which indicates puberty. Ejaculatory competence is rather widely considered to be the milestone of puberty, but, like menarche, the first ejaculations precede fertility by a year or more. Live spermatozoa and androgens in the urine are indicators of reproductive capacity,[21] but for obvious reasons these diagnostic tests are not done on most adolescent males, and hence the time at which puberty (fertility) occurs goes unmarked. The prostate, seminal vesicles, and bulbourethral glands enlarge and develop to form seminal fluid. American boys experience their first ejaculation, either spontaneously or as a result of masturbation, at an average age of just under 14 years.[22]

The primary and secondary sex characteristics continue to develop through late adolescence in many boys. The period of rapid growth in height and weight lasts longer in males than in females, and, in addition, boys grow at a greater rate during the growth spurt than girls do. This faster, longer-lasting growth is responsible for the usually greater size of adult males in spite of the fact that they are generally later than females in beginning their pubescent growth. On the average, boys in the United States reach full physical maturity between 17 and 18 years of age. The last secondary sex characteristic to develop is indentation of the hairline above the temples.

PSYCHOSOCIAL DEVELOPMENT

Developmental Tasks

Psychologically and socially, as well as physically, adolescents must make the substantial changes which cause them ultimately as adults to be very different from 10- or 12-year-olds. Relinquishing a child's life-style and attaining an adult life-style is the overall developmental task of adolescence. More specifically, the developmental tasks of this phase of the life span include (1) becoming able to provide for one's own requirements (food, shelter, recreation, clothing, etc.), (2) selecting and preparing for a vocation, (3) establishing one's own integrated set of values and beliefs, (4) participating in intimate (mutually self-disclosing, not necessarily sexual) relationships, and (5) pulling together, after the uncertainties about oneself that pervade early and middle adolescence in particular, a stable sense of personal identity. Obviously, these tasks are not all-or-none phenomena that adolescents (or even adults) master entirely or once and for all. But it is useful, for the following discussion, to consider them as

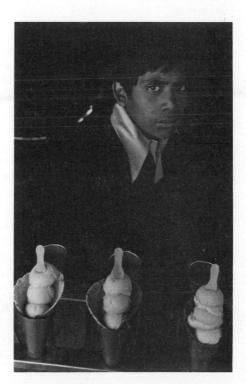

Sociocultural factors heavily influence the age by which the adolescent developmental tasks are undertaken and accomplished. (*Copyright © 1980 by George Lazar.*)

"destinations" toward which adolescents move, for much of the behavior that characterizes teenagers is directly related to their seeking the destinations and can be best understood in that light.

The age at which the developmental tasks are undertaken and accomplished varies enormously from person to person. Also, there is often considerable variation within one young person in the degree to which the several tasks have been achieved at any one time; for example, an adolescent may be quite independent about finances and living arrangements but not equally mature in interpersonal relations. Sociocultural differences may be the major determinants of the age by which developmental tasks are mastered. Living independently from parents typically occurs sooner in low-income families, for example, and occupational preparation is often a longer process among upper-income groups. Health status is also a highly important determinant of the rate and extent of accomplishment of the adolescent developmental tasks, because illness or handicap can complicate independence, identity, sexuality, peer group experience, and the other aspects of psychosocial development (see later chapters).

Sturm und Drang

G. S. Hall described adolescence as comparable to the *Sturm and Drang* ("storm and stress") movement in eighteenth century German literature—a literary movement characterized by idealism, rebellion, self-expression, and suffering. Since then the adolescent years have very often been written about as a period of turmoil and emotional instability. Adolescence is even regarded as "a normal psychosis" by some psychiatrists. These views are believed by others to be the skewed observations of psychotherapists who work with an atypical youth population or who "see" what they expect to see because of their theoretical viewpoint, psychoanalysis.

Many adolescents demonstrate emotional extremes and exaggerated reactions which would be deemed peculiar in either school-age children or adults under the same circumstances but which are normative for teenagers. This extremism is largely attributable to the facts that adolescence does present the growing person with a great many stressful situations and that those situations are often of a kind with which he or she has had little or no previous experience. Hence, behavior often lacks the steadiness that either children or adults show in their interactions with a less rapidly changing world in which they have had longer experience. Under the circumstances, most adolescents actually cope quite well. Those who do demonstrate signs of maladaptation must not be left without mental health intervention because of the mistaken suppositions that it is normal for teenagers to be disturbed or that intervention should be delayed until the developmental stage of "ego fluidity" passes.

Peer Groups

In order to make the transition from childhood to adulthood, adolescents call into question a great many of their old ideas and practices and "try on" many new ones. Because the old ways have been largely acquired from parents and other influential adults, it is a developmental inevitability that adolescents exhibit a certain amount of resistance to parents and most other adults as well as to old ways of thinking and behaving. They do not, however, proceed with their development in isolation; they use one another as the sources and/or evaluators of values, attitudes, and behavior. The peer group thus serves the essential function of enabling young people to lessen their reliance on parents for guidance and approval by providing a kind of social laboratory in which experimentation and new learning can take place. Practice with same-sex peers helps establish confidence to venture into opposite-sex relationships later.

Young and middle adolescents usually demonstrate considerable fervor in their need to be with their friends. When they are not together, they stay in close telephone contact in order to share in what's going on, see how everybody feels about it, and find out how they themselves fit in. Conformity and loyalty to the group are strong, although factions can develop as group members, in the process of testing who they are and what they like, identify and reject behavior they disapprove. Peers are major sources of "feedback regarding normality, . . . emotional support in the struggle for independence, . . . companionship for shared activities, and . . . models of age-appropriate behavior."[23]

Position in the peer group structure has great influence on self-concept. Being different is not generally valued by adolescents. It is important to do the "in" things, such as wearing the popular style of clothing and going to the current hangout. The peer group often defines appropriate behavior quite differently than adults do. In fact, behavior such as doing what everybody else does, considered immature by adults, may be highly regarded and considered mature by peers.[24] By late adolescence, as identity becomes established and young people become more certain about what they believe and how they wish to behave, their need for the peer group lessens and they progress to more adultlike self-reliance and interdependence with one person or a small number of others.

Manaster[25] presents an excellent discussion of aspects of peer group structure and function not covered here, including differences between boys' and girls' groups, subculture groups such as delinquent gangs, socioeconomic differences, and friendship couples.

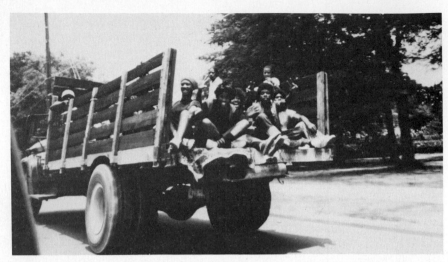

The peer group is the primary social "laboratory" in which adolescents practice and select or reject social roles, values, and specific types of behavior. This young tobacco field crew is no doubt also learning some things about employment that may serve them either well or badly in the future. (*Copyright © 1980 by Patricia Yaros.*)

Early Adolescence

The physical changes of pubescence are accompanied by changes in emotional control and response. Late childhood is generally a rather stable period. The school-age child has reached the peak of childhood development. Prepubescent children are confident about what they can do with their bodies. Their world is dependable and their place in it well established. Pubescence, and especially puberty, disrupt their well-structured world. Their bodies look different to them and react in unfamiliar and unexpected ways. They are no longer children but are unready to function as adults. People respond differently now and have different expectations. As youngsters grow up at different rates, even best friends may develop new interests that separate them from one another and make the things they have shared seem childish.

   In response to all these changes, early adolescents are characterized by wide mood swings. They may be up, up, up one moment and down, down, down the next. Young teenagers are prone to intense daydreaming, and they may take instant exception to any opinion expressed by anyone else. The first year or so of adolescence can be the hardest as far as parent-child conflict is concerned,[26] but the teenager's greatest push for emancipation and hence the low point in parent-child relations is more likely to occur in middle adolescence (about age 14 to 18).[27]

   Twelve-year-olds may retain much of the stability of late childhood. They use humor effectively to criticize friends and family. They generally keep their moods and feelings to themselves but may lash out with name-calling and cutting remarks when their feelings are hurt. Activities are shared mostly with others of the same sex. Girls are beginning to be interested in boys, but mostly as objects of conversation within their small group of girlfriends. They like to meet in someone's bedroom and talk about boys, clothes, boys, makeup, and boys. Boys' activities center around sports and games involving much physical activity. They talk mostly about sports and know the records of heroes in every sport. Youngsters of both sexes value group activities, but it is common to have one special friend of the same sex with whom interests are shared and confidences are exchanged. Pets also may play a very important part in the young adolescent's life, although parents may still have to assume some responsibility for care of the pet. Young adolescent girls are infamous for their fondness for horses.

By 13 or so, most teenagers become more introspective. When their feelings are hurt or they are otherwise upset, they tend to withdraw. Feelings are confided only to special friends. Worry about schoolwork is common and is often expressed either by studying harder or by not completing assignments out of fear of failing to meet one's own or teachers' standards. Certain school subjects may also be rejected as appropriate only for persons of the opposite sex: Boys may consider English, poetry, and French as feminine, and girls occasionally consider themselves unable or "too feminine" to do well in mathematics. As at other ages before college, girls tend to receive better marks in school than boys, probably because girls are generally better socialized to meet the school's expectations.

Throughout early adolescence, television continues to be a popular activity: It entertains, appeals to young teenagers' fantasies of adventure, and gives young people something to do together that does not require social skills they may lack. Many also enjoy reading. Both boys and girls like mysteries; boys also like adventure stories, and girls enjoy romances and biographies of women. Movies are popular with both sexes as group activities, especially films about conflict between generations. Transistor radios are constant companions of many young adolescents, who listen while carrying on almost all activities. Even in study halls there is frequently a radio hidden in someone's lap and an earplug attached. A radio plugged into the ear and inaudible to others can be played at sound levels which cause permanent hearing loss.

School sports activities occupy much of the time of many young adolescents as well as older ones. Until recently, girls have been involved mainly as spectators or cheerleaders. New federal requirements for increased spending for girls' athletic programs are changing this, and court decisions are opening Little Leagues to girls. It will be interesting to see what effects these changes may have on young women's physical strength, skill, and health, and on social behavior.

Another favorite activity is talking with friends. Particularly in early adolescence, and to a lesser extent throughout the teenage years, experiences happen almost constantly which the adolescent feels a need to report to a friend or group of friends. This seemingly endless conversation includes a great deal of both explicit and implied exchange about what is and is not appropriate behavior, and talking in this manner helps orient young people to social norms and expectations and hence increases their self-confidence. Opinions and ideas are exchanged and critiqued by peers. Conversational skills are practiced and improved, and this too enhances confidence and social competence. Much of this talking is done by telephone, which can create strain among parents and their teenage children. Parents may be helped by knowing that this genuine need to be in contact with friends is a developmental trait not unlike others that have caused annoyance in past years and that it, too, will pass. In the meantime, families and their adolescents need to devise ways to solve the problem of family members' never being able to make or receive telephone calls when the teenager is at home. In some households, the teenagers have their own telephone. Other families set definite limits on the number of calls and length of each. If there is more than one adolescent in the family, they are likely to set limits for one another.

By age 14 or so, more activities involve the opposite sex. Boys are beginning to be interested in girls; the girls, however, are likely to be interested in older boys. The first dates are occasions of high anxiety. Boys worry about how to ask for dates and whether they will be accepted. Girls are concerned about being asked and about how to behave during the date. For each, these problems tend to smooth out with practice. Kissing and petting are very likely to ensue if a young couple dates over a period of time, with the extent of sexual activity being related to both partners' cultural and personal values. Girls who date older boys are more likely to become sexually involved than girls who go out with young adolescents.

Sexual maturation is a cause of much anxiety in early adolescence. Youngsters of both sexes experience concern that their bodily changes are going awry and that the outcome will be unsatisfactory. In addition to this general anxiety that they are and will be too small, too large, disproportionate, or otherwise unattractive, young adolescents worry about the functioning of their bodies. Girls may feel that something is wrong if their menstrual periods are irregular. They may fear that they have become pregnant, whether or not they have had intercourse. Even some girls who have had sex education may believe that pregnancy can result from deep kissing or heavy petting, and the fantasies of less well informed girls can be practically limitless. The notion that others can tell when she is having her period can cause a girl embarrassment and uneasiness. Few girls reportedly masturbate in early adolescence, but, whether or not they do, sexual fantasies may be a cause of alarm and guilt.

For boys, erections in public may be a major source of embarrassment, and keeping other people from noticing can become a preoccupation. Boys may be disturbed by the possibility that their mothers will notice that they have had seminal emissions during sleep. Most boys masturbate, and many experience guilt about it or fear that it may damage their health. Information they are likely to read or hear to the effect that masturbation is normal and harmless ''unless carried to excess'' is not very reassuring since ''excess'' is undefined. Adolescents are highly interested in the process of sexual intercourse, and even young adolescent boys worry that they may not be able to perform sexually when the time comes. Size of the penis is another source of anxiety, and jokes about penis size are frequent. Boys also may be alarmed if one testicle is larger than the other or if the two sides of the scrotum do not hang at the same level, both of which are common and normal conditions. One young adolescent reported acute concern about a difference in size of his testicles; he was horrified that a favorite female teacher might read a notation to this effect in his school health record.

Both boys and girls are concerned about the impression they make on members of the opposite sex. Advertisements that imply that certain toothpastes, cosmetics, mouthwashes, scents, or soaps can ensure one's appeal find a prime target in teenagers. The contradictory messages given by advertisements (''You must make yourself attractive'') and by parents, school, and church (''Not yet, you're too young'') contribute to the young adolescent's uncertainty.

Middle and Late Adolescence

The intense narcissistic concerns about physical changes and about entrance into postchildhood sex roles and other social relationships diminish as the adolescent grows and gains experience. Physical growth nears completion, and the earlier questions about whether one's body will attain acceptable height, weight, and sexual characteristics are resolved (although it is usual for adolescents to feel dissatisfied about some aspects of their appearance even if they are objectively well within the norms). Height and weight increase more slowly than in early adolescence, awkwardness and disproportion correct themselves, and eventually adult body configuration is achieved. The secondary sex characteristics are usually mature before the teen years end, but the sex organs themselves may not be fully mature until several years later. Skin problems such as acne and excessive oiliness of the hair usually subside by late adolescence.

If all is going well, the young person is now beginning to assume adult roles quite comfortably so that, by the end of late adolescence, he or she will have mastered the adolescent developmental tasks and will be competent to begin functioning as an adult. Relationships in the family usually improve markedly by late adolescence, both between adolescents and parents and among siblings.

Automobiles often are *not* a focus of family harmony. In most states drivers' licenses can be obtained by 16 years of age. Both boys and girls are eager to acquire this symbol of adulthood. Boys especially feel the need of a car. Despite some softening of sex role delineations in recent years, adolescents still expect boys to provide transportation for dating activities. Having a particular kind of car, whether an expensive late model or an individualized "crate," may carry high prestige. Many boys enjoy tinkering with their cars and developing the knowledge and mechanical skills involved. Automobiles also represent freedom, provide privacy, and give young people access to people and events at some distance.[28] Family members may experience conflict about who will use the family car at a particular time, but on the other hand an adolescent who is licensed to drive can provide a valuable service by running errands such as transporting younger children to and from their after-school activities. Parents' worry about accidents to teenage drivers and their passengers is not without justification: Car accidents are by far the leading cause of death in adolescence.

Many high-school-age youngsters have some sort of summer and/or after-school job. The money they earn may be used to buy longed-for items such as a car, to finance activities, or to save for some future project such as college. Some teenagers pursue earning at the expense of school achievement and needed rest. One young friend of mine, anxious to own both a horse and a car, worked evenings at one job and Saturdays at another in addition to driving a school bus each morning and afternoon. The horse and car were obtained, but little time was left for enjoying them.

The jobs available to adolescents frequently serve mainly as a source of money and do not offer prospects for advancement or long-term employment. Sometimes, however, teenagers can try out parts of a role that attracts them to see if it is an area they wish to pursue. Examples of such jobs include being a nurse's aide, assisting a veterinarian, and doing minor automobile work for a service station. Even jobs without future can be valuable. By being employed, young people glimpse the kinds of effort, responsibility, and cooperation that are involved in working for a living; develop feelings of self-confidence and autonomy; gain practice and appreciation regarding the value of money and the rudiments of money management; gain experience with various kinds of people in various situations; learn more about work's relationship to the other aspects of life and begin to see what kinds of work may and may not be personally satisfying to them; and accrue the enjoyments of having their own money to spend. However, young people may encounter disappointment and disillusionment as they undertake the work role. Jobs may be scarce, especially for the young and unskilled and for members of minorities. Idealized expectations of a particular job, of working in general, or of oneself as a worker may not materialize.

Love relationships either with peers or with others may be painful or ecstatic or both. Adolescent attachments, sometimes dismissed by adults as "puppy love," in fact serve important developmental functions and are very important to the persons experiencing them.

It is not unusual for an adolescent to develop a "crush" on some adult. This older person, perhaps a teacher or a friend, seems to the adolescent to embody all the most desired characteristics and in addition is perceived to understand when parents do not. Peak ages for crushes are 15 to 19 for boys and 13 to 18 for girls.[29] A crush ordinarily lasts from one to six months, but some last longer. This kind of attachment poses no problem unless the adolescent becomes involved with the older person to the point where the adolescent's romantic and/or sexual interests are explicit. Rejection of the youngster's amorous intentions (or failure to recognize them) can lead the young person to depression and extreme behavior. In those rare instances where the older person reciprocates, the situation can become difficult indeed. Adolescent crushes are not to be laughed at; the feelings are intense and, while they last, real to the young person. Crushes can help in the process of selecting characteristics desired in a potential mate. In many societies such relationships are encouraged as a way of learning roles in sexual interaction.

Heterosexual relationships within the peer group move from group dating, in which groups of girls just happen to show up where there are groups of boys, to pairing off at social events after arriving with a group of the same sex, then to group dating in which boy-girl couples participate in social activities with one or two other couples, and finally to single-couple dating. The first two types of group dating are especially favored in middle adolescence because they facilitate getting together for those who do not have cars and for girls who are not permitted by parents to ride with recently licensed drivers. The far less desirable alternative is to be brought by parents, which most adolescents consider highly embarrassing.

Characteristics desired in a dating partner by boys include physical attractiveness, good personality, concern for others, and dependability. Girls value manners, neatness, and ability to carry on a conversation. Of course, there are other qualifications, particularly as adolescents get older and become more diversified in their tastes.

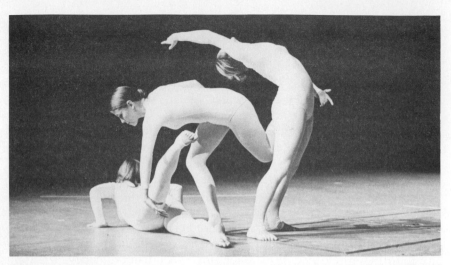

Physical skill, coordination, strength, and beauty are highly desired in adolescence and strongly influence both self-esteem and acceptance by other adolescents. (*Copyright* © *1980 by Anne Campbell*.)

Adolescents tend to see steady dating at an early age as desirable because it provides social security and group acceptance. Parents, on the other hand, are likely to disapprove, partly because they fear that the increased time the couple spends together will lead to sexual intimacy.

Each partner in a dating relationship is concerned about the other's sexual expectations. There may be little discussion between them about this topic. Girls still carry the special burden of the double standard. Boys still as a general rule distinguish "good" from "bad" girls according to their willingness to participate in sexual activity, and they expect the girl to set the limits. Girls, however, wish to avoid being rejected as prudish. Boys may feel that they themselves have a dilemma to deal with because, while they may fear hurting the girl or making her pregnant if they engage in intercourse, they may also fear that they are sexually inadequate if they do not proceed or that they will not meet the girl's expectations.

Pregnancy and sexually transmitted disease are real dangers for sexually active teenagers, and failure to take contraceptive precautions is common. It is not unusual for each partner to think that the other is using some form of contraception. In one such pregnant couple, even though they had planned on marriage at some future date, the young man said, "I don't know her well enough to talk about things like birth control." Both partners also said they had progressed to intercourse because they believed the other expected it. Even among college-age young people, decisions about sexual intimacy and communication about it remain difficult. The following exchange occurred in a university discussion group.

Boy: Look, you girls should know we don't want you to get pregnant
any more than you want to. Why don't you just go to the clinic and
get the pill, or else tell us you aren't so we can do something?

Girl: You just don't know how hard it is to do that. It's going and saying
that we expect to go all the way, that we're planning on it. That's
against all we've been taught. It's supposed to just happen because
you get carried away.

Boy: That doesn't make sense.

Girl: It may not, but that's the way I feel.

Steady dating at an early age, with or without sexual intimacy, unfortunately encourages many young couples to marry before they are
developmentally mature enough to sustain a marriage relationship. Adolescent marriages, especially if contracted to legitimize a pregnancy,
have a high divorce rate. Marriage or pregnancy (or both) markedly disrupts a high school girl's peer relationships and may bring her formal
education to at least a temporary close. Marriage during high school also
ordinarily interferes with a boy's education and career development by
severely limiting his options.

Emotionally, older adolescents are somewhat less labile than when they
were younger. They have achieved more mature ways of interpreting their
experience and expressing their feelings. However, these new responses
and means of expression are more reliable and appropriate, by adult
standards, in some situations than in others.

Anger is a common response to frustration and may be expressed by
moodiness and temper outbursts. Anger is less likely to be expressed by
physical displays (e.g., throwing things) than at earlier ages, but name-
calling and other verbal insults remain common methods of expressing
anger. Anger may be held in and built up longer before it is displayed.
Parents, especially, may be the recipients of temporarily concealed anger
and are often left to guess what their offense has been.

Grief may be deeply felt but concealed as a private emotion. A family
that experiences the loss of a loved one may feel that the adolescent is
untouched because he or she does not cry or show other recognizable
evidence of grief. The adolescent may seek to hide feelings of loss by
making light of the responses of others. This "I'm not too involved"
facade may hide deep hurt. The loss of a loved pet, particularly one that
has been a childhood companion, can also induce grief. Adolescents may
be very concerned about their own inability to show grief in the same
ways as others in their family or group.

Because feelings of inadequacy are common, jealous accusations frequently play a part in affectional relationships. Jealousy between dating
partners may also be interpreted by each as a sign of caring and conse-

quently may be encouraged. In this instance, jealousy may be intentionally provoked and may create difficulties if it is maintained as a pattern for future expectations.

Feelings of personal inadequacy, while practically universal among adolescents, are concealed by many. Worries about career goals, boy-girl relationships, achievement potential, personal behavior, and myriad other things are often hidden behind an apparent "I couldn't care less" attitude, and worried teenagers can have difficulty asking for help. They may approach adults with indirect questions, often about "a friend" who has a problem. Adults who wish to help must be alert to cues while allowing adolescents to state the problem in their own way.

COGNITIVE DEVELOPMENT

The developmental changes that occur in the way children think from infancy through childhood and adolescence have been described by Piaget and his co-workers and followers.[30, 31] The *quality* of cognition changes during early and middle adolescence, and gradually—not all at once—the teenager's thinking becomes free from the cognitive errors and inflexibilities that limit children. By about age 14 or 15[32, 33] the final stage of intellectual maturation is attained and the young person becomes capable of thinking in an adult manner. School-age children (except during excursions into fantasy) are restricted to thinking about things which, from experience, they know to be real or true, but adolescents become able to think hypothetically and deductively and to deal with abstractions.

Piaget labeled this final stage of cognitive growth the period of *formal operations*, because it is characterized by the ability to work intellectually with the *form* or *structure* of a situation or argument rather than being restricted to dealing only with its content. Thus, in the formal operations stage it is possible to reason and make predictions about things beyond one's actual experience or knowledge or even about situations believed to be contrary to fact. Adolescents and adults can think about what *might be* ("What if . . . ," "Suppose that . . .") rather than only about what *is*. Scientific laws and principles become understandable, and the scientific method of forming hypotheses and proceeding logically to test them becomes possible for the first time.

This new quality of thought has several behavioral consequences that are familiar to persons who observe adolescents. Teenagers are able for the first time to be introspective, to think about their own behavior and to "think about their thinking." This inward-looking is no exception to the developmental truism that newly developed abilities are practiced or exercised extensively when they first become part of the developmental repertory, and middle adolescents are typically quite introspective. Elkind[34] has pointed out that adolescents who are thus focused on themselves readily assume that other people are equally interested in them.

During this stage of developmental egocentrism, adolescents thus create an "imaginary audience"[35] and erroneously believe that the people around them are aware of and intent upon the adolescents' every flaw (of character, appearance, etc.) and every strength. This belief accounts in part for the ease with which teenagers become embarrassed over what would seem to adults to be small things. The imaginary audience also explains the ebullience with which an adolescent who is temporarily pleased with himself or herself expects that others also will be quick to admire. The same egocentrism leads to feelings of separateness and even of isolation; adolescents are prone to believe that no one else has ever felt as strongly as they do—been so in love, so embarrassed, so discouraged—and that no one can understand them. These (false) beliefs about being distinctive have been called "the personal fable."[36] The personal fable is credited with some of the risk-taking in adolescence, such as driving recklessly or experimenting with addictive drugs, because an attitude of "it can't happen to me" is part of the fable.

When adolescents become able to conceptualize things as they might be rather than as they are, they easily become intolerant of things as they are and idealistically think up many grand schemes for bringing about change in practically any aspect of life. They may be quite opinionated, overbearing, and irritable as they attempt to bring others' thinking into agreement with their own. On the other hand, partly because formal thinking enables one to envision many alternative possibilities, the rigid and judgmental moral code of middle and late childhood and early adolescence usually gives way by late adolescence to a situational ethic that takes into account mitigating circumstances and tolerates individual differences.

The back side of the coin of adolescent idealism is vulnerability to disillusionment. Seeing that people and institutions fail to live up to all their own principles, teenagers may reject those people and institutions and in some cases more or less completely sever their ties to them.

EARLY AND LATE MATURATION

The age at which a particular child begins the growth spurt and reaches puberty depends on a number of factors including nutrition, body build, and heredity. Early and late development show strong familial patterns. Age ranges for beginning and completing the development of secondary sex characteristics are so broad that the early maturers in any sizable group attain adult body configurations before the late maturers even begin the growth spurt. Adolescents whose bodies undergo pubescent changes much earlier or much later than most of their age-mates are placed in the difficult position of being different at a time in life when differences are poorly tolerated. The timing of maturation is generally more important, psychosocially, for boys than for girls.

The early maturing girls are the first children in their age group to begin the changes of adolescence. Some welcome their approaching womanhood, while others feel conspicuous and embarrassed and may try to hide their new height and breast development by slumping and wearing loose-fitting clothing. Early maturers have the advantages and disadvantages of being regarded as "older" by adults and peers alike. Among age-mates, early maturing girls may be awarded prestige and/or may be talked about and questioned about their experiences with brassieres, menstruation, etc. Early maturing girls tend to associate with older girls who share their new interests and with older boys who are nearer their own maturation level than are the prepubescent boys in their grade at school. These interactions with somewhat older adolescents can enhance a girl's maturity, but she can also "get in over her head" because she is unready to participate in some of their activities and feels pressured to defer to their judgment because they are older. Dating and sexuality may be particularly difficult for early maturing girls to manage because, although they attract the attentions of sexually mature males, they themselves are still psychosocially nearer to childhood than appearances suggest and usually feel little or no sexual urgency and do not understand it in others.

Early maturation is usually considered almost entirely advantageous, and strongly so, for boys. Early maturers tend to excel at the physical activities that are important in the peer-status hierarchy and hence are likely to be popular with other boys (and with girls). Consequently, they take leadership roles and, having done so, tend to retain leadership even after age-mates catch up in growth. Early maturing boys do not experience the embarrassment or ambivalence that early maturing girls may, both because large size and physical maturity are probably universally desired in males and because some of their age-mates (the early developing girls) have already set the precedent for the growth spurt. Early maturing boys relate better to pubertal girls than do less mature boys, and, although they may have to compete with older boys for the attentions of those girls, they do get a head start on later maturing boys of their age. Adults tend to allow early developers more responsibility and independence than they grant less well developed boys the same age. The hazard for early maturing boys is that, because social and intellectual skills usually keep pace with chronologic age rather than maturing as rapidly as physical appearance, other people may expect too much and a boy may be labeled "dumb." Contributing to this difficulty is the possibility that rapid physical growth and psychologic adjustment to it (including perhaps preoccupation with athletics) can use much energy and leave little for school achievement.

Late developing girls certainly may suffer from impatience and anxiety about when they will ever stop being little girls and become more womanly, but late maturity is not nearly the stressor for girls that it is for boys. Late maturing girls are not seriously stigmatized for being small and undeveloped, and they generally get along well both with mature girls their age and with boys who have not yet developed. These girls avoid the awkward phase of being bigger and taller than everybody else in the class. By observing others, they learn a great deal about physical maturation and the social changes that go with it before they have to become involved for themselves. Dating and sexuality are deferred until the girl is older and emotionally better able to adapt to these new experiences, and by that time there is also likely to be somewhat less parent-child conflict about dating. When she is ready to date, there are boys her own age, usually boys she has grown up with and knows, who are ready to go out with her.

Boys whose physical growth and secondary sex characteristics appear late may suffer greatly. Small stature and childish proportions and voice cause great dismay to the boy who sees all the other boys, and the girls too, surpass him in size and maturation. Even younger children pass him by. Since many of the peer group activities involve athletics, in which he cannot compete on an equal basis, and boy-girl interactions, for which he feels ill-prepared and has limited interest, the late maturing boy is likely to be cut off from other boys and girls in his school class. To make matters worse, the more mature boys and sometimes also the girls, because they are still insecure, may make him the object of their teasing. Peers and adults generally regard him as younger than he actually is. Late maturing boys are likely to be acutely concerned about their failure to develop. They may refuse to participate in physical education classes because they feel ashamed of their bodies or because bigger boys make fun of them in the locker room. They may also believe that there is something drastically wrong with them physiologically and may sincerely fear that they will never develop. Nurses should assume that late maturing boys are concerned about their delayed development, whether or not the boys mention it. All such boys need to know that the normal age range for onset of puberty is wide and that final adult height has very little to do with age at which growth occurs. Since age at pubescence and puberty tends to be consistent from one generation to the next within families, it may be very helpful to have late maturers inquire about growth patterns of older relatives; often it is discovered that now-mature men of good stature were also late developers.

RELATIONSHIPS WITH PARENTS AND OTHER ADULTS

The relationships between adolescents and their parents are frequently marked by conflict. Elkind,[37] as well as many others, has described both adolescents and their parents as ambivalent about the adolescent's attainment of the developmental tasks. For example, the teenager wants and does not want to be independent of parents, wants and does not want to be an adult, wants and does not want to be sexually functional, and so forth. Hence, while adolescents eagerly seek some adult privileges and prerogatives, they expect their parents to provide cooking and housekeeping services and pay most of their expenses. They may not want parents to offer advice (except on request) or make demands, and they may wish adults in general to keep out of their affairs, but they may at the same time be unwilling or unable to assume responsibility for the outcomes of their independent actions.

Parents can be quite ambivalent, particularly about their children's developing independence. Parents know that if they have done their job well, eventually their child will largely prefer others as confidants, companions, and sources of support. Adults in their middle years may look forward to completing the period of greatest financial and emotional responsibility for their children and may be pleased that their adolescents, like the parents themselves, are continuing their developmental progress and moving on to a new relationship with one another and new opportunities for personal growth. But, at the same time, something is lost that parents may be quite reluctant to let go. They also are somewhat fearful about entrusting adolescents to their own judgment and giving them freedom to make their own decisions and, inevitably, some mistakes.

Relationships between mother and daughter and between father and son may be particularly strained. Daughters may think their mothers' expectations are unrealistic and unfair. "You don't trust me!" is a frequent accusation. Often there seems to be no correct course for the mother to take. If she dresses according to current style she can be condemned for not acting her age. My sister still remembers her rage when she returned from a visit to discover that in the interim she and our mother had purchased dresses of similar style. The mother who adheres to more conservative styles may be deemed hopelessly old-fashioned. Not long ago I heard a teenager complaining about her mother's purchase of wire-rimmed glasses: "People as old as that don't look right in 'granny' glasses." If her mother asks about her activities, a daughter may think her nosy. If she doesn't ask, she's perceived as not interested.

Fathers and sons also disagree about many things. This is not new: It has been some time since Mark Twain remarked about his amazement

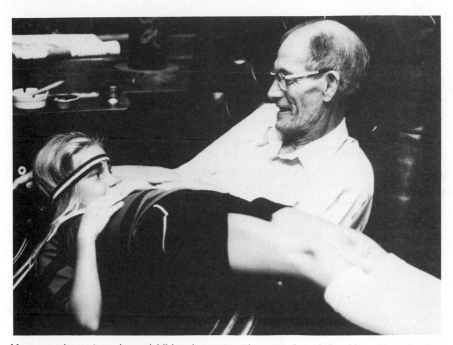

Many grandparents and grandchildren have strongly supportive relationships with each other during these years, when one or both are likely to be at odds with the child's parents over such issues as independence from the middle generation's protection and advice. (*Copyright* © *1980 by Patricia Yaros.*)

at how much his father had learned between the time the son was 17 and the time he reached 21. The family car is a particularly touchy area. Fathers, aware of the high accident rate among males under 25 and worried about the safety of their children and companions, may express concern and set curfews and other regulations. Boys interpret these misgivings as lack of trust in their judgment and ability. Choice of friends and attention to schoolwork are other common topics of disagreement.

Parents read of accidents, alcohol and other drug abuse, teenage pregnancy, and venereal disease among adolescents, and they worry about their children. Their influence on the young people's decisions seems small. They have high aspirations for their children's achievement and opportunity in the world, and they worry that high school grades will be too low to ensure acceptance into college or the job market. They worry about dating patterns. Will their son or daughter be popular? Is he or she settling too early into relationships that may lead to early marriage or pregnancy? Where will the money for college come from? In short, although the specifics vary among subcultures, parents worry about their effectiveness in the difficult job of parenting.

Moreover, the job of parenting children during the "difficult" stage of adolescence often comes at a time in parents' lives which is difficult in itself. During the middle years many men (and women who have careers outside the home) are reaching the peak levels of career advancement and earning power. They are coming to grips with the reality of what that peak is, and it may be lower than their earlier aspirations. They may feel confined by their life circumstances and think restlessly of things they would have liked to do. Those who have built their lives around their children face the time when the children will no longer need them or fill the roles they now do. Already the teenagers are moving more into non-family social groups, and soon the nest will be empty. At this same time in their lives, parents often are faced with their own parents' decline in health and in independence.

But the idea that parents and adolescents are chronically and seriously in disagreement has been exaggerated, for the differences in point of view between the generations are not actually as great as has commonly been supposed. Leichtman[38] notes that the things parents and teenagers quarrel about are generally rather superficial matters, such as hair style, while they in fact share the same basic major values. In those instances in which parent-adolescent conflict *is* more pervasive, Leichtman believes the differences stem from earlier childhood rather than arising in adolescence.[39] Manaster's discussion of family and peer influences[40] includes a review of the pertinent research literature, which indicates that adolescents hold quite closely to their parents' views about issues of major importance although they subscribe to contradictory peer opinion about some of the more transient and less important matters. He summarizes, "It would appear that the great generation gap is really not very great at all."[41]

During adolescence most young people at times turn to an adult friend for advice. They feel a need to discuss things with an adult who cares about them but has less emotional investment, and hence can be more objective, than a parent. If the adult can listen without passing judgment, the adolescent can frequently come to a very reasonable and responsible solution. Siding *either* with the teenager against parents *or* with the parents against the young person must be absolutely avoided if the adult wishes to maintain a relationship with the teenager. Mutual trust is also an essential ingredient of such a relationship, and confidential information must not be shared with parents or others except with the prior knowledge of the teenager. Guidelines for establishing and maintaining effective professional relationships with young people are discussed in detail in the remaining chapters of this book.

REFERENCES

1   G. S. Hall, *Adolescence*, 2 vols. New York: Appleton-Century-Crofts, 1904.
2   D. Rogers, *The Psychology of Adolescence*, 3d ed. New York: Appleton-Century-Crofts, 1977.
3   Ibid.
4   F. Falkner, "Physical Growth," in H. L. Barnett (ed.), *Pediatrics*, 15th ed. New York: Appleton-Century-Crofts, 1972.
5   J. M. Tanner, *Growth at Adolescence*. Oxford: Blackwell Scientific Publications, 1962.
6   Ibid.
7   Ibid.
8   L. Zacharias, W. M. Rand, and R. J. Wurtman, "A Prospective Study of Sexual Development and Growth in American Girls: The Statistics of Menarche," *Obstetrical and Gynecological Survey*, **31**(supplement):325–337, 1976.
9   R. M. Malina, "Adolescent Changes in Size, Build, Composition, and Performance," *Human Biology*, **46**:117–131, 1974.
10 Tanner, op. cit.
11 H. Katchadourian, *The Biology of Adolescence*. San Francisco: W. H. Freeman and Co., 1977.
12 Ibid.
13 J. M. Tanner, "Growing Up," *Scientific American*, **229**(3):34–43, September 1973.
14 Tanner, 1962, op. cit.
15 R. E. Frisch and R. Revelle, "Height and Weight at Menarche and a Hypothesis of Critical Body Weight and Adolescent Events," *Science*, **169**:397–399, July 24, 1970.
16 C. A. Cowell, "The Female Reproductive System," in R. A. Hoekelman et al. (eds.), *Principles of Pediatrics: Health Care of the Young*. New York: McGraw-Hill Book Co., 1978.
17 W. A. Schonfeld, "The Body and the Body Image in Adolescence," in G. Caplan and S. Lebovici (eds.), *Adolescence: Psychosocial Perspectives*. New York: Basic Books, 1969.
18 Ibid.
19 Cowell, op. cit.
20 Ibid.
21 Schonfeld, op. cit.
22 Ibid.
23 S. R. Leichtman, "Psychosocial Development of Adolescence," in R. A. Hoekelman et al. (eds.), *Principles of Pediatrics: Health Care of the Young*. New York: McGraw-Hill Book Co., 1978, p. 639.
24 R. Zosselson et al., "Phenomenological Aspects of Psychosocial Maturity in Adolescence. Part I. Boys," *Journal of Youth and Adolescence*, **6**(1):25–62, 1977.

25   G. J. Manaster, *Adolescent Development and the Life Tasks*. Boston: Allyn and Bacon, 1977.
26   Leichtman, op. cit.
27   A. D. Hofmann, R. D. Becker, and H. P. Gabriel, *The Hospitalized Adolescent: A Guide to Managing the Ill and Injured Youth*. New York: The Free Press, 1976.
28   Leichtman, op. cit.
29   G. Kaluger and M. F. Kaluger, *Human Development: The Span of Life*. St. Louis: C. V. Mosby Co., 1974.
30   J. Flavell, *The Developmental Psychology of Jean Piaget*. New York: D. Van Nostrand Co., 1963.
31   D. Elkind, *A Sympathetic Understanding of the Child—Birth to Sixteen*. Boston: Allyn and Bacon, 1974.
32   Flavell, op. cit.
33   J. D. Douglass and A. C. Wong, "Formal Operations: Age and Sex Differences in Chinese and American Children," *Child Development*, **48**(2):689–692, 1977.
34   D. Elkind, "Egocentrism in Adolescence," *Child Development*, **38**(4): 1025–1034, 1967.
35   Ibid.
36   Ibid.
37   Elkind, 1974, op. cit.
38   Leichtman, op. cit.
39   Ibid.
40   Manaster, op. cit., pp. 235–237.
41   Manaster, op. cit., p. 237.

BIBLIOGRAPHY

American Academy of Pediatrics, Committee on Youth: "A Model Act Providing for Consent of Minors for Health Services," *Pediatrics*, **51**(2):293–296, February 1973.
Bayley, N., and S. R. Pinneau: "Tables for Predicting Adult Height from Skeletal Age, Revised for Use with the Greulich-Pyle Hand Standards," *Journal of Pediatrics*, **40**:423–427, 1952.
Coleman, J., et al.: "Identity in Adolescence," *Journal of Youth and Adolescence*, **6**(1):63–75, 1972.
Elkind, D.: *Children and Adolescents: Interpretive Essays on Jean Piaget*. New York: Oxford University Press, 1970.
Erikson, E.: *Identity: Youth and Crisis*. New York: W. W. Norton, 1968.
Flavell, J.: *Cognitive Development*. Englewood Cliffs, N.J.: Prentice-Hall, 1977.
Frisch, R. E.: "Critical Weight and Menarche: Initiation of the Adolescent Growth Spurt, and Control of Puberty," in M. M. Grumbach et al. (eds.), *Control of the Onset of Puberty*. New York: John Wiley and Sons, 1974.
Gallagher, J. R., et al. (eds.): *Medical Care of the Adolescent*, 3d ed. New York: Appleton-Century-Crofts, 1976.

Grinder, R. E.: *Studies in Adolescence: A Book of Readings in Adolescent Development*, 3d ed. New York: Macmillan, 1975.

Guthrie, D.: "The Endocrine System," in *McGraw-Hill Handbook of Clinical Nursing*. New York: McGraw-Hill Book Co., 1979.

Kagan, J., and R. Coles: *Twelve to Sixteen: Early Adolescence*. New York: W. W. Norton, 1972.

Klerman, L. V., and J. F. Jekel: *School-Age Mothers: Problems, Programs, and Policy*. Hamden, Conn.: Shoe String Press, 1973.

McAnarney, E. R.: "Adolescent Pregnancy: A Pediatric Concern?" *Clinical Pediatrics*, **14**(1):19–24, January 1975.

Muuss, R. E.: *Theories of Adolescence*, 2d ed. New York: Random House, 1968.

Peel, E. A.: "Intellectual Growth during Adolescence," *Educational Review*, **17**:169–180, 1965.

Schwartz, P., and J. Lever: "Fear and Loathing at a College Mixer," *Urban Life*, **4**(4):413–431, January 1976.

Seig, A.: "Why Adolescence Occurs," *Adolescence*, **6**:337–347, 1971.

Tanner, J. M.: "Sequence, Tempo, and Individual Variation in the Growth and Development of Boys and Girls Aged Twelve to Sixteen," *Daedalus*, **100**(4):907–930, Fall 1971.

Walker, D. K.: *Runaway Youth: An Annotated Bibliography and Literature Overview*. Washington, D.C.: Office of Social Services and Human Development, U.S. Department of Health, Education, and Welfare, May 1975.

Wettenhall, H.: "Growth Problems," in J. R. Gallagher et al. (eds.), *Medical Care of the Adolescent*, 3d ed. New York: Appleton-Century-Crofts, 1976.

Whisnant, L.: "A Study of Attitudes toward Menarche in White Middle-Class American Adolescent Girls," *American Journal of Psychiatry*, **132**(8):809–814, August 1975.

Yaros, P. S.: "The Adolescent," in G. M. Scipien et al. (eds.), *Comprehensive Pediatric Nursing*, 2d ed. New York: McGraw-Hill Book Co., 1979.

Chapter 2

The Nurse-Adolescent Relationship

Rita Bayer Leyn

The nurse's goal in relation to the adolescent is to assist the young person in maintaining or restoring physical and emotional well-being. A trusting relationship is a prerequisite to attaining this objective. This chapter discusses ways to form a productive alliance by appealing to adolescents' natural developmental narcissism, by enhancing their receptivity, and by supporting their autonomy. Clinical anecdotes taken from the writer's experiences at an inner-city neighborhood health center* are used to enrich the discussion.

APPEALING TO THE ADOLESCENT'S NARCISSISM

During adolescence, young people become intensely preoccupied with their own bodies and emotions. They hardly recognize their bodies because

*This small ambulatory clinic is operated by nurses. A physician participates in the clinic one day each week and is available by telephone the other days. Patient appointments are scheduled so that persons the nurses believe need to see the physician come on the day he is there.

of the rapid growth and intense reaction to physical stimuli. Surges of aggressive and sexual impulses buffet them. These feelings are difficult for an adolescent to label, and even more difficult to control. The adolescent dwells upon his or her inner tensions in an attempt to understand them and to discover satisfactory means of relieving them. Adolescents focus a great deal of attention upon their bodies and examine their multiple new sensations in an attempt to regain a firm self-image.

This egocentricity need not be a hindrance to the establishment of a productive relationship between adolescent and nurse. Nurses can actually use teenagers' narcissism to advantage, drawing the adolescent into an alliance by stressing their mutual interest: Nurse and adolescent alike are concerned about the adolescent's body and emotions, and the nurse, as a health professional, is committed to preserving the adolescent's physical and emotional well-being. Moreover, the nurse can help adolescents in very tangible ways to care for their bodies and cope with their emotions. If the nurse can convey to the adolescent the benefits to be derived from their interactions, the adolescent will want to maintain their relationship. This appeal to the adolescent's narcissism should not be construed as an act of condescension. The only way to get adolescents involved in their health care is to reach out to them where they are, namely, within themselves. One example of this approach is described below.

> The majority of the adolescents living in the area served by our neighborhood clinic were reluctant to come for routine health maintenance. They ignored my repeated personal invitations to come for yearly physical examinations. Their parents also felt that health care was not a high priority, so they did not insist that their children come for preventive care. I calculated that those who declined to come for physical exams would eventually be forced to do so, because most teenagers wish to drive a car, participate in organized sports, or get a part-time job, and, for all these activities, adolescents in Pennsylvania must have verification of their good health. As anticipated, most of the teenagers who had previously resisted my overtures contacted the clinic for these required physicals. I realized I might have only this single opportunity to engage them in an alliance. Therefore, I decided in this initial interaction to concentrate on areas of health they would find meaningful because of their stage of development. I focused on ways I could help them improve their appearance, augment their physical strength, and be more knowledgeable about their sexuality. Detailed instructions about skin care were given, as was nutritional information appropriate to each adolescent's particular situation, either for gaining or reducing weight. If the adolescent was anemic, and many of these inner-city youths were, the physician prescribed iron medication. I initiated a discussion about sexuality and distributed sex education booklets. The adolescents responded positively to this concentrated attention to their needs. They became more receptive to the clinic's offerings and were willing to return for ongoing health care.

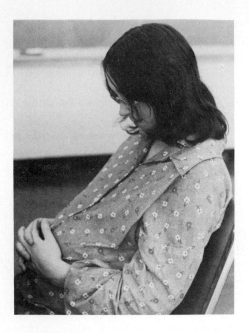

If health care is to be successful, it must focus first on the concerns *the adolescent* thinks are important. Teenage clients must be approached where they are, which is not necessarily where the professional would wish them to be. (*Copyright* © *1980 by Patricia Yaros*.)

The nurse can *arouse* adolescents' interest in health care by pointing out the beneficial aspects of their relationship but can *sustain* adolescents' interest only by supplying some immediate gratification of their needs. It is necessary to help adolescents obtain relief for symptoms and concerns *as quickly as possible*, because they are intensely present-oriented. They feel their needs are urgent and have but slight tolerance for long-term solutions. It is of little consequence to a teenager that a troublesome situation may have existed for some time; the teenager wants it alleviated now. It is not realistic to expect that all the adolescent's problems can be quickly resolved by nursing intervention, but the nurse should be able to draw upon clinical skills to offer some temporary relief. The following clinical anecdotes highlight ways the adolescent's sense of urgency can be placated.

> Judy, 15 years old, came to the clinic with a complaint of acne. She said her skin problems had existed for some time. She was distraught about her appearance because she had an important social event in a few days and wanted help to look more attractive. The physician prescribed a course of antibiotics for this severe case of acne. I instructed Judy about long-term skin care, but I also told her about a special makeup she could apply to cover her blemishes until her skin cleared.
>
> Seventeen-year-old Jackie had severe headaches that, following a thorough diagnostic evaluation, were determined to be the result of tension. Jackie was embroiled in making decisions about his career following high

school graduation, and the headaches occurred when he thought about his plans. He said he had been having the headaches for months, but they had recently gotten worse and he could not tolerate them. I cautioned Jackie that his headaches would probably not go away completely until his plans were finalized, but I also emphasized that there were ways to moderate the intensity of the headaches when they did occur. I taught him methods of relaxation, such as reclining postures and deep breathing, and the physician prescribed analgesics.

To summarize this discussion about appealing to adolescents' narcissism: When the nurse is trying to form a relationship with an adolescent client, it will be found most effective to concentrate on those health needs that are most meaningful to young people at their stage of development. Also, the nurse must supply the adolescent with some immediate benefits as a result of intervention to sustain the adolescent's interest during the initial phase of their relationship.

ENHANCING THE ADOLESCENT'S RECEPTIVITY TO HEALTH CARE

The nurse is knowledgeable about adolescent health and can suggest to the teenager means for improving the teenager's well-being. Nothing is accomplished, however, if these recommendations are not followed. So the plan of care must be presented in a manner that will enhance the adolescent's receptivity to it.

Having worked with the young person to identify objectives for the health care program, the nurse can increase the probability of active participation in working toward their goals by giving the adolescent a detailed explanation of the therapy. This intellectual approach, explaining the rationale behind the care plan, is in alignment with the adolescent's cognitive development. Adolescents can think abstractly and reason inductively and deductively. The nurse demonstrates respect for the adolescent by appealing to the adolescent's intellectual capabilities. This approach also encourages the adolescent to react in a rational manner and to follow the plan of care because it is logical.

It is unwise for the nurse to expect a teenager to adopt recommendations solely on the basis of trust or respect. Such an approach can succeed only if the adolescent forms a strong interpersonal bond with the nurse. Such a tie is not always possible or, of course, in the best interests of either of them. Adolescents may not be highly invested in the relationship with the nurse because of involvement in other interactions, such as realigning their positions with their parents and developing alliances with their peers. It is poor policy to expect compliance from an adolescent based upon emotional commitment. The nurse is on safer (and more ethical) ground when encouraging the adolescent to follow suggestions because they make sense.

Appealing to adolescents on an intellectual level to obtain the adolescents' cooperation in caring for themselves does not mean that the nurse should refrain from expressing personal feelings. Sharing these feelings with teenage clients conveys the nurse's commitment to their relationship and stimulates them to reciprocate by expressing their own viewpoints. Patience is a necessity because adolescents often do not readily confide in adults. However, most adolescents eventually respond with trust to a nurse who authentically cares about their well-being.

Adolescents respond particularly well to an enthusiastic, upbeat approach. Humor can be used effectively with teenagers because they are developmentally capable of understanding sophisticated nuances. Teasing is, of course, not appropriate, but teenagers generally appreciate jokes about such things as mutual misunderstandings. For example, when examining a boil on Donna's face, I asked, "Did you ever have this before?" "Yes, and I couldn't sit down," responded Donna. We both laughed at her reply, and she added, "Sounds like I'm a pretty mixed-up kid."

There are times when the nurse cannot be cheerful in interactions with an adolescent. Frustration and disappointment naturally arise if their relationship is at a stalemate. The nurse should not be reticent about revealing those feelings to the client, but diplomacy is important. Nothing will be gained if the adolescent is made to feel angry or guilty. The nurse should then explain that this concern is caused by caring about the adolescent and feeling frustrated about being unable to be more helpful. A frank encounter can reassuringly show the teenager the depth of the nurse's commitment. The following example shows how the expression of frustration helped to resolve an impasse in interactions with one client.

Sam, age 15, came to tell me that he was having spells during which he felt slightly dizzy, his heart beat rapidly, and his mind went blank for a few seconds. He had had the spells at school on several occasions during the previous weeks. Sam appeared depressed but would not admit to any problem with his family, friends, or teachers. A thorough examination revealed no physical abnormalities. Sam was not relieved when told he was in good health. He felt something was wrong. I agreed with him that he did have a problem. I said I suspected the spells were caused by anxiety and that it would be helpful if he shared his concerns with me. Sam did not respond to the invitation to confide in me, but he did agree to return for another appointment. He came back a number of times, reporting that the spells were still occurring and insisting they were caused by some physical disorder rather than by anxiety. I told Sam I was convinced he was worried about something and that his unwillingness to reveal his concerns was very upsetting and frustrating to me. I said I wanted very much to help and felt angry because he would not allow me to do so. I explained that I felt Sam had something on his mind he had wanted to share with me or he would not have kept coming back week after week, and I emphasized that anything he might say would be kept confidential. Sam then revealed that his first spell had occurred the only time he had smoked marijuana. Because the spells kept returning, Sam felt he was having flashbacks of his drug experience and feared he had permanently damaged his brain. I explained that a single use of marijuana could not cause brain injury and that the symptoms he described were body responses caused by his worrying about the drug rather than by the drug itself. Sam was relieved by the explanation, and, as anticipated, when he stopped worrying about his experimentation with marijuana, his spells ceased.

To enhance the adolescent's receptivity to services, the nurse must take into account the client's family dynamics, because the nurse-patient interactions are in some ways similar to a parent-child relationship, and approaches and responses will be colored by family experiences. The nurse assumes the role of an adult authority figure who both pleases and angers the adolescent client. The adolescent is pleased because the nurse provides the means for maintaining or improving well-being but angry because the therapeutic measures suggested have unpleasant components. The therapy may involve physical discomfort or be time-consuming, and it may require unwelcome self-control. So a certain amount of ambivalence tinges the adolescent's responses to the nurse. The experience of having a love-hate relationship with an adult is not new to the adolescent: The adolescent and the adolescent's parents have been involved in this type of alliance for many years. Therefore, it is highly important for the nurse to gather information about the parent-adolescent relationship. Knowing whether the teenager has been experiencing trustful or distrustful interactions with these other significant adults will provide insights for adaptation of the nurse's role to maximize effectiveness. The nurse should have little difficulty developing a productive alliance with an adolescent who has a trusting relationship with parents if the nurse emulates the parents' methods of interacting with their child. The following anecdote illustrates this point.

Leslie, 13 years old, had a good relationship with both his parents. They openly expressed their affection for him. They fostered his intellectual skills and encouraged him to be self-reliant. He was a patient at our clinic because of numerous allergies. I was outgoing in my encounters with Leslie. I gave him detailed explanations about his allergies and the medications that had been prescribed for him. I encouraged Leslie to assume responsibility for administering his own medications, which he did willingly. He was very responsive to approaches patterned after his positive parent-child interaction.

If an adolescent has a highly conflictual relationship with parents, the nurse can learn from an analysis of the parent-child interaction what pitfalls to avoid in encounters with the adolescent. The following case describes a situation in which interactions with one teenager were successful because they differed from the approach used by the parents.

> Charlene, 16, had a very stormy relationship with her parents. Her natural mother had died when Charlene was a toddler, and her father had remarried shortly afterward. The father took little interest in his daughter, and her stepmother resented this child who was not her own. The parents described Charlene as very negativistic and constantly testing limits. She, in turn, complained that her parents had no affection for her and always criticized her. She came to the clinic complaining of back pain. Her stepmother, who accompanied her, stated that Charlene was probably faking an ailment in order to be excused from swimming class. It was discovered that Charlene had a urinary tract infection, and a course of antibiotics was begun as part of her treatment. She was delighted that her stepmother was wrong and that she had a justifiable complaint. The stepmother countered by saying Charlene would probably not cooperate in taking her medicine. Wanting to be a neutral figure, I avoided denigrating either Charlene or her stepmother and took the positive approach of saying I was confident that Charlene would want to care for her body properly. Charlene and I agreed that I would phone her periodically to be sure she was obtaining relief from her symptoms. From these phone contacts, I learned that she was not taking all the medication prescribed for her. She was not having any adverse reactions from the medicine; she simply didn't remember to take every dose. I did not criticize her, but I explained that she would notice she was not improving and that she would soon realize she could feel much better if she did take all her medicine. Within a few days Charlene phoned to say she was following my advice, and she cooperated further by bringing in a series of urine samples to be tested.

To summarize this discussion about enhancing the adolescent's receptivity: The nurse is best able to elicit cooperation from adolescent clients by giving them a detailed explanation of the therapy; by conveying commitment to the adolescent by being honest when displeased by their progress; and by adapting the approach to the client in light of the adolescent's prior experiences with other adult authority figures.

SUPPORTING THE ADOLESCENT'S AUTONOMY

The nurse tries to present a therapeutic plan that will be agreeable to the adolescent, but a crucial fact to keep in mind is that adolescents should and do have ultimate control over their health care. During adolescence, the young person must abandon a dependent position in relationships with adults in order gradually to achieve a separate identity. Independence is not acquired easily or quickly, because teenagers are impulsive in their behavior and vacillating in their goals. They need support from understanding adults who encourage them to strive for autonomy. The nurse can assist adolescent clients in attaining self-reliance by urging them to assume responsibility for controlling their emotions and caring for their bodies. The nurse supports adolescents' autonomy by making them equal partners in devising plans for their health care and placing with the clients the primary responsibility for carrying the health plan to fruition.

When young people take primary responsibility for their health care, they may exercise their right not to comply with therapy. The nurse, if truly respectful of the adolescent's autonomy, must refrain from using intimidation when the adolescent disagrees with the nurse and should try to identify the reasons for the noncompliance and attempt to resolve the problem; this will not always be successful. Although frustrated by an adolescent's failure to do what is felt to be in the adolescent's best interest, the nurse should not present ultimatums or threaten to discontinue care. It is appropriate to inform the client that although disappointed by the client's decision not to cooperate with the care plan at this time, the nurse is willing to reconsider the situation in the future. The nurse who works with adolescents cannot indulge in carrying grudges. The nurse must put aside the client's previous rejections and offer a relationship free of recriminations. The following reports a nurse-adolescent situation that involved the patient's refusal of recommended treatment.

> My first contact with 16-year-old Marsha was very unsatisfactory. She was being seen for a routine yearly physical. During her entire examination she was extremely negative. She questioned my every action and protested vociferously when her finger was pricked for blood studies. She was deficient in her immunizations but flatly refused to allow me to administer any vaccines, saying she hated needles. Marsha's mother, who accompanied her, did not attempt to exert any control over her daughter. The mother seemed amused and bewildered by Marsha's behavior. Despite Marsha's rejecting attitude, I tried to relate positively to her. I said I could understand her hatred of needles, that I respected her right to refuse treatment at this time, and that she would not be forced to do anything against her will. I explained that I wanted Marsha to remain in good health and that that was why I wished to give her the protective vaccines. I suggested that we could discuss the situation again at her next appointment. Marsha listened but made no reply. Several months later, Marsha returned on her own to have forms signed so she could participate in school sports. She seemed pleased that I greeted her by her nickname. Again I recommended that she be given her immunizations, especially since she would be participating in rough outdoor sports. Marsha admitted she was still frightened of needles. I suggested that she would probably be able to tolerate the experience of getting injections if she sat upright and held someone's hand for support. After some discussion she

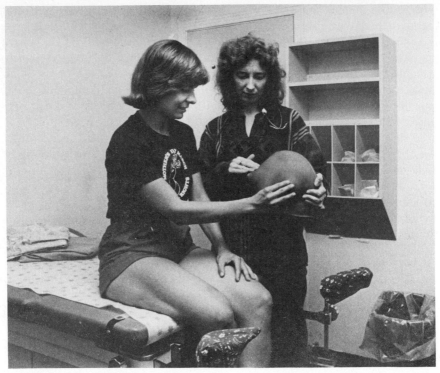

Adolescents are generally responsive to nursing approaches that utilize their cognitive maturity. Furthermore, intellectualization is a functional method of coping that many teenagers use to deal with stresses of actual or threatened illness. Both factual information and sensory data are being provided for this young woman, who is beginning to learn breast self-examination with the aid of a plastic model that has simulated breast lumps. (*Copyright* © *1980 by Anne Campbell.*)

decided this plan was agreeable. She clutched the hand of my assistant while I administered the vaccines to her, but she was able to sit still. Marsha was proud of her ability to maintain control and seemed complimented by my acknowledgment of her ability to cope with a frightening experience.

The nurse's goal is to support the adolescent's autonomy, but it is important to be aware that there will be fluctuations in the adolescent's ability to be independent. When experiencing psychological stress or afflicted with a physical ailment, the adolescent will be more dependent. The nurse can be extremely helpful during these periods of distress by explaining that the adolescent should not be ashamed of this increased reliance on others, because it is a sign of maturity to accept help when a problem is too difficult to solve alone. While the nurse offers assistance, autonomy can still be encouraged by suggesting to the teenager a number of possible solutions to the problem and allowing him or her to choose the one that is most agreeable. Care must be exercised not to engulf the adolescent during periods of illness or stress, when the adolescent is vulnerable to domination. There is a danger that the nurse will be seen as omnipotent because the nurse has a more fully developed sense of identity and is more competent in health-related matters than the adolescent. If the nurse fosters excessive dependency in the adolescent client, their therapeutic relationship will be damaged because the adolescent will eventually resent this secondary position. On recovery from the physical or emotional disorder, the adolescent will gain in confidence and competence. The nurse must be sensitive to recognize and encourage this increase in ability to be independent when it occurs. The teenager's movement away from temporary dependency and resumption of health care is an indicator of the nurse's success and should not be misinterpreted as a rebuff.

As the nurse fosters autonomous behavior in the adolescent client, the adolescent's parents should also be encouraged to become involved in their child's health care. The young person needs assistance from understanding adults as he or she strives for independence. By encouraging parents' interest, the nurse enhances the adolescent's access to the benefits of multiple support systems. Including parents helps keep communication open among all parties and makes information available from which to design the plan of care that will be most beneficial to the teenager. Nurses can demonstrate to parents, by interactions with their child, that adults can act as advisers rather than as authoritarian figures attempting to control the adolescent's behavior. Many parents are eager for their teenagers to be self-reliant and readily agree that adolescents should be responsible for their health care.

At times the nurse encounters a parent who does not encourage autonomous behavior. This situation needs to be handled carefully to avoid alienating either the parent or the child while attempting to reduce the intense degree of parental control. The following case study illustrates one method of interacting with an overprotective parent and a dependent adolescent.

> Fourteen-year-old Bill was the only child of older parents. Bill's father was minimally involved with him because he had a drinking problem and was in ill health. Bill's mother, in an attempt to compensate for her husband, showered Bill with attention. He was seen regularly at our clinic for routine well-child care. Bill's mother always accompanied her son to his appointments. It was the mother, not Bill, who reported about his health status. When he needed treatment for an ailment, both he and his mother always expected me to be able to do something that would quickly and almost miraculously solve the situation. For example, Bill was overweight and wanted to reduce so he could be eligible to play in school sports. When I explained that he

must limit his intake of food in order to reduce, he and his mother were disappointed. They had hoped I would be able to give him diet pills that would melt away his fat.

I attempted to encourage Bill's autonomy by suggesting that he was old enough now to come alone for his appointments, but he declined. My approach then, in my interactions with Bill and his mother, was to focus more on the son, encouraging him to describe his symptoms himself and asking him for his opinions. I told Bill I knew he had the potential to solve some of his problems on his own. On those occasions when he did assume a more active role, I commended him. I was cautious not to ignore or undermine Bill's mother. I asked for her perceptions and recommendations, but I also gently conveyed to her that Bill could and should be the one to control his plan of health care.

While it is appropriate to urge adolescents to assume responsibility for their health, it is obvious that the minor child cannot do so independently of his or her parents. Parents are financially and legally responsible for their teenage children's health care. Consequently, it is usually necessary and appropriate for parents to be informed about the professional treatment their teenager is receiving. Usually, adolescents are not reticent about sharing details of their health care with their parents. However, most adolescents feel their parents should not know everything about them, and there are situations in which teenagers request that information not be relayed to parents. The nurse must grant the request for confidentiality whenever possible, or else the adolescent may not come for health care the adolescent really needs. Young people should be encouraged to confide in their parents about matters they need to be aware of. There are, of course, some kinds of information which cannot ethically or legally be kept confidential. The laws regulating rights of minors and disclosure of information to parents or other authorities vary considerably from state to state. Each nurse must find a personal ethical stance and become aware of the laws in his or her practice area.

To summarize this discussion about supporting the adolescent's autonomy: The nurse must respect and encourage adolescents' rights to have control over their bodies and health care. At the same time, the nurse needs to be sensitive to the times when the adolescent needs help and to offer assistance in a nonthreatening manner. Parental involvement in health care can be very valuable and should, under ordinary circumstances, be sought.

BIBLIOGRAPHY

Blos, Peter: *On Adolescence*. New York: The Free Press, 1962.
Freud, Anna: "Adolescence," *Psychoanalytic Study of the Child*, **13**:255–278, 1958.

Group for the Advancement of Psychiatry: *Normal Adolescence*. New York: Charles Scribner's Sons, 1968.

Josselyn, Irene: *Adolescence*. New York: Harper and Row, 1971.

Laufer, Moses: "Preventive Intervention in Adolescence," *Psychoanalytic Study of the Child*, **30**:511–528, 1975.

The Health Assessment

Leona J. Haverkamp

The nurse who is to make a health assessment of an adolescent has a challenging task. The roughly ten-year span between the time the earliest developers begin their growth spurt and the time the latest developers complete theirs is in itself sufficient to make assessment somewhat complicated, and the complexity is made greater by large individual differences in psychologic, physiologic, and social maturity.

KNOWLEDGE NEEDED FOR MAKING A HEALTH ASSESSMENT

Health assessment of adolescents requires a broad range of background knowledge. *Health*, of course, encompasses much more than physiologic status, and understanding the biologic developments that take place during this phase of life is but a starting point in the assessment. Psychosocial and cognitive development as well are obviously and intrinsically tied to health, since they involve mental health, numerous social and environmental influences on health, and learning necessary for self-care and health-seeking behavior. Nurses must be especially aware of the effects of culture on adolescents' physical and mental health: Sociocultural factors such as laws, customs, and practices related to ethnicity, socioeconomic group membership, peer group membership, rural or urban residency, and so forth affect present and future health. Finally, nurses need a good base of knowledge about the health problems that are common in adolescence.

This chapter deals primarily with the health history as it pertains to adolescence. Common health problems of this particular age group are also discussed and interventions are identified. A word is in order at this point about what the chapter does not do. The basic principles and facts about physical growth and development, presented in Chapter 1, are not repeated here, although they constitute essential background information. Psychosocial assessment procedures are presented in greater detail elsewhere in the book, particularly in Chapters 9 and 11. Finally, no attempt is made to teach physical assessment skills. Such techniques can be learned only in clinical practice, and written materials to guide or supplement that practice are already widely available.

PURPOSES OF THE HEALTH ASSESSMENT

A health assessment serves various short-range purposes. It may be used to identify reasons for symptoms, to make a follow-up evaluation of some previous treatment, or to screen certain individuals or populations for particular problems (e.g., newborns are tested for phenylketonuria and hypothyroidism). It is important to realize, however, that in clinical practice *the ultimate purpose of the health assessment is to obtain information from which to develop an individualized plan for health care and health teaching.* That is, the assessment is not an end in itself but a means toward the end of health care *delivery.*

If an adolescent is found to be well, the plan of care is designed to enable him or her to maintain health and includes such items as (1) teaching about immunizations, nutrition, utilization of the health care system, and avoidance of health hazards; (2) anticipatory guidance about growth and development; and (3) reassurance that growth and health are proceeding normally. The care plan for persons whose assessment reveals some health problem is geared toward restoring normality wherever possible, helping the teenager adjust to the treatment regimen and to the disorder if full recovery is not anticipated, and teaching for general health promotion and maintenance.

THE PATIENT'S ROLE IN THE ASSESSMENT

The adolescent whose health is being evaluated must be an *active* participant in the nurse-adolescent relationship. This is both an ethical require-

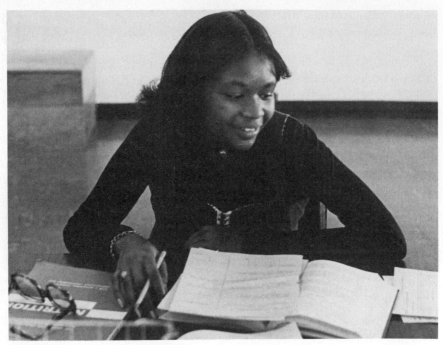

Health is broader than physical development and function; it resides also in the young person's psychosocial and intellectual adequacy. *Health assessment* includes these three major areas and in addition explores for sociocultural and environmental factors that may affect health and health practices. (*Copyright* © *1980 by Patricia Yaros.*)

ment and (particularly with teenagers) a pragmatic necessity. It has been recommended[1] that the professional and the client draw up a contract during their first meeting to specify what they hope to achieve together and what responsibilities and activities each person will contribute toward reaching the goals. Malasanos et al.[2] suggest that the contract should clarify where, when, how often, and for what length of time they are to meet; how the adolescent will be expected to participate in the assessment; each person's responsibilities concerning any confidential information that may be required or disclosed by the assessment; ground rules about including other persons (parents, professionals, or patient advocates); and fees involved, if any. Igoe's recommendations for a counseling contract (Chapter 11) are similar. The contract reduces "misconceptions, fears, or fantasies [the adolescent] may have had concerning what might happen during the interview and examination" and "establishes norms and role behavior."[3] Especially until the public becomes familiar with the nurse's role in physical assessment, it is helpful to clarify for patients how the nurse functions in assessment and treatment and how and when a physician will be involved. A further advantage of the contract is that it makes clear that the adolescent will be an active participant in the assessment and in subsequently designating goals and working toward them. In this way it encourages mature responsibility for self and at the same time eliminates the power inequity that leads some teenagers to resist health professionals' recommendations in more traditional patient-professional relationships.

COMPONENTS OF THE HEALTH ASSESSMENT

A complete health assessment consists of a health history, a physical examination, and related laboratory studies. The history, which is emphasized here, is a subjective report obtained from the adolescent (and sometimes supplemented by other informants) about past and present phenomena that are pertinent to health status. Topics included in the health history, each of which will be elaborated on in the following pages, are:

1 Past health and development
2 Family data
3 Social history
4 Review of systems and present illness

The physical examination and laboratory studies are not described here. However, the section about the review of systems includes a discussion of problems often found in physical examinations of adolescents, as well as those they commonly report in the history. This combined presentation of review of systems and physical examination is done in order that the information presented may be useful to readers who do not perform physical examinations as well as to those who do.

THE HEALTH HISTORY

Symptomatic screening leads to a commonsense rather than a brilliant diagnosis. . . . There is no alternative to the traditional long history, short examination, and selective investigation, supplemented by [laboratory findings].[4]

A health assessment will be inadequate unless it includes a good history. The health history is an organized record of events in a person's life which have relevance to mental and physical health. Even in its most abbreviated form, it is a necessary precursor to making even a provisional plan of care or a referral. The nurse who responds to patients' telephone calls, the nurse in an emergency room, the nurse practitioner in a clinic setting, and a public health or school nurse all need to be skilled in asking an organized set of questions to obtain the information that will enable them to evaluate the patient's situation. History taking is a skill learned by repeated practice.

In addition to its data-gathering function, the history is an excellent health education tool to use with adolescents. It also allows the nurse to demonstrate availability as a professional resource with a caring, concerned attitude and an organized approach toward evaluating one's well-being.

Many factors contribute to success in obtaining a health history. Whether the young person comes for care of an illness or for routine care, the skill of the nurse in planning, organizing, and interviewing will affect the adequacy of the history. Adolescents are eager to explore their own personal history and want to know the importance of all that is discussed. The quality and quantity of information exchanged depends on the nurse's and the adolescent's attitudes toward each other and on whether the situation is crisis-oriented or preventive. It also depends on the amount of time both persons have to spend. Skill in interviewing is a basic requirement for obtaining the history, and the nurse must also have a good understanding of growth and development and an empathic sense about the young person in each situation in order to have rapport. An open, honest approach is very important, as are willingness to listen and interest in what is said. It is necessary to be nonjudgmental, or teenagers may withdraw. Adults need to remember that adolescents, as a result of their developmental self-consciousness, may easily be offended or embarrassed by the nurse's real or imagined amusement, shock, or other evidence of judging their appearance or behavior. It is also important to remember that the young person's original reason for coming to see the nurse needs to be addressed to the adolescent's satisfaction, even though other matters may seem more pressing to the nurse.

Confidentiality is a major concern to most teenagers when they seek health care, and the thoroughness with which a nurse provides for it affects the adequacy of the health history. Adolescents generally will not (and should not be asked to) disclose personal information unless they are assured of privacy: protection against being overheard and against having the information passed on to other persons without their prior knowledge and consent. It should be standard procedure with every new patient to explain that all information the nurse obtains about the adolescent will be kept in confidence and used only to help the teenager improve his or her health. Patients need to know the nurse's policies about referral and the attendant sharing of personal data and should be assured that they will be involved in planning any referral. Exceptions to confidentiality must also be understood by adolescents *before* they disclose information that the nurse is legally or ethically obligated to report; generally this kind of material involves impending, serious danger to the informant or to others.

Clinicians disagree about the desirability of having patients complete a written questionnaire. A questionnaire inhibits the exchange of ideas and feelings and is not to be considered as reliable as a personal interview. However, a printed questionnaire or interview schedule may provide the format for the interview. Its use protects the interviewer against inadvertently omitting something and may give the adolescent assurance that there is no hidden agenda. Such an interview guide also facilitates record keeping. Furthermore, it is only realistic to recognize that, in a busy practice setting, a written questionnaire may be a needed time-saving device. A questionnaire completed by the adolescent before meeting with the nurse may efficiently provide information and may then be used as an aid to discussion and teaching.

The ideal situation for obtaining a health history is one in which the adolescent comes voluntarily for preventive health care. Time is scheduled but nurse and patient are unhurried. The teenager is in no apparent physical distress. Privacy is provided, and parents are asked only for that information which the adolescent cannot provide.

It is very important to put all adolescents at ease about terminology by stating that you will be using some terms that may be unfamiliar to them. Encourage questions and voluntarily clarify as you go along. Much of the language health professionals use as a matter of course is not familiar to laypersons, particularly young people. On the other hand, teenagers tend to have their own vocabulary and word usage patterns that adults do not understand. It is not possible to keep abreast of their language nor wise to try to use it. Simply use clarifying statements or questions so that you will be sure you understand each other.

Adolescents who upon interview or observation are found to exhibit physical, emotional, or social problems need to be selected for an extended history (interviewed in greater depth than others). This group includes teenagers whose stature is greatly different from that of peers; the obese; those with frequent illnesses (especially headache and abdominal pain); students with adjustment or relational problems at home or school such as depression, absenteeism, or stealing; adolescents who have acne, use drugs alone, have no friends, or are sexually active; and those with precursors of adult conditions, such as hypertension.

School is often the place where many of these problems are first noticed. School nurses have the unique advantage of seeing teenagers with peers and school authorities, and often they know something about their families. Many students return repeatedly to the nurse's office with vague or changing complaints but are not forthright enough to say what is really bothering them or ask for the nurse's help. The astute nurse recognizes these behaviors as indicative of some problem and pursues opportunities to further assess these youngsters in order to identify and intervene in their unexpressed needs.

There is a standardized sequence for taking a health history, which differs only slightly from one practitioner to another. Readers are encouraged to adapt their own format to fit the needs of their clients.

PAST HEALTH AND DEVELOPMENT

The past history of an adolescent's health is usually best obtained by sending a questionnaire home or from family records. Few adolescents have discussed their birth history with their parents, nor do they know what immunizations they have had and when. It is imperative that a record of rubella immunization or disease be obtained. If the reliability of this information is questionable, the adolescent girl should have a rubella titer done. The preventive aspect of rubella immunization should be explained. Many students will know if there was anything unusual about their birth. Be prepared to explain your interest by telling them that the way in which their life began often gives clues to understanding what's happening to them at their present growth state. Talking about birth history also affords the opportunity to educate young people about the effects on the fetus of a mother's poor nutrition or use of tobacco, alcohol, or medicines. Adolescents should know that venereal diseases, German measles, and other viruses can also affect the unborn child.

Adolescents do not usually know when they attained the various developmental milestones, but variations from normal, such as "faster than" or "slower than" others, may be known from conversations in the family. Nevertheless, this section of the history should be included because the adolescent, perhaps soon to be a parent, is able to grasp the concept of building one developmental skill upon another and the child's normal progression through stages. Examples of sitting before crawling and then walking, and the language sequence of babbling, using simple words, and then speaking in sentences may be given.

Developmental disorders to be discussed may include bed wetting, sleep disturbances, and nail biting. Some of these may have been present only in childhood, but a surprising number of adolescents still suffer with these conditions. A simple statement that these kinds of problems occur among adolescents may help young people to acknowledge their own concerns.

Illnesses and Accidents

Illnesses, accidents, emergency room visits, and hospitalizations reported in the history provide clues to the adolescent's general health and to crisis situations that may have been experienced. Teenagers who have had repeated illnesses may also have school problems because of absences. Questions about driving a motorcycle or car, ability to swim, and use of firearms help to establish accident risk factors and indicate areas for counseling. Repeated accidents may indicate a need for thorough neurological screening. Information about past hospitalizations or operations can help the nurse assess an adolescent's response to stress and the parents' response to crisis situations.[5,6]

Allergies

The history of allergies should include questions about asthma, hay fever, food, medications, and insect bites or stings. It is especially important to determine what medications the client may take for relief and what medications, if any, are being taken at the present time, as well as medications which have produced allergic responses.[7,8]

Nutrition

Nutritional assessment of the adolescent can be a difficult task. The history should provide information about how many meals are eaten each day and where, what kinds of snacks are eaten, and what foods are usually included in the daily food intake (see Chapter 5, Table 5-3, for a food intake questionnaire, which is recommended in place of a 24-hour recall of foods eaten). The nurse should estimate amounts by questioning. Using the recommended amounts for the four food groups as a criterion, it is then possible to decide whether a more detailed food record is needed. The physical assessment will provide further data to indicate whether referral for laboratory data such as metabolism, BUN, or others is needed. Detailed assessments should be made of adolescents who are more than 20 percent overweight or below the fifth percentile. Also assess more completely those who have frequent illnesses, learning problems, or acne, those who use oral contraceptives or tobacco, and those who are pregnant. Nutritional intervention is challenging, because eating habits are part of the peer culture and of long-standing family patterns. Adolescents may respond to innovative approaches to obtaining nutrients if this is acceptable to their peers. They are not going to change their life-style in order to get the proper food. A nutrition lecture will probably be ignored.[9] Chapter 5 presents nutritional assessment, dietary needs, and interventions in detail.

Sexual Development

Sexual development is of great importance to adolescents. Their primary concern is whether or not they are normal. The nurse must provide an opportunity to discuss this concern by asking both boys and girls about their development. Too often girls are asked only about menstruation and boys are ignored altogether. It is not difficult to say to an adolescent, "A very important part of health evaluation at this time in your life is how you are developing sexually. There are many changes taking place in your body and in your feelings and thoughts. Have you been wondering about these changes? Do you feel you are developing like other boys/girls? Have you thought about how to handle your feelings about being sexually mature? What alternatives have you thought about? Do you know about masturbation? Have you heard anyone talk about sublimation? Are you sexually active? What do you know about contraceptives? What do you know about venereal disease?'' In the review of systems (genitourinary), questions will be asked regarding abnormalities.

Nurses who work with adolescents in a clinical situation have excellent opportunity for complete observation of body changes. School nurse clinics and indeed some hospital situations may not provide for full body inspection. Keen observation and questioning will help to determine the stage of growth. I believe it is extremely important to compare growth stage to chronological age for a better understanding of the social problems the adolescent may be experiencing. Visible body changes, which are very important to the adolescent, occur in a predictable order (described in Chapter 1). This fact affords the nurse an opportunity for anticipatory guidance.

Whenever the body changes occur, you may be sure that they cause great concern for the youngster. Boys are concerned about the size of their genitalia, believing that this determines potency or virility. Girls are concerned about the size of their hips and breasts. Both sexes may experiment with masturbation and worry about that. Persons of either sex may develop physical characteristics more typical of the other sex; these changes are usually temporary and a normal part of adolescent hormonal regulation, but they can be intensely disturbing to teenagers themselves. All adolescents avidly compare their own bodies to those of peers, and their resulting self-evaluation profoundly affects self-esteem.[10] The nurse should be sensitive to these feelings and, by recognizing the relationships of the events of puberty, be able to assure the youth about his or her development.

Family Data

Adolescents are either very open about their families or are reluctant to discuss them at all. Those who are disinclined to talk about their families will need explanations that help them see how family life relates to health. Information should be obtained about parents' ages, occupations, and health, as well as siblings' ages and health. Wherever indications of possibly hereditary conditions are found, the teenager should be given appropriate screening tests. Heritable disorders also indicate a need for genetic counseling from a qualified physician or nurse practitioner at another time.

Significant problems of inadequate or crowded housing, insufficient income, crowded sleeping arrangements, family disputes, parental illness or alcohol abuse, and other family difficulties can all affect the teenager's coping style. A thorough family history helps the nurse learn how the family handles discipline and how family members and the teenager respond to crisis.

Social History

Sometimes also called personal history, this part of the history is done in order to assess the adequacy of the adolescent's personal and social adjustment and to identify aspects of personal life that may either predispose to poor health or affect responses to health problems or health care. The social history may include such items as employment, daily routine, marital status, recreational patterns, housing arrangements, friendship affiliations, patterns of substance use (i.e., use of cigarettes, alcohol, and other drugs), religion, temperament, and self-description. The interview reveals areas in which teaching and counseling may be given to ease the young person's movement toward maturity and promote self-understanding. The adolescent may gain a new perspective from the nurse's questions regarding independent actions, responsibilities as a family member, allowances, parents' expectations, and plans for self. The discussion of the teenager's personality and interpersonal relationships is important. One can ask the youngster, "How would you describe yourself? How do you think your parents would describe you? How do you get along with your siblings? Who are your friends? What do you and your friends do together during your free time? How do you get along with other students, if you are in school? With teachers?" The nurse should also ask about school attendance or absenteeism and causes for it. Has the adolescent been in trouble with the law?

Habits and life-style have much to do with the adolescent's state of health. Like adults, adolescents experience self-induced illness as a result of poor nutrition and use of alcohol, tobacco, and other drugs. Accidents and injuries may be a result of poor habits and unsafe behavior patterns. Why some people practice these habits, why some try them and discard them, and why some never try them at all is poorly understood.[11]

Methods for assessing the complex behavior of adolescents to determine whether it falls outside normal bounds and requires referral to a mental health specialist are presented elsewhere (Chapters 9 and 11), as are types of intervention (Chapters 11, 17, and 21 particularly). Fine's[12] organized system of analyzing behavior around developmental tasks and substages of adolescence is also a very helpful assessment tool. *Family relationships* at adolescence are usually strained. Most young people are trying to loosen the emotional ties with parents, and this causes unrec-

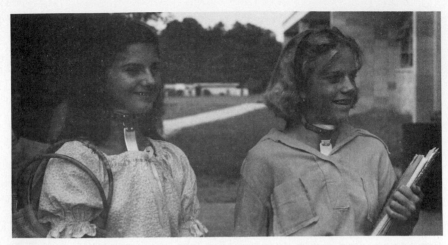

Health assessments are used (1) to screen populations known to be at risk for certain problems (e.g., young adolescent girls for scoliosis), (2) to identify reasons for signs or symptoms of illness, (3) to evaluate outcomes from any previous interventions, and (4) to obtain the information with which to develop an individualized plan for health care and health teaching. (*Copyright © 1980 by Anne Campbell.*)

ognized guilt and depression. This natural aspect of leaving childhood behind is not always understood by parents either, which further complicates the problems. Typically, parents feel rejected and adolescents feel restricted. Interpretation of the normalcy of this stage is needed by the parents as well as the child, and in many settings the nurse can find ways to provide developmental information and anticipatory guidance to both. *Peer relationships* are especially important for establishment of identity. An adolescent without friends is an adolescent in trouble. *School attendance and performance* often are the first indications that a teenager is having problems. Failure to function in an age-appropriate manner in school, at home, and with peers requires more intensive appraisal. Mental health services, family service agencies, or private therapists provide both assessment and therapy.

REVIEW OF SYSTEMS AND COMMON DISORDERS (PRESENT ILLNESS)

The systems review and description of the present illness is considered to be the heart of the diagnostic history. Weed[13] has been developing and refining an organized questionnaire to provide the best and most complete information. For each body system, current, past, and potential problems are identified. A plan of action is then made for every problem. Frequently, this plan includes obtaining more information by means of a present illness survey. Weed's questionnaire is excellent for use in offices for initial preventive examinations or for a client who has had a series of continuing complaints. Its disadvantage is its length and fairly complicated instructions for measuring symptoms. It requires interpretation, and sometimes it might be necessary for the client to wait for recurrence of symptoms in order to describe them accurately.

Another approach to the systems review is presented by Kugelmass.

Constitutional systems are discussed in terms of genetic, nutritional, musculoskeletal, and neoplastic disorders. Personality systems are unravelled in terms of mental, sensory, psychological, and psychosocial disorders. Behavior systems are viewed in terms of antisocial, psychosomatic, and psychiatric disorders. Adaptive systems are presented in terms of alimentary, respiratory, cardiovascular, and renal disorders. Defensive systems are interpreted in terms of skin, blood, immunologic, connective tissue, and allergic disorders. Cybernetic systems are described in terms of neurological, endocrine, and metabolic disorders. Reproduction systems are viewed in terms of sexual disorders.[14]

This systems concept arrangement is useful to nurse practitioners who work with adolescents, particularly from the cause-effect standpoint.

The more traditional approach to the systems review as organized by Silver, Kempe, and Bruyn[15] or the DeGowins[16] can also be used effectively with adolescents. The following conglomerate of the several methods of systems review has provided the author with a workable format. Although this format appears lengthy, it does not take a great deal of time when it is memorized and used repeatedly. At the beginning of the review of systems, adolescents must again be assured that the information sought is necessary to help the nurse recognize areas of concern and that it is confidential and will be used only to help them improve their health. Nurses who will do a physical examination may choose to do the review of systems at that time rather than as part of the interview preceding the physical.

For nurses who perform a physical examination, the objective data obtained from it are added to the subjective data collected by the health history, and the problem list is derived from the combination. For nurses who do not do physical examinations, the history, including review of systems, provides the basis for the problem list, from which health teaching and other interventions are designed. The first decision to be made is whether additional information is needed about any problem before interventions can be planned. Some nurses will refer to a physician or other professional or agency those problems needing further analysis. Nurse practitioners, depending on their practice setting and role parameters, may take a present illness history for presenting problems and plan interventions on the basis of established protocols that are mutually agreeable to the nurse and the prescribing physician. All nursing plans should make provision for patient education, which must include an explanation of the reasons and procedures for any referrals, relief of anxieties about the interview and/or examination and findings, and plans for an ongoing program to manage problems. The essence of the nursing function is to recognize variations from normal, to provide for needed intervention, to increase the patient's awareness of the dynamics of his or her condition, and to provide alternatives for action.

The body systems to be reviewed are listed below. Items to be explored in the review of each system are identified, and conditions commonly occurring during adolescence and some suggested nursing interventions follow each systems heading.

Integument   *Skin: color, pigmentation, eruptions, scaling, bruising. Hair: color, texture, distribution. Nails: ridging, pitting, color changes.*

Skin problems, because of their ready visibility, bring numerous complaints, not only from the affected adolescents but also from those closely associated with them. Concerns include repulsion because of appearance, fear of contagion, and self-consciousness of the affected teenager. Adolescents can have a great number of skin disorders. Among the common problems are acne, erythrodermas, bacterial infections, viral infections, fungal infections, contact dermatitis, pigmentation defects, and nevi.

Acne Vulgaris   is a serious condition to the teenagers who are afflicted. Yet many parents and some physicians defer treatment, believing it will be outgrown. Nurses are expected to be able to provide helpful treatment plans. The profusion of lay beliefs and advertisements about acne care tends to confuse teenagers, and an adequate explanation of the disorder is very important. The following information, taken from Sauer, is written as it might be used in talking to adolescents.

> Acne is a skin disorder in which the oil glands are overactive. It usually occurs on the face, chest, and back where there are a lot of oil glands. Blackheads or whiteheads are called comedones and are caused by plugged oil gland openings. Some of the plugged glands become irritated and red, causing pustules or pimples. If these infections are deep and severe they may cause scarring. The tendency to develop acne runs in families. It is aggravated by poor skin care, certain foods, nervous tension. In girls, it is usually worse before a menstrual period. Even in boys, acne flares on a cyclic basis. There are at least two important reasons to get medical care. The first is to prevent scarring from severe pustules and cysts. The second is to improve appearance, especially if this is causing you embarrassment and worry. Treatment will depend on how much you are concerned with controlling this condition.[17]

The nursing care plan depends as much on the adolescent's concern for controlling "pimples" as on the severity of the condition. Treatment which may be planned by nurses for mild acne includes the following measures. Wash affected areas twice a day with antibacterial soap. It is not desirable to perform ritualistic scrubbing, but every effort should be made to make the skin dry, not red and uncomfortable. Girls may use face powder, dry rouge, and lipstick, but no face creams of any kind. Boys should shave regularly but should avoid hair tonics or oils. If the hair is very oily, suitable shampoos will help to keep oiliness under control. Plenty of rest is important. Some foods do aggravate acne and should be restricted. These include chocolate in any form, nuts, whole milk, excesses of sweets, and fatty foods. There are a number of over-the-counter preparations that may be used successfully. These include Resulin lotion, Rezamid lotion, Liquimat, Komed lotion, and Microsyn lotion.[18] Follow-up visits with the adolescent are advised in order to watch the progress of the condition. Referral to a dermatologist is advised for the more severe cases: Surgical procedures and an antibiotic regimen minimize scarring.

Erythrodermas are skin inflammations with desquamation. *Psoriasis* is a chronic papulosquamous disease characterized by white, scaly patches, most commonly on the elbows, knees, and scalp. Psoriasis is a chronic condition. Patients need to know that there is no "cure." They may get better for a time but should not be discouraged or feel the doctor is not treating them adequately if lesions recur over and over. Psoriasis is considered genetic, and it is often disfiguring. Medical management varies according to the proportion of the body that is involved. Topical measures used successfully by some physicians include Lubath, Keri lotion, and Nivea cream. Scalp scaling is treated with Selsun, Zetar, or "P&S" Liquid. Coal tar cream is rubbed into the patches at night, and they are exposed to ultraviolet radiation after the bath in the morning. Cordran tape can be cut to size and applied occlusively.[19, 20] Adolescents generally need a great deal of support to carry out the treatment regimen. They must be reassured that psoriasis is not contagious or infectious, and many need encouragement to continue social activities. Good health habits are very important, because psoriasis is exacerbated by trauma, anxiety, drugs, and infection. Arthritis is a complication. Genetic counseling is recommended so that patients will understand the heredofamilial tendency.

Pityriasis rosea is a noninfectious, papulosquamous eruption occurring on the trunk and extremities. There is usually a preliminary lesion, the "herald patch," which looks like ringworm. Following the herald patch, new lesions appear for two to three weeks. The rash usually disappears in six weeks. Itching varies from none to severe. The nursing care plan includes assuring the adolescent that this is not a blood disease and not contagious. If the eruption does not itch and the patient is reassured of the mild nature of the disease, then no treatment is necessary. Itching may be relieved by colloidal baths using one-half of a small box of cornstarch (for laundry or cooking) or one packet of Aveeno oatmeal preparation to a tub containing 6 to 8 inches of water. The patient should bathe 10 to 15 minutes every other day and avoid soap as much as possible. Moderate itching may be relieved by antihistamines.[21] A patient who has severe itching should be under a doctor's management, and the itching may be treated with ultraviolet therapy and/or drugs, which may include corticosteroids.

Seborrheic dermatitis is a chronic inflammatory scaling of the scalp, eyebrows, eyelids, nasolabial folds, axilla, submammary folds, and groin. It is a nuisance and embarrassment to the adolescent. Nursing care again involves constant interpretation of the nature of the condition, i.e., it is not infectious or contagious, and it is not a "disease" but a "condition" that the patient can manage. There is no cure, but remissions can occur for varying amounts of time. The best management is by shampooing with Selsun suspension or any of the tar shampoos such as Ionil T., Sebutone, Head and Shoulders, or Sebulex. Pragmatar ointment is helpful on lesions not controlled by shampoo and on other locations of the body.[22, 23]

Bacterial Infections   range from superficial to deep ones involving the dermis and subcutaneous tissue. In management of pyodermas, certain general principles must be followed. Improve bathing habits by use of bactericidal soap. Remove crusts or pustules to allow penetration of medication. Clothing and bedding should be changed frequently. Washcloth and towel should not be used by anyone else. Chronic or recurring incidents require diet management as for acne. Rule out drug ingestion, which can cause lesions that mimic pyodermas, such as ingestion of iodides and bromides. Rule out diabetes, particularly for recurrent boils.[24]

Impetigo is a superficial infection caused by either β-hemolytic streptococcus or *Staphylococcus aureus*. It is contagious, and the general principles outlined above apply. In addition, many physicians feel systemic antibiotics should be administered to prevent glomerulonephritis.[25, 26] Impetigo is a nuisance disease among school children, and nursing plans include educating students and their families regarding cleanliness and inspection of close contacts.

Folliculitis is a common infection of the hair follicles. Most infections clear up with use of hot packs and improved bathing. Recurrences, however, usually cause the patient to seek preventive help. A *furuncle* or boil is a deep infection of the hair follicle, often caused by friction, diet rich in sugars and fats, and poor hygiene or diabetes. The nursing plan is to teach the adolescent how to apply hot packs and how to prevent spreading the infected matter to other parts of the body and to other persons. Severe or recurring cases should be referred to a doctor for incision of the "ripe" lesion, followed by antibiotics systemically. In addition, it may be necessary to rule out a focus of infection in teeth, tonsils, genitourinary tract, or gallbladder. Preventive teaching includes the general principles above.

A *carbuncle* is an extension of the furuncle to several hair follicles which drain onto the skin surface through multiple openings. It is a much more serious infection and is treated as a furuncle is, but with more emphasis on systemic antibiotic therapy and rest.

Cellulitis is often seen following athletic injury to the skin. It produces red, hot, swollen tissue along with lymphangitis and lymphadenopathy. Status of tetanus immunization should be checked. Cool compresses relieve the local pain. Systemic antibiotic therapy is indicated.

Paronychia caused by yeast is a painful, red swelling around the nails. Treatment is to avoid constant exposure to soap and water. Topical and systemic antibiotics are effective. Hot applications may give relief from pain.[27, 28]

Virus Infections   of the skin are not uncommon. *Herpes simplex*, commonly called fever blister or cold sore, is characterized by a single group of blisters. It is caused by Herpesvirus Type I and can affect the mouth, genitalia, and central nervous system. It is somewhat painful and can be spread through intimate contact. A serious herpes infection is caused by Type II virus and now ranks as the second most common venereal infection, gonorrhea being first.[29] Nursing care involves instructing adolescents about avoiding spread of the disease and informing them that no specific treatment is available to shorten the natural course of the infection. Most patients want to try something, and some relief from pain may be obtained by use of antibiotic ointments. Petrolatum lessens cracking and crusting. Xylocaine ointment or idoxuridine may be prescribed by a physician for relief from burning.[30, 31]

Warts are autoinnoculating viral tumors of the skin. Spreading is increased by irritation produced by clothing, picking, shaving, or other injury to a wart. Probably no one escapes this infection. Warts can occur anywhere, depending on their type. Common warts appear most often on hands; filiform warts on the eyelids, face, and neck; flat warts on the forehead and dorsum of the hand; and plantar warts on the feet. Treatment varies from home remedies using castor oil applied to the wart for six weeks, to liquid nitrogen therapy, to corticosteroid creams. The nursing plan includes educating the teenager regarding spread and helping with aspects of selecting treatment and interpreting the results. The necrotic tissue and inflammation resulting from treatment are a concern to adolescents.[32, 33]

Fungus Infections   most commonly occur on the skin but may also invade the lungs, brain, and other organs. Superficial fungi live on the dead horny layer of the skin, hair, and nails. Common terms for the more common disorders are ringworm, athlete's foot, and jock itch. Athlete's foot and jock itch are prevalent in adolescents and frequently result in school absence because of pain and discomfort. Ringworm of the scalp occurs less frequently after puberty, partly due to the higher content of fungistatic fatty acids in the sebum. The nurse should be aware of the following: *Correct diagnosis of fungus infection is very important and often difficult.* Griseofulvin is the drug of choice for treating fungus infection but is of no value for treating atopic eczema, contact dermatitis, psoriasis, monilial infections, pityriasis rosea, impetigo, or even tinea versicolor. The affected youth and the youth's parents and teachers should be instructed regarding contagion and methods of prevention.[34]

Athlete's foot (tinea pedis) is mildly contagious to susceptible persons and apparently spreads from feet to groin. Preventive measures include drying the feet last when toweling after baths and not reusing towels. General cleanliness in showers and dressing rooms, especially the benches, is important. Stockings should be changed daily.[35]

Ringworm of the smooth skin (tinea corporis) is highly infectious. It is commonly due to contact with infected kittens and puppies or with children who usually also have scalp infection. Affected persons should be excluded from gymnasiums and swimming pools and from activities likely to lead to exposure of others. Preventive measures also include examination of pets and thorough washing of clothing and towels, which should not be used by others.

Ringworm of the scalp (tinea capitis) is highly infectious and is spread by the backs of theater seats, barber clippers, combs, caps or other contaminated clothing, or hair. Prevention and control depend on locating the source of infection. Nurses, particularly in schools, should use a Wood's light to examine any suspicious scalp lesion and to check the scalp of any child with suspected ringworm of the smooth skin. Tinea of the scalp fluoresces a bright yellow-green. Keep infected persons out of public places and under treatment, which usually takes six to eight weeks. They may attend school if a cotton cap is worn and sterilized frequently and if they adhere to the treatment regimen. Wash hair after every haircut.[36]

Ringworm of the groin and of the nails does not seem to be very infectious, but the general precautions outlined above should be followed.[37]

Drug therapy for fungus infections should be under the direction of a doctor who is skilled in differential diagnosis. Griseofulvin is not recommended for mild infections. Mild cases of athlete's foot may be managed by the patient through use of boric acid crystal soaks and/or Tinactin. Minor fungal infections of the smooth skin may also respond to Tinactin. Resistant cases may have to be treated with griseofulvin, which is also used for scalp, beard, groin, fingernails, and hands but is not recommended for toenail infections.[38] Superimposed bacterial infections require a physician's attention.

Contact Dermatitis   is commonly seen in adolescents. It is an inflammation of the skin caused by irritant substances such as soaps, metals, cosmetics, or allergenic substances such as poison ivy resin. The nursing plan is to take a good present illness history in order to help the student determine what the causative agent is and to avoid future contact with it. The location of the rash helps identify the cause, as does the activity of the young person just before the rash appeared. The season of the year is frequently of diagnostic importance. The affected adolescent and friends need to be assured that oozing lesions will not spread to another person, unless the allergen (such as poison ivy resin) is present on the skin. A general rule for contact dermatitis is to "cool it" with boric acid solution (2 percent) wet packs. Antihistamines relieve itching, and calamine promotes drying. Contact dermatitis of the hands is aggravated by soap and water. Rubber gloves should be worn and mild soaps used for bathing. In severe cases of contact dermatitis corticosteroid-antibiotic therapy will be prescribed by the doctor, but injured skin must be pampered and drugs alone will not relieve the condition.[39,40]

Pigmentation Defects also cause adolescents much concern, particularly for black teenagers affected with hypopigmentation. The psychologic effects for both white and black youth can be severe, and the nurse must be alert to the youth's feelings. The nursing plan may include referral for mental health counseling, but it most surely will be a supportive plan including pragmatic instruction regarding use of cosmetics to cover exposed areas. More specific treatment by a doctor may include psoralen derivatives, but their effectiveness is disappointing. Hyperpigmentation causing brown spots is seen in some pregnancies and is increasing in incidence among women using contraceptive hormones.[41]

Nevi are pigmented or nonpigmented tumors of the skin. There are two questions concerning nevi, or moles, that must be answered: (1) When and how should they be removed? and (2) What is the relationship between nevi and malignant melanomas? Strauss and Pochi[42] say it is imperative that bathing trunk nevus or large congenital hairy nevus elsewhere be referred for total surgical excision. Sauer[43] says *never* remove a nevus in a child by electrosurgery; remove only by surgical excision. Also to be excised only are flat pigmented nevi, particularly on the palm, sole, or genitalia. Adolescents' concern regarding potential malignancy of a mole can be relieved by pointing out that most people have these and that observation for changes in color and size, bleeding, and ulceration is a more practical safeguard than unwarranted surgery. These signs are cause for seeking medical care.

Sensory System *Eyes: double image, loss of vision, injury, inflammation, styes, glasses. Ears: frequent earache, ringing, vertigo, discharge, last audiometric examination, use of firearms, frequency of exposure to rock music, other loud noises. Nose: frequent colds, stuffiness, discharge, nosebleed, obstruction.*

Because vision and hearing are so important in communication, the adolescent with deficiencies in either sense has very real and complex difficulties. Nurses who assess for problems in vision and hearing should recognize that it is painful for adolescents to acknowledge any body defect. Consider the student with vision problems. Detection of deficiencies is often difficult because students who do not want to wear glasses find many ways of "passing the eye test." Students who do want to wear glasses sometimes go to great lengths to fool not only the screener but also the ophthalmologist or optometrist. Adolescents with common refractive errors who have worn glasses since early childhood without any resistance may suddenly believe glasses make them "different." Boys may feel wearing glasses is not manly. Girls may think glasses make them ugly. Parents and teachers are concerned that adolescents will injure their eyes if they don't wear their glasses. The nurse can help in several ways to resolve the conflict that may develop. First, students who say they don't need to wear glasses all the time should be taken seriously. Rather than testing to find out what they cannot see on a chart, ask them to demonstrate what visual tasks they can accomplish. Most students who really need their glasses will wear them. If refractive errors are minor, not wearing glasses is not going to hurt the eyes. Astigmatism does not seem to become worse if glasses are worn only for reading, television, or any activity requiring that the eyes be used at a fixed distance. Muscle imbalance may be helped if glasses are worn all the time, but when the eyes are directed to objects of varying distances, naked vision may help the student use visual clues and interpret blurs. The nurse should know the visual deficiency of every adolescent counseled about vision. What are the physician's recommendations about wearing glasses? When was the last examination? Determine whether there are signs of eyestrain, such as squinting, rubbing, blinking, and frowning. Students who will be taking driver education classes should be counseled regarding the importance of using glasses as necessary to ensure good vision while driving. Referrals for ophthalmologic evaluation should be made for every adolescent who has a considerable refractive error and has not been reexamined in two years, who has symptoms of eyestrain, who has visual acuity less than 20/30 in one or both eyes, or who complains of vision problems but passes all screening tests. Remember to consider the whole person, not just the eyes.[44]

Adolescents with severe vision deficiencies must expend a great deal of energy to accomplish what normally sighted persons do easily. Sight saving classes, print enlargers, and special books all emphasize the differentness of the visually handicapped adolescent, and this is damaging to the self-concept. The nurse should suggest to these students that they physically place themselves in the best position for visual tasks, e.g., near the blackboard, under the light, or wherever they can see best. Most students with severe deficiencies can safely be encouraged to hold reading material as close to their eyes as they need to and to read as much as they want to. They will not "use their eyes up." Students who need vision devices usually adapt to them and become enthusiastic users with a little encouragement. Teachers must be cautioned not to emphasize handicaps by overprotection.[45]

Contact lenses may be worn because of severe visual problems or injury, or for cosmetic reasons. Problems associated with contact lenses include corneal irritation, often due to improper care, and displacement within the conjunctival sac. Lenses worn during vigorous activity are often pushed up under the upper lid. This is the first place to look for a lost lens since injury to the conjunctiva occurs if it is not removed. Adolescents with frequent irritations of the eye should be referred immediately to their eye doctor. The importance of frequent checkups will be more apparent to teenagers if the nurse uses sketches or anatomical models of the eye to demonstrate the relationship of the contact lens to the eye and explains proper care and safety.

The number of adolescents with hearing problems is increasing. Hearing loss creates problems in communication and is often complicated by other handicaps. Hearing-impaired adolescents expend a great deal of energy paying attention, trying to read lips, trying to cope with background noises in the classroom, or simply visiting with a group of peers.

Hearing depends on sensitivity, discrimination, and recognition. Sensitivity depends on intensity and frequency of sound reaching the tympanic membrane. Intensity is measured by decibels, with normal speech being in the 60-decibel range. Discrimination depends on being able to distinguish the sounds of speech either alone or in sequence. Some people do not hear beginning sounds or ending sounds. Recognition, or perception, involves the brain and the meaning of sound. Interference here causes the most deleterious effect of hearing loss. A loss of acuity is classified as either conductive or sensorineural. Conductive losses involve sensitivity. A loss of 20 decibels is marginal. A youth with a loss of 30 decibels or more should be able to profit from the use of a hearing aid but should be so advised after full consideration of medical and surgical treatment. Sensorineural loss, on the other hand, has no "cure" or surgical treatment. Persons with this type of loss require patience and a thoughtful plan of long-term management. They can benefit enormously from learning to lipread and, in severe cases, learning to sign. Perception is an integrative function and depends on memory, attention, and relating to previous experience. When these functions are disturbed, problems with learning usually occur. Nursing plans for hearing-impaired adolescents include teaching them the anatomy and functioning aspects of hearing, interpreting a youth's particular loss in terms of educational needs and physical care,

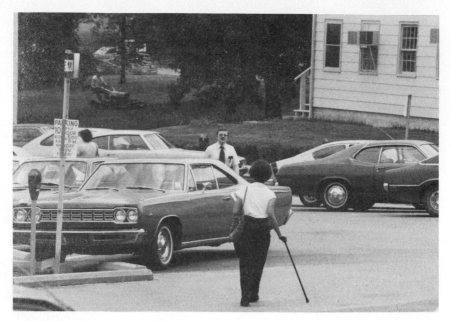

The health history is an organized record of events in the client's life that have relevance to mental and physical health. The history may include such items as employment, daily routine, marital status, recreational patterns, housing arrangements, friendship affiliations, patterns of substance use, religion, temperament, and self-description. (*Copyright © 1980 by Anne Campbell.*)

and providing emotional and social support.[46] Adolescents with hearing difficulties need a good understanding of their condition. An explanation, using charts or models, of the anatomy and physiology involved will improve a teenager's interpretation of (and attitudes about) his or her impairment.[47]

Ear infections are common among adolescents. Complaints of pain in the external meatus may be caused by a furuncle, trauma, a foreign body, or infection. Acute external otitis is usually very painful. It is usually caused by streptococcus or staphylococcus, and often swimming in contaminated water initiates it. Chronic external otitis is usually pruritic and accompanied by discharge. There is insensitivity to pain. The causative agents are usually bacteria or fungi. Pyogenic infections should be treated with antibiotics, irrigation, and ear drops. Swimmers need to be excluded from swimming until healed and subsequently should wear earplugs when swimming.[48,49,50]

Cerumen may also cause pain and interfere with hearing. The adolescent should be cautioned about inserting anything in the ear to try to remove the wax. Rather, a softening preparation such as glycerine and peroxide should be used to soften the wax and allow natural drainage.

Finally, acute otitis media is not uncommon, with symptoms of throbbing earache, nausea, dizziness, impaired hearing, and fever. Prompt antibiotic therapy is essential. Nursing plans should place special emphasis on teaching the effects of infection on hearing. Much support must be given for adherence to the treatment plan.[51]

Exposure to loud noises is a recognized cause of hearing loss. Rock music, motorboats and snowmobiles, and gunshots are all hazards to which more and more adolescents are being exposed. The increasing numbers of persons who are choosing jobs in construction and industry may be exposed to loud noises for eight-hour days, five days a week. Effects of these hazards are not immediate, and counseling adolescents about long-term effects does not always bring about behavior change, but educational efforts should be persistently continued.[52,53]

An adolescent may be more concerned about the effect his or her nose has on appearance than about any discomfort it causes. Nosebleed may be to the adolescent just an embarrassing situation. It may also be a sign of serious local or generalized disease. Local causes include sneezing, injuries, ulcerations, acute infections such as folliculitis or furunculosis, and fissures. Generalized causes include exertion, hypertension, blood coagulation disorders, or infections such as influenza, scarlet fever, mononucleosis, and rheumatic fever. The nurse should examine the nasal passages for infection, obstruction, or injury. Persons with infections should be referred to a physician for treatment. A simple treatment for nosebleed is to apply direct pressure on the nose for five minutes. After bleeding has stopped, the adolescent should keep quiet in a sitting position leaning forward. It is important not to blow the nose, laugh, or in any other way disturb the clot for three or four hours. Take the teenager's blood pressure and interpret it and reassure him or her about this. Referral for medical care should be made if the bleeding is not controlled with three attempts, properly carried out. Fracture, injury that causes difficulty in breathing, history of bleeding or blood disorders, and lacerations to the skin on the outside of the nose also necessitate referral to a physician. Deformities that affect appearance may be congenital or acquired, but whatever the cause the adolescent will experience extreme psychologic trauma, and nurses can provide mental health resources. Obstruction to breathing may be caused by allergies, infections, or a deviated septum and can be alleviated by proper treatment.[54]

Mouth and Throat; Neck and Lymph *Soreness of tongue, canker sores, poor dental hygiene, poor dental care, loss of taste. Tonsillitis, sore throats, hoarseness or other voice changes. Swelling of neck, goiter, stiffness, limitation of motion. Enlarged lymph nodes, pain.*

The most common problem of the mouth is dental disease. In a great many adolescents, carious teeth are not repaired and oral hygiene is poor. Nurses should be involved intensively with correction of these problems. Schools employing a dental hygienist are able to provide for many of the dental needs of youth. Malocclusion may also be a source of embarrass- ment, especially with severe overbite or underbite. Orthodontia for the underprivileged is often difficult to obtain. Nurses and hygienists spend much time and effort in the health advocate role in order to make dental care possible for these students.[55]

Other conditions of the mouth which are troublesome to the adoles- cent are canker sores and herpes simplex, which was discussed under dermatitis. *Cheilosis* is seen frequently in adolescents. It is an ulceration of the skin at the corners of the mouth with crusting and fissuring. Cheilosis is associated with riboflavin deficiency and indicates a need for a nutrition history and dietary counseling. Good sources of riboflavin are milk, cheese, eggs, beef, and leafy green vegetables. Bleeding gums may be caused by a number of general disorders, such as trauma from brushing or flossing teeth, infections, Hodgkin's disease, hemophilia, or other blood dyscrasias. *Vincent's stomatitis*, often called trench mouth, produces in- flamed gums and ulcers of the mucosa. *Gingival hyperplasia* is often seen in adolescents who take Dilatin and in those with leukemia.

Soreness of the tongue is frequently the presenting symptom for a number of disorders. Skilled observation for dryness (dehydration), en- largement (acromegaly), tremor, glossitis (extreme vegetarian diets), strawberry tongue (scarlet fever), canker sore, or sublingual mass (salivary gland obstruction) will improve the referral for medical care. Any per- sistent pain with or without any recognizable signs should be referred to a physician.[56]

Throat pain may be caused by acute pharyngitis and is a common complaint of adolescents. The infection is caused by either bacteria or viruses, and therein lies the difficulty of diagnosis. The DeGowins[57] believe that a good history and physical findings provide the best diagnostic base. If the infection is thought to be bacterial, the throat should be cultured and treated with antibiotics until the laboratory report is received. Nurses who assess sore throat should take a present illness history to elicit per- tinent information about trauma, irritants, or contagion. The oral cavity should be examined, lymph nodes palpated, and temperature taken. Gen- eral rules for a nursing plan are to refer to a physician any person with a temperature over 38.3°C (101°F); a bright red, swollen, exudative phar- ynx; tender, swollen cervical lymph nodes; or a history of exposure to strep throat or mononucleosis. The patient should be instructed regarding warm water gargles, throat lozenges, increased fluid intake, aspirin, bed rest, humidifier at night, and adherence to a medication plan. Viral in- fections are usually not accompanied by fever, and the above palliative measures will provide relief from discomfort.[58] Mononucleosis is frequently a cause of acute pharyngitis and disproportionately large cervical lymph nodes. Axillary and inguinal lymph node involvement may also be seen. Further discussion follows under lymph examination.

Hoarseness may be caused by overuse of the voice, upper respiratory infections, chronic inflammation of the vocal chords, goiter, and many other conditions. A present illness history and referral for medical care are indicated if the condition has existed for longer than two weeks or if there is interference with breathing.[59]

Assessment of pain in the neck may be improved by determining if movement increases the symptoms. Chewing, swallowing, and head or shoulder movements may enhance pain and localize its origin. It is especially important to observe for signs of stiffness, which may indicate meningitis. Brudzinski's sign (passive anteflexion of the neck causes the patient to flex hips, knees, and ankles) indicates meningeal irritation and calls for immediate referral for medical intervention.

Lymph glands should be examined systematically by groups. A localized cervical lymphadenitis is commonly caused by infection of the scalp, face, mouth, teeth, pharynx, or ears. A search for generalized enlargement of nodes elsewhere in the body should follow. This is especially important during adolescence, because the incidence of mononucleosis is high. Cervical lymph nodes are enlarged in 99 percent of patients with mononucleosis, splenic enlargement is detected in 75 percent, and enlargement of axillary and other lymph nodes is found in a majority. Laboratory tests show atypical lymphocytes in the blood smear and a positive agglutination test. Many adolescents have liver damage. Unfortunately, the course of this disease is misunderstood by many young people and their parents. Nursing plans need to take into account previous energy levels of the adolescent, as well as attitudes of the parents and teenager toward fatigue and illness. Bed rest is essential only until the temperature is normal, usually within 10 days. Activity does not affect the course of the disease. If there is spleen enlargement, care must be taken to avoid a blow to the abdomen, but routine activity may be resumed. Depression is not uncommon among students whose schooling is interrupted, and both psychological and academic support for these patients is indicated.[60,61]

Hodgkin's disease is characterized most often by chronic localized cervical lymphadenopathy, although it may occur in other lymph nodes. The incidence in adolescent boys is twice as high as in girls. Besides lymph node involvement, signs and symptoms include anorexia, fever, weakness, weight loss, and night sweats. Teenagers with Hodgkin's disease often have pruritis, cold intolerance, and anemia. Diagnosis is made by extensive blood analysis, biopsy of the node and of the bone marrow, or laparotomy with liver biopsy and spleenectomy, as well as numerous other tests and procedures. The nursing plan is based on current approaches to oncology and, of course, growth and development. "Living with" rather than "dying from" cancer is a suitable approach for the adolescent's sense of immortality. Long-term treatment, however, is a difficult management problem. First, the separation from peers (for hospitalization) and interruption of schooling or future plans are hard to accept. Most adolescents become intensely introspective, seeking to learn causes for their condition and reasoning whether it is just or unjust that they should bear it. The surgical procedures and physical results of treatment may produce severe personality changes and alteration in body image. Constantly open involvement of the doctor and nurse with the adolescent can help to provide hope, an essential stimulant to life.[62]

Thyroid disorders occur frequently at the onset of adolescence. A nursing assessment must give careful attention to observation and history for signs and symptoms related to these disorders. Genetic factors are thought to be involved, with more girls than boys being affected. The major function of the thyroid gland is to concentrate iron from the blood and return it to the peripheral tissues in a hormonally active form. Tissue respiration and most metabolic processes concerned with growth, development, and maturation are determined by the available quantity of hormonal iodine. Thyroid hormone also influences mental growth, body resistance to infection, nervous system activity, and circulation.[63,64]

Enlargement of the gland is called goiter and may occur with hypofunction or hyperfunction, the most common cause among adolescents being chronic lymphoid thyroiditis (Hashimoto's struma). Signs and symptoms are nervousness, tachycardia, and other indicators of thyrotoxicosis (without exophthalmos). The thyroid is usually about twice regular size, firm, and of rubbery consistency. Serum thyroglobulin antibodies are present in about 80 percent of these patients. Surgery should be avoided since it may accelerate progression of the autoimmune process and increase hypothyroidism. Diagnostic laboratory studies should include T_4 and a number of other thyroid function tests. Diagnosis may be easily confirmed by needle biopsy. Therapy for most forms of chronic lymphoid thyroiditis requires thyroid hormone suppression. Hypothyroidism in adolescence usually presents classic symptoms of sluggishness; weight gain despite loss of appetite; puffy face and eyes; coarse, brittle hair; dry skin; and thick tongue. The heart is quiet and the pulse slow. Puberty may be delayed or there may be menorrhagia. Treatment is by replacement with thyroid hormone.[65]

Juvenile thyrotoxicosis is a diffuse thyroid hyperplasia. The most common form in adolescence is Graves' disease, which affects girls six times as frequently as boys. It evidently results from a disturbance in the immunochemical systems of the body. Signs of Graves' disease are usually striking. There is a marked hyperkinetic state, often seen in school gym classes as poor coordination. The adolescent experiences increased appetite and weight loss, heat intolerance, irritability, behavioral difficulties, and poor schoolwork. Cardiac signs include tachycardia (especially at rest), murmurs, and wide pulse pressure. Eye signs in adolescence include staring, blinking, redness, and mild exophthalmos. The goiter becomes very large. Treatment is by drugs, surgery, or, if these are not successful, radioactive iodine. A so-called combined antithyroid-thyroid therapy seems to be the most beneficial program. The second treatment choice is subtotal thyroidectomy. The nursing plan[66] should include helping the young person, parents, and teachers to understand the adolescent's actions until he or she is regulated by treatment. The teenager needs to eat more and rest more than usual. Reduction of stimulating foods and environment will help to reduce tension. The eyes may need to be protected from infection, dust, and glare. If exophthalmia is noticeable, there may be a loss of self-esteem. Good grooming and dark glasses help maintain appearance. The long-term use of drugs will require continuing explanation and support from the nurse. Antihistamines are contraindicated in all thyroid disease.

Neuromuscular System   *Headache, nervousness, dizziness, convulsions, tics, gait irregularities, weak or wasting muscles, facial weakness, temperature or pain sensitivity.*

There are many diseases of nerves and muscle which may first appear during adolescence. These diseases are characterized by weakness and fatigability; myasthenia gravis and muscular dystrophy are two classical, well-known conditions. However, I have chosen Bell's palsy for this discussion, because it appears more frequently.

Bell's palsy is a sudden, unilateral paralysis of the seventh cranial (facial) nerve. Frequently the first symptom is pain in the ear. The adolescent may shortly complain of numbness of the lips and tongue. The mouth draws to one side, and there is difficulty closing the eyelid. Eventually all the muscles innervated by one facial nerve are affected. Taste is usually diminished, and noises seem louder in the homolateral ear because of weakness of the stapedius muscle. Nursing assessment depends on a present illness history and examination of all cranial nerves. Although the disease may be self-limiting, early medical referral and treatment may provide fuller recovery of function. The nursing plan should include education about the cause of the palsy and the self-limiting nature of the disease. There is often fear that this disorder may be caused by a brain tumor. The young person will need reassurance and support as long as the paralysis causes facial changes, because family, peers, and teachers will make him or her conscious of the disfiguration.[67]

Bones and Joints   *Fractures, sprains, dislocations, joint pains, postural deformities, night cramps.*

Adolescents probably spend more time practicing and playing sports and games than any other age group in American society. The participation of girls, especially, has increased greatly during the last five years. Every sport has some potential for injury, and unsafe acts lead to accidents and injuries. The school nurse in particular makes assessments of all kinds of sports injuries and must make decisions not only about the severity of injury and proper referral for care but also about return to participation. It is imperative, therefore, that nurses in schools and other sports settings develop assessment skills and master first-aid and emergency treatment procedures. Assessment begins with the health assessment to determine whether the adolescent may safely participate in sports. This assessment should include history of previous illness and injury, especially heart ailments, head injury, and injury to extremities. It is very desirable also to do some cardiovascular fitness tests, such as the recovery-step test or Balke's 15-minute run. Some coaches or teachers are qualified to do these. Evaluation of developmental stage and somatotype can be done by the nurse and may result in counseling for appropriate choice of activity. Any student who is injured repeatedly should be evaluated for cerebellar function.[68]

Every school should have an established plan for the first-aid treatment of injuries. Written designation of responsibilities, location of equipment, and procedures for parent notification all help to provide better care and treatment and reduce further injury and anxiety.

Poor posture is common among adolescents, partly due to rapid skeletal growth and lagging muscular growth. Adolescents with poor posture should be evaluated through history and examination to determine if there are skeletal problems. Persistent backache in adolescence is generally due to some underlying pathology, the most common being kyphosis and spondylolisthesis, a forward slipping of one vertebral body on another. Exercises, braces, and sometimes surgery are treatment modalities and should help to prevent deformity and back problems later in life.[69,70]

Scoliosis is defined as one or more lateral-rotary curvatures of the spine. Eighty percent of adolescent scoliosis occurs in girls, and most curves are to the right. A flexible curve will correct when the client bends to the convex side, and it is called nonstructural. The curve is called structural when it fails to straighten on side-bending. If detected early, the deformity can be successfully treated with a Milwaukee brace and exercises.[71,72] Scoliosis screening of students in grades six through nine is being done routinely by school nurses in many schools throughout the

Standing erect: One shoulder may be higher than the other. There is an unequal distance between the arms and the sides of the body. The shoulder blade is usually elevated on the side of the convexity of the curve.

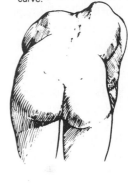

Bending forward: A rib hump or an elevation in the lumbar area will be observed on the side of the convexity of the curve.

Figure 3-1 Scoliosis can easily be detected by observing the teenager from the back in the two positions shown. (*Drawing from G. Scipien et al. [eds.]*, Comprehensive Pediatric Nursing, *2d ed., McGraw-Hill Book Company, New York, 1979.*)

country. The best procedure is to examine the student from behind while the student stands firmly on both feet and with the upper trunk completely exposed. Figure 3-1 illustrates the points to be observed: level of shoulders, scapula, and hips; unequal distance between arms and the sides of the body; or a rib hump seen when bending forward from the hip with arms dangling. Referral should be made for orthopedic examination with x-rays for bone age as well as spinal defects whenever any of these indications of scoliosis is observed. Nursing plans are based on the adolescent's feelings about the body deformity, even though it may not be very noticeable. If a Milwaukee brace is prescribed, talking with another adolescent who has made an adjustment to the condition will often help to alleviate anxiety. Shared information about clothing styles to wear while in braces and support for the exercise routine are also helpful. If scoliosis is diagnosed but bracing is not needed, follow-up visits to watch the progress of the curve are essential.[73]

Osgood-Schlatter disease, inflammation of the tibial tubercle, is assessed by history of pain and a lump on the tubercle. Pain is aggravated by squatting as well as running, kneeling, and stooping. Rapid growth of legs and knees causes stretching of the patellar tendon and occurs most frequently in boys during the period of rapid growth (Tanner's Stage 3). Mild involvement is treated by limitation of activity and local heat. More severe cases may require use of a plastic cylinder cast for six weeks. This is a self-limiting condition which will heal without treatment but may then leave a very large and tender tubercle. The nurse should follow the progress of adolescents with Osgood-Schlatter disease to help guide a course between overtreatment and undertreatment.[74]

Juvenile rheumatoid arthritis is a connective tissue disease, but the most easily observed signs and symptoms involve joints. Therefore, I have included this condition in the review of bones and joints. Juvenile rheumatoid arthritis may be grouped into three broad categories: systemic (Still's disease), pauciarticular, and polyarticular. Still's disease onset is characterized by high fever, rash, lymphadenopathy, splenomegaly, and leukocytosis. Arthritis may not be present at first, but eventually all the large and small joints become involved. Unlike other forms of juvenile arthritis, this acute systemic disease appears more often in boys than in girls. The outcome is unpredictable. In a small number of patients the disorder may clear up in 6 to 18 months, but a larger percentage develop a polycyclic course. This development causes the youth much anxiety because it mimics the initial onset. In the majority of patients, the arthritis becomes chronic and in about 25 percent results in severe permanent disability. It seems from studies in England and Scandinavia that the older the child is at onset of the disease the poorer the prognosis.[75]

Pauciarticular rheumatoid arthritis is limited to five or fewer joints. Girls are more often affected than boys. Large joints of the lower extremities are most commonly involved. An important complication that occurs late in the disease is iridocyclitis. It is suggested that all children and adolescents with juvenile rheumatoid arthritis should have six-month or yearly ophthalmologic examinations as long as the joint disease is active and for four to five years thereafter.[76]

About one-third to one-half of all juvenile rheumatoid arthritis patients have polyarticular arthritis resembling the adult type, which involves small joints of the hands and feet as well as large joints. This type affects girls twice as often as boys.[77]

The prognosis for recovery from juvenile rheumatoid arthritis is more promising today than in the past. Prompt treatment, range of motion exercises, planned rest periods, and heat applications all help to relieve pain and prevent flexion deformity. The nursing plan should be coordinated with the medical plan in order to give the patient the necessary support for following the treatment regimen. Teaching should help increase understanding of the disease and the treatment plan. Adjustment of the school program should be planned by the nurse and the adolescent with teachers. Morning stiffness makes physical education class difficult at that time. Painful hands cause writing difficulties. The adolescent's necessarily slower gait and need for rest periods should be recognized and the patient's schoolday schedule adjusted accordingly. Aspirin is the drug of choice for treatment and is used not as an analgesic but as an anti-inflammatory agent. Large doses are given regularly in order to maintain high blood levels of salicylate. These levels are near toxicity, and the nurse should teach the youth the symptoms of toxicity: tinnitis, lethargy, and gastrointestinal symptoms. If gold therapy is used, the nurse must know the preparation being used in order to monitor the adolescent for side effects. Rash, urticaria, renal disease, and weakness are a few of the toxic reactions experienced, and the drug should be discontinued if they arise.[78]

Endocrine System *Stature variations; abnormal weight and body configuration; abnormal size of hands, feet, and head; abnormal hair distribution or skin pigmentation; goiter; exophthalmos; dryness of skin and hair; intolerance to heat or cold; tremor; excessive thirst, hunger, and urination.*

Endocrine disorders become apparent when the normal control mechanisms for hormone production are not functioning adequately and there is increased, decreased, or untimely secretion of hormones. Observable manifestations include delayed puberty, precocious puberty, dwarfism, gigantism, short stature, tall stature, thyroid disorders, Cushing's syndrome, Addison's disease, and diabetes mellitus. Two of these conditions, growth disorders and diabetes mellitus, will be discussed here.

One of the most difficult adjustment problems for adolescents arises from differences in stature. All boys presumably want to be tall, and nearly all girls prefer being short. Linear growth involves an interplay of growth hormone, thyroxine, and sex hormones. Nurses in schools are in a good position to make growth assessments because they see adolescents regularly and have growth records available. Familial short stature and slow maturation are common causes for short stature. Undernutrition and metabolic, cardiac, respiratory, or bone disorders are also causes. A detailed history about stature of near and distant relatives should be obtained. Other history to be sought is age of onset of puberty of parents, pregnancy and birth events, developmental milestones, and nutritional history. In addition, physical examination and laboratory tests including radiologic bone age, chromosomal testing, and endocrine function are necessary for correct diagnosis. Therefore, medical referral is essential. Growth failure can usually be treated if recognized early, which will prevent the psychological difficulties of short stature in adolescence.[79]

Tall stature presents no social problems for boys unless height is excessive. It may, however, cause exquisite torture for girls. Severe psychological problems may arise in some girls and are a sufficient reason to consider hormone therapy. The best results are achieved when treatment is begun before menarche, but girls may also benefit after menarche. The decision to initiate treatment involves a long discussion with the girl, her parents, the nurse, and the physician. A prediction of adult height can be made quite accurately using the girl's present height and hand-wrist skeletal age and comparing them to Bayler-Pinneau prediction tables. Girls who are predicted to grow taller than 178 cm (70 inches) are likely to request therapy. Details of treatment, side effects, outcomes, controversies about estrogen therapy, and length of treatment should be discussed thoroughly.[80]

Whether diabetes mellitus develops before or during adolescence, its effect at this stage of life requires special consideration. Adolescent diabetes is characterized by rapid onset, early remission lasting many weeks or months, and later development of what appears to be complete diabetes with a tendency to acidosis, labile blood sugars, and nocturnal hyperglycemia. Teaching the young person how to manage the disease is initially done by nurses during hospitalization while control is being established. Thereafter, the office, school, or public health nurse will be expected to help the adolescent attain the management goals that have been set. These goals most likely will include: no acetone in the urine, a 24-hour glycosuria not to exceed 10 to 15 percent of carbohydrate intake, near normal blood sugar before meals, normal growth and weight, freedom from symptoms of uncontrolled disease, and a satisfactory emotional development.[81] If these goals are to be accomplished, diabetic adolescents must be taught a great deal about their disease.

A simple explanation about failure of the pancreas to produce insulin will often not be enough information for adolescents. They need to know that this disease prevents normal metabolism and storage of carbohydrates. They need to be taught the reasons for and the symptoms of ketoacidosis, which results from insufficient insulin. Dry skin, flushed face, thirst, nausea, vomiting, abdominal pain, rapid pulse, blurred vision, and deep (Kussmaul) respirations are signs that immediate administration of insulin is necessary. Diabetic teenagers also need to learn how to replace the missing insulin by injecting proper dosages for the body's needs. Most are willing to learn about insulin mixing, doses, aseptic techniques for injections, and rotation of sites. They need to learn the symptoms of insulin shock, caused by too much insulin. Shock may occur when meals are delayed, when the adolescent has exercised more than usual, or in periods of emotional stress. Pallor and sweating, nervousness, fatigue, headache, hunger, tremor, faintness, diplopia, and often irrational behavior indicate a need for more sugar, which can be given in fruit juices or sugar cubes.[82,83]

Diet management is essential for a stable course. Diabetics need to understand calories and exchanges. They need to be taught how to select foods at restaurants or in school cafeterias. They need to know that the social aspects of life that include food do not have to be avoided, but that a few careful substitutions will allow them to be free of reactions and therefore to be more "normal." Consideration should be given to individual likes or dislikes, cultural and racial background, and habits.[84]

Diabetic adolescents should be taught how and when to test their urine for sugar and acetone. They should be able to correlate urine testing and insulin need. They should learn that infections heal more slowly and that therefore careful attention to injuries and illnesses is important. They must always take their insulin when sick, sometimes will need more, and should convert to a full liquid diet. Tooth decay is more frequent in teenagers with diabetes, and regular visits to the dentist should be scheduled.[85]

Adolescents' needs for independence and peer recognition are key aspects for satisfactory emotional development of the young person with diabetes. The nurse's patient explanations, reasonableness, and willingness to listen will gain the adolescent's trust without impairing independence. Teenagers need confidence that the nurse knows as much as they do about their disease, but they also need recognition that they are the best observers of their own symptoms and that they are the ones who have the greatest control. They should be enabled to express resentments and hostilities about having diabetes, but they should be reminded that good control of the disease brings them very close to the normal state of their peers. Adolescents really do welcome some rules that they understand, and this is true for diabetics also. Unnecessary restrictions, however, should not be imposed. The youth should be encouraged to have normal exercise and even to engage in competitive sports. Nurses must be astute in their observations of adolescents with diabetes. There are many social situations that may cause the teenager to skip a dose of insulin or eat too many high-carbohydrate foods. There will be times of despair and depression that should be responded to. Any insulin reaction should be reported to parents so that there may be follow-up and dosage or dietary adjustment, although contacting parents must be done carefully so as not to make the adolescent feel that he or she is losing control. Good communication among school, parents, and physician and continued education of the adolescent can enable the diabetic to manage satisfactorily and to come very close to being a normal young person.[86,87,88]

Adaptive Systems   *Gastrointestinal: Appetite change, difficulty swallowing, pain or distress, nausea or vomiting, pyrosis, flatulence, unusual color and form of stools, food intolerance, unhealthful eating patterns (e.g., gulp, nibble, eat and run, fast and feast). Liver: Alteration of color of urine and stools, history of hepatitis, yellow sclerae. Respiratory: Dyspnea, pain, cough, wheezing, cyanosis, hemoptysis, tuberculosis contact, last chest x-ray. Cardiovascular: Pain, dyspnea, edema, heart consciousness, cyanosis, abnormal blood pressure. Kidney: Enuresis, dysuria, polyuria, hematuria, kidney infections.*

This section in the review of systems is what Kugelmass[89] calls the adaptive systems. He believes that good health depends on how well a person adjusts to the stresses, strains, and crises of everyday life. The physiological response mechanism is determined, he believes, by constitutional disposition. The person's reactions may be automatic and may result in psychosomatic illness and anxiety disorders. The psychological mechanism depends on the personality pattern, the appraisal of threat, and frustration or challenge. Responses may be defective performance, emotional dissonance, or neurosis. The grouping of gastrointestinal, liver, respiratory, cardiovascular, and kidney disorders provides a good means of assessing how well the adolescent is coping with experiences and how well the body's restorative processes are working.

Gastrointestinal disorders are often reflectors of the emotions. Signs and symptoms of inflammatory disease of the bowel (Crohn's disease) include diarrhea with cramps and bloody, mucous stools. Relief of stress, careful diet control, and reasonable rest are the first modes of treatment. Records indicate that greater than 50 percent of these patients are eventually advised to have surgery.[90] Upper gastrointestinal symptoms include heartburn, nausea, vomiting, distension, and pain. These can collectively be classified as peptic disorders, since pepsin and hydrochloric acid are always present. However, the amount present is not as important as many other rather poorly understood factors. Heredity, physical or mental stress, and commonly ingested chemicals such as coffee, alcohol, and salicylates are factors. If a trial of antacid gives relief, it confirms the suspicion that the symptoms indicate peptic disorder. In mild cases where there is no bleeding, symptoms are usually relieved by frequent feedings of bland protein foods such as milk and fermented cheeses. Diet may include cooked vegetables and fruits and simple meats. Coffee, alcohol, citrus fruits, leathery fried foods, spices, and seasonings are to be avoided. Supportive assistance to adjust life-style to reduce stress is an important nursing function (see Chapters 9, 11, and 18).

Liver disorders most commonly seen in adolescence are the various forms of hepatitis. Acute viral hepatitis is caused by the two different viruses which produce infectious hepatitis and serum hepatitis. Both may be transmitted orally or parenterally. However, adolescents at greater risk for contracting serum hepatitis are those in the drug culture. Skin tattooing and ear piercing also can cause serum hepatitis. Infectious mononucleosis is frequently complicated by liver involvement, and adolescents with mononucleosis must be watched closely for signs of hepatitis. Before the jaundice which accompanies hepatitis is observed, there may be fever, chills, headache, arthralgia, and urticarial rash.[91,92]

Respiratory disorders include streptococcal pharyngitis, the common cold, chronic sinusitis and chronic bronchitis, bacterial pneumonia, and asthma. Asthma presents one of the most complicated management problems in adolescence. Two complicating attitudes of asthma victims often make assessment of the severity of an attack difficult. Some adolescents suppress symptoms and ignore the disease, while others have a tendency to exaggerate subjective complaints in order to get attention. These attitudes and the life-threatening possibilities make it difficult for parents as well as teachers and school nurses to plan effectively for some youth. In general, however, adolescents with asthma should be encouraged to maintain nutrition, to continue normal physical activities, and to adhere to and regulate their drug therapy. Nebulizers, if used in single doses and in anticipation or in the early stages of an acute attack, are very effective. Daily medications, in fact, are considered preventive. One of the most effective nebulizers uses cromolyn sodium, which protects against offending allergens.[93]

Cardiovascular disorders in the adolescent are complicated by the many physiologic changes of this age. Any adolescent who has had a cardiac problem since childhood will now require some new nursing approaches. Adolescents want to know more about their disease and what it means to them now and for the future. The developmental needs for peer identity are especially difficult for young people with cardiac problems. The self-restrictions that prevented overexertion during childhood are no longer used reliably and symptoms are ignored. Differentiating symptoms from fears is also a difficult task. School nurses often see students whose symptoms are causing them great anxiety. It is important to get them to a quiet place to rest where they can then talk about their fears without their peers observing. If the physician has not supplied the information the adolescent needs in order to understand his or her condition, the young person should be encouraged to make an appointment for this purpose. Health habits, nutrition, and life-style should be discussed in a way that is not restrictive but which promotes a preventive attitude. Any teenager who had rheumatic fever or has congenital heart defects should be on an endocarditis prevention program. This means that any dental or surgical procedure should be preceded by prophylactic antibiotic coverage. Many rheumatic fever patients, whether or not there was cardiac damage, are placed on a lifetime prophylactic program. Compliance with this program is often poor during the adolescent years, but it must be encouraged. Birth control methods and pregnancy risks should be thoroughly discussed with girls and plans made on the basis of the individual diagnosis. Other problems for adolescents with cardiac conditions are employment and insurance. Rehabilitation services provide for the most thorough evaluation of employment possibilities and also provide good counseling, guidance, and training. Students should be referred early during their high school years.[94,95,96]

The identification of hypertension in adolescents is a challenge for nurses, since it is they who most commonly take blood pressure readings. Their knowledge and alertness regarding norms will improve evaluation and referral. Loggie,[97] who has conducted studies of adolescent hypertension at Cincinnati Children's Hospital, uses the following criteria for borderline hypertension: any male whose supine systolic pressure is usually between 130 and 145 mmHg, or whose supine diastolic pressure is usually between 75 and 82 mmHg; any female 12 to 15 whose supine systolic pressure is usually between 135 and 140 mmHg, or whose supine diastolic pressure is usually between 75 and 88 mmHg. Supine diastolic pressure of 90 or greater in teenagers 16 to 21 is considered systemic hypertension. If diastolic readings above 90 mmHg are found, they should be repeated at least three different times. The nurse should then obtain the following patient information and family history: incidence of headaches, dizziness associated with headaches, chest pain, and shortness of breath; edema of legs, ankles, hands, and face; menstrual history, pregnancies, diet, drug use; hypertension, stroke, coronary insufficiency, diabetes, kidney disease, or kidney tumors in blood relatives.

School nurses have the opportunity to conduct blood pressure screening clinics for students, and this is especially important in areas where the adult population is known to have a high incidence of hypertension and among the black population. Repeated readings and the compiling of historical information will make any subsequent referral to the family doctor especially meaningful. Follow-up and reinforcement of the medical plan will provide the adolescent with needed support. It is difficult for an adolescent to internalize the fact that the average duration of life after the onset of primary hypertension is only 20 years. Adhering to a medication plan is also a very difficult thing for teenagers to do, especially when the side effects make them feel worse than before. The management plan for adolescent hypertension is time-consuming and demands patient and continued counseling.[98]

Kidney disorders or genitourinary problems may result from streptococcal infections, errors in tubular absorption, and structural abnormalities. Problems range from enuresis to urinary tract infections to acute glomerulonephritis, which is believed to be caused by streptococcal infections. For this reason penicillin treatment of all streptococcal infections is very important. Subjective symptoms of glomerulonephritis are rare, and diagnosis depends on laboratory findings of proteinuria, hematuria, and pyuria. Such findings should be followed by more thorough laboratory work including creatinine clearance and intravenous pyelogram. Long-term treatment of any genitourinary disorder is common.[99,100]

Reproductive System   *Girls: menstrual history—age of onset, frequency of periods, regularity, amount of flow, dysmenorrhea, date of last* *period. Breast sensitivity, trauma, or changes in size. Sexually active? Pregnancy? Abortion? Vaginal discharge? Boys: gynecomastia, abnormalities of penis and testicles, circumcision. Both: venereal disease history; chancre, bubo, discharge, treatment.*

The assessment of the reproductive system is really not complete without an accurate evaluation of the young person's stage of sexual development. Tanner's pictorial stages[101-104] simplify this task in situations in which the nurse can visually inspect the breasts of female clients and the external genitals of both males and females. A consideration of the young person's chronological age plus a comparison to Tanner's photographs or equivalent pictures provides the most accurate assessment of sexual development.

Disorders of the reproductive system are especially troublesome to the adolescent in the establishment of a positive self-image. When the changes that are taking place are poorly understood, there is fear of nonacceptance, fear for the future, and many doubts about self. The physical changes may be extremely upsetting, as when the facial bones enlarge or when a boy develops gynecomastia. A sensitive handling of the questions in the review of the reproductive system will convey to the young person that you realize how important this aspect of growth is.

The most common gynecologic disorders that adolescent girls complain about are dysmenorrhea, amenorrhea, and vaginal discharge. *Dysmenorrhea* is often a perplexing condition because physicians generally believe that there is a psychological component. Every girl who has severe cramps which cause her to interrupt her usual routine should be referred to her doctor for a thorough pelvic examination, and her attitude toward her sexuality should be evaluated. The complaint could be due to a pelvic inflammatory disease, dermoid cyst of the ovary, adhesions, or endometriosis. In most cases there is no evidence of pathology, but the very real pain must be dealt with. Because administration of hormones generally alleviates this condition, the belief that it is of psychologic origin has come under suspicion. Reaction to pain differs in every individual, and the tendency to treat the complaint lightly does nothing to relieve the pain. Sturgis,[105] after careful examination to rule out secondary dysmenorrhea, assures his patients that he can provide relief from pain. He says that if he gives estrogen throughout one cycle to prevent ovulation, there will be no primary dysmenorrhea. His very careful plan of relief of pain through hormone use and monthly consultations for 8 to 10 months usually alleviates the problem.

Amenorrhea is normal during the first few years after menarche. Irregular periods may persist for several years and are brought about by stress, malnutrition, and seasonal and environmental changes. The most common cause for amenorrhea, however, is pregnancy, and this possibility must always be discussed when counseling with a concerned adolescent. Amenorrhea is considered to be primary if a girl has never menstruated by the end of her seventeenth year. There are many causes for primary amenorrhea, including pituitary lesions, uterine disorders, thyroid disorders, and chromosomal abnormalities such as Turner's syndrome. The anxiety of the girl and her parents demands a thorough examination to determine the reason.[106,107]

Vaginal discharge is troublesome to adolescent girls, but rarely do they find courage to ask anyone about it. Nurses can explain the normalcy of a discharge by explaining about the effects of hormonal activity on the cervix and vagina. Good personal hygiene should be stressed. The irritations that can be caused by colored toilet tissue, tight panty hose, and vaginal tampons should be discussed. If the girl is sexually active, a smear for gonorrhea should be done. The warning signs of an abnormal discharge are itching, burning, and foul odor. Monilia produces a white, sometimes cheesy exudate and should be treated with mycostatin. Trichomonas vaginitis is caused by a protozoan parasite and produces thin, yellow, very irritating discharge. It is usually curable with the use of Flagyl.[108,109]

Differences among boys in size of penis and testicles may be simply developmental and apparent because of the wide age range during which this development occurs. Small genitals may also be a sign of gonadal disorder. Delayed puberty, hypogonadism, and Klinefelter's syndrome are all possibilities when there are small testicles. A thorough history and physical examination should be followed by gonadal function tests. Hormone therapy is usually beneficial.

No review of the reproductive system is complete without discussing venereal disease with the client. Most adolescents are aware that gonorrhea and syphilis are sexually transmitted diseases, but they are hardly aware of the significance of the epidemic in which adolescents and young adults are involved. Furthermore, many have never heard of the other sexually transmitted diseases, some of which are also of epidemic proportion: genital warts (condyloma acuminatum), genital Herpesvirus Type 2 infection, Trichomonas infestation, and Candida (Monilia) vaginitis. (The last-named two infections are transmissible by sexual contact, although most persons who develop these disorders do not acquire them that way.) Education, early treatment, and follow-up of contacts are still regarded as essential weapons against the venereal disease epidemic, even though it is obvious that the incidence of infection has continued to rise.

Gonorrhea is difficult both to diagnose and to treat. About 75 percent of infected females have no symptoms, and the percentage of asymptomatic males may now be as high as 6 percent. Therefore, all sexually active persons should have a gonococcus culture at regular intervals (and persons with gonorrhea should be tested for syphilis). The currently recommended treatment for both of these diseases is procaine penicillin with probenecid. Adolescents who are infected are thrust into coping with parental horror, peer reactions, management of their physical symptoms, and the community of health care providers. The tortuous route from infected sexual partner to sympathetic friend to diagnostician to treatment center can be very taxing. Not only is the first treatment visit difficult, but also adherence to follow-up instructions is very poor among teenagers. I believe nurses must be very clear, very specific, and very firm in dealing with adolescents about treatment. This does not imply moralizing, but abstinence, which is as important as the proper drug regimen, can certainly be emphasized as a part of the treatment plan.

REFERENCES

1 L. Malasanos, V. Barkauskas, M. Moss, and K. Stoltenberg-Allen, *Health Assessment*, St. Louis: C. V. Mosby Co., 1977.
2 Ibid.
3 Ibid., p. 12.
4 I. N. Kugelmass, *Adolescent Medicine: Principles and Practice*, Springfield, Ill.: Charles C Thomas, 1975, p. 10.
5 E. L. DeGowin and R. L. DeGowin, *Bedside Diagnostic Examination*, 3d ed. New York: Macmillan Co., 1976.
6 H. K. Silver, C. H. Kempe, and H. B. Bruyn, *Handbook of Pediatrics*, 12th ed. Los Altos, Calif.: Lange Medical Publications, 1977.
7 Ibid.
8 DeGowin and DeGowin, op. cit.
9 E. Getchell and R. Howard, "Nutrition in Development," in G. Scipien et al. (eds.), *Comprehensive Pediatric Nursing*, 2d ed. New York: McGraw-Hill Book Co., 1979.
10 Group for the Advancement of Psychiatry, *Normal Adolescence: Its Dynamics and Impact*. New York: Charles Scribner's Sons, 1968.
11 K. W. Sehnert and H. Eisenberg, *How to Be Your Own Doctor—Sometimes*. New York: Grosset and Dunlap, 1976.
12 L. L. Fine, "What's a Normal Adolescent? A Guide for the Assessment of Adolescent Behavior," *Clinical Pediatrics*, 12:1-5, January 1973.
13 L. L. Weed, *Your Health Care and How to Manage It*. Essex Junction, Vt.: Essex Publishing Co., 1975.
14 Kugelmass, op. cit., p. ix.
15 Silver, Kempe, and Bruyn, op. cit.
16 DeGowin and DeGowin, op. cit.
17 G. C. Sauer, *Manual of Skin Diseases*. Philadelphia: J. B. Lippincott, 1973, pp. 92–94.
18 Ibid.
19 Ibid.
20 Kugelmass, op. cit.

21 Sauer, op. cit.
22 Ibid.
23 Kugelmass, op. cit.
24 Sauer, op. cit.
25 Ibid.
26 Kugelmass, op. cit.
27 Ibid.
28 Sauer, op. cit.
29 A. J. Nahmias et al., "Genital Infection with Type 2 Herpesvirus Hominis: A Commonly Occurring Venereal Disease," *British Journal of Venereal Disease*, **45**:294–298, December 1969.
30 Sauer, op. cit.
31 Kugelmass, op. cit.
32 Ibid.
33 Sauer, op. cit.
34 Ibid.
35 Ibid.
36 Ibid.
37 Ibid.
38 Ibid.
39 Ibid.
40 J. S. Strauss and P. E. Pochi, "Acne and Some Other Common Skin Disorders," in J. R. Gallagher et al. (eds.), *Medical Care of the Adolescent*, 3d ed. New York: Appleton-Century-Crofts, 1976.
41 Sauer, op. cit.
42 Strauss and Pochi, op. cit.
43 Sauer, op. cit.
44 A. E. Sloane and J. A. Kraut, "Problems Relating to Vision," in J. R. Gallagher et al. (eds.), *Medical Care of the Adolescent*, 3d ed. New York: Appleton-Century-Crofts, 1976.
45 Ibid.
46 W. G. Hardy, "Problems Relating to Hearing," in J. A. Gallagher et al. (eds.), *Medical Care of the Adolescent*, 3d ed. New York: Appleton-Century-Crofts, 1976.
47 Ibid.
48 Ibid.
49 DeGowin and DeGowin, op. cit.
50 Kugelmass, op. cit.
51 Ibid.
52 Ibid.
53 Hardy, op. cit.
54 DeGowin and DeGowin, op. cit.
55 Ibid.
56 Ibid.
57 Ibid.
58 American Academy of Pediatrics, *Standards of Child Health Care*. Evanston, Ill.: American Academy of Pediatrics, 1972.

59 DeGowin and DeGowin, op. cit.
60 Kugelmass, op. cit.
61 W. Dalrymple, "Infectious Mononucleosis," in J. R. Gallagher et al. (eds.), *Medical Care of the Adolescent*, 3d ed. New York: Appleton-Century-Crofts, 1976.
62 Kugelmass, op. cit.
63 Ibid.
64 J. C. Hallal, "Thyroid Disorders," *American Journal of Nursing*, 77(3):417–432, March 1977.
65 H. A. Selenkow and T. Himathongkam, "Thyroid Disease in Adolescence: Diagnosis and Therapy," in J. R. Gallagher et al. (eds.), *Medical Care of the Adolescent*, 3d ed. New York: Appleton-Century-Crofts, 1976.
66 Hallal, op. cit.
67 G. M. Fenichel, "Neuromuscular Disorders," in J. R. Gallagher et al. (eds.), *Medical Care of the Adolescent*, 3d ed. New York: Appleton-Century-Crofts, 1976.
68 R. Whittemore, "A General Consideration of Cardiovascular Problems," in J. R. Gallagher et al. (eds.), *Medical Care of the Adolescent*, 3d ed. New York: Appleton-Century-Crofts, 1976.
69 Kugelmass, op. cit.
70 A. W. Trott, "Posture and Other Musculoskeletal Problems," in J. R. Gallagher et al. (eds.), *Medical Care of the Adolescent*, 3d ed. New York: Appleton-Century-Crofts, 1976.
71 DeGowin and DeGowin, op. cit.
72 H. A. Keim, "Scoliosis," *Clinical Symposia*, vol. 24, no. 1, Ciba-Geigy Corporation, 1972.
73 Ibid.
74 Trott, op. cit.
75 N. J. Zvaifler, "Arthritis in Adolescents," in J. R. Gallagher et al. (eds.), *Medical Care of the Adolescent*, 3d ed. New York: Appleton-Century-Crofts, 1976.
76 Ibid.
77 Ibid.
78 Ibid.
79 H. N. Wettenhall, "Growth Problems," in J. R. Gallagher et al. (eds.), *Medical Care of the Adolescent*, 3d ed. New York: Appleton-Century-Crofts, 1976.
80 Ibid.
81 C. C. Bailey, "Diabetes," in J. R. Gallagher et al. (eds.), *Medical Care of the Adolescent*, 3d ed. New York: Appleton-Century-Crofts, 1976.
82 Ibid.
83 DeGowin and DeGowin, op. cit.
84 Bailey, op. cit.
85 C. N. Hudak et al.: *Clinical Protocols*, Philadelphia: J. B. Lippincott, 1976.
86 Ibid.
87 Bailey, op. cit.
88 Kugelmass, op. cit.

89 Ibid.

90 W. W. Point, "Inflammatory Bowel Disease: Regional Enteritis and Ulcerative Colitis," in J. R. Gallagher et al. (eds.), *Medical Care of the Adolescent*, 3d ed. New York: Appleton-Century-Crofts, 1976.

91 DeGowin and DeGowin, op. cit.

92 Kugelmass, op. cit.

93 Ibid.

94 Ibid.

95 Whittemore, op. cit.

96 K. D. Rose, "Cardiovascular Fitness," in J. R. Gallagher et al. (eds.), *Medical Care of the Adolescent*, 3d ed. New York: Appleton-Century-Crofts, 1976.

97 J. M. Loggie, "Systemic Hypertension," in J. R. Gallagher et al. (eds.), *Medical Care of the Adolescent*, 3d ed. New York: Appleton-Century-Crofts, 1976.

98 Ibid.

99 Kugelmass, op. cit.

100 C. E. Hollerman, E. H. Jenis, and P. L. Calcagno, "Renal Disease in Adolescents," in J. R. Gallagher et al. (eds.), *Medical Care of the Adolescent*, 3d ed. New York: Appleton-Century-Crofts, 1976.

101 J. M. Tanner, "Sequence, Tempo, and Individual Variation in the Growth and Development of Boys and Girls Aged Twelve to Sixteen," *Daedalus*, **100**(4):907–930, Fall 1971.

102 W. A. Marshall and J. M. Tanner, "Variations in Pattern of Pubertal Changes in Girls," *Archives of Disease in Childhood*, **44**:291–303, June 1969.

103 W. A. Marshall and J. M. Tanner, "Variations in Pattern of Pubertal Changes in Boys," *Archives of Disease in Childhood*, **45**:13–23, February 1970.

104 W. A. Daniel, Jr. et al.: "Diseases of the Reproductive System," in R. A. Hoekelman et al. (eds.), *Principles of Pediatrics: Health Care of the Young*, New York: McGraw-Hill Book Co., 1978.

105 S. H. Sturgis, "Menstrual Disorders," in J. R. Gallagher et al. (eds.), *Medical Care of the Adolescent*, 3d ed. New York: Appleton-Century-Crofts, 1976.

106 Ibid.

107 Kugelmass, op. cit.

108 Sturgis, op. cit.

109 Sehnert and Eisenberg, op. cit.

BIBLIOGRAPHY

Barness, L. A.: *Manual of Pediatric Physical Diagnosis*. Chicago: Year Book Medical Publishers, 1972.

Bates, B.: *A Guide to Physical Examination*. Philadelphia: J. B. Lippincott, 1974.

Bowens, B.: "The Nervous System," in M. Armstrong et al. (eds.), *McGraw-Hill Handbook of Clinical Nursing*. New York: McGraw-Hill Book Co., 1979.

Elkind, D.: *A Sympathetic Understanding of the Child: Birth to Sixteen*. Boston: Allyn and Bacon, 1974.

Farrell, H.: "Communicable Diseases," in M. Armstrong et al. (eds.), *McGraw-Hill Handbook of Clinical Nursing*. New York: McGraw-Hill Book Co., 1979.

Frauman, A. and C. Gilman: "The Urinary System," in M. Armstrong et al. (eds.), *McGraw-Hill Handbook of Clinical Nursing*. New York: McGraw-Hill Book Co., 1979.

Gallagher, J. R.: "The Care of Adolescents," in J. R. Gallagher et al. (eds.), *Medical Care of the Adolescent*, 3d ed. New York: Appleton-Century-Crofts, 1976.

Greene, P. and C. Hall: "The Hematologic System," in M. Armstrong et al. (eds.), *McGraw-Hill Handbook of Clinical Nursing*. New York: McGraw-Hill Book Co., 1979.

Guthrie, D.: "The Endocrine System," in M. Armstrong et al. (eds.), *McGraw-Hill Handbook of Clinical Nursing*. New York: McGraw-Hill Book Co., 1979.

Harris, P.: "The Integumentary System," in M. Armstrong et al. (eds.), *McGraw-Hill Handbook of Clinical Nursing*. New York: McGraw-Hill Book Co., 1979.

Havelock, R. G.: *The Change Agent's Guide to Innovation in Education*. Englewood Cliffs, N.J.: Educational Technology Publications, 1973.

Hazinski, M.: "The Cardiovascular System," in M. Armstrong et al. (eds.), *McGraw-Hill Handbook of Clinical Nursing*. New York: McGraw-Hill Book Co., 1979.

Lewis, M.: *Clinical Aspects of Child Development*. Philadelphia: Lea and Febiger, 1973.

Marren, E. and Burton, L.: "The Gastrointestinal System," in M. Armstrong et al. (eds.), *McGraw-Hill Handbook of Clinical Nursing*. New York: McGraw-Hill Book Co., 1979.

Point, W.: "Peptic Disorders and Functional Digestive Disorders," in J. R. Gallagher et al. (eds.), *Medical Care of the Adolescent*, 3d ed. New York: Appleton-Century-Crofts, 1976.

Scipien, G. M. et al. (eds.): *Comprehensive Pediatric Nursing*, 2d ed. New York: McGraw-Hill Book Co., 1979.

Snow, J.: "The Respiratory System," in M. Armstrong et al. (eds.), *McGraw-Hill Handbook of Clinical Nursing*. New York: McGraw-Hill Book Co., 1979.

Chapter 4

Responses to Illness and Disability

Patricia S. Yaros
Jeanne Howe

Any particular health problem may elicit different responses in some people than in others who have the same affliction. Furthermore, illness, injury, or disability may affect one person differently at one time than at another time. The reasons for these differences among people and within the same person from time to time are highly complex; no doubt the manner and adequacy of any individual's adjustment to a health problem are affected by many factors. This chapter discusses selected factors which are believed to be influential during adolescence and which suggest directions for nursing intervention.

DEVELOPMENTAL LEVEL

Illness and disability are particularly potent influences when they arise during a period of already existing rapid change. An organism undergoing rapid transition is relatively unstable and is therefore particularly vulnerable to disruptive influences that impinge upon it during that period of time. The embryo's susceptibility to malformation is a familiar example.

Adolescence, like the preschool period, is considered to be a period of high vulnerability to psychosocial difficulty if illness, injury, or disability occurs.[1]

Health problems, and some aspects of treatment as well, can conflict with the activities and ideals that adolescents pursue with great urgency and can readily make more difficult the already complicated business of maneuvering through adolescence and mastering its tasks. Self-esteem, social skills and acceptance, vocational preparation, sexual identity, and many other basic developmental components of the adolescent period can be impeded by loss of physical or intellectual function, relinquishment of self-care to parents or health professionals, deviation from peers in appearance, social isolation, interrupted schooling, or limited experience imposed by a health problem. In fact, the impact an illness or disability may have on development can be more taxing for an adolescent than the health problem itself. As will be discussed later, health problems can also have positive effects on the adolescent's resolution of the developmental tasks.

Developmental level is probably the most important single influence on an adolescent's response to illness, injury, or disability, because the developmental tasks demand resolution in the midst of virtually any circumstances and regardless of other influences. For this discussion, three stages of adolescence—early, middle, and late—serve as convenient divisions in order to examine the developmental context in which health problems may have predictable effects.

Early Adolescence—Am I Normal?

In the preteen or early teen years, the young person's body is greatly changed by the growth spurt and the development of male or female contours. Thought and behavior also undergo the usually pronounced changes that distinguish early adolescents from younger children. (Physical, cognitive, and emotional growth and development are described in Chapter 1.) Adolescents themselves are highly attentive to their physical changes and are often absorbed in their new thoughts. The biological and psychological selves are not distinctly segregated, and bodily changes and sensations are prominent in the early adolescent's thought.

This high degree of interest in one's body is accompanied by anxiety about normality. Young adolescents fear that their physical development will not turn out the way it should and that some of their new thoughts and feelings are "weird." These fears combine with the relative ignorance of youngsters this age about the changes that constitute normal adolescence, and concern about what is normal and how one compares to that standard is typical of early adolescence.

Fears of physical illness are common. "Psychosomatic" symptoms such as headache and abdominal pain are often reported by pubescent youngsters, particularly girls, in the absence of detectable pathology. Numerous and varied physical complaints and suspicions of illness are manifest. This phenomenon is sometimes described in the literature as a degree of hypochondriasis, but at this age it is normative and normal rather than pathological. Those youngsters whose physical development begins much earlier or much later than their age-mates' seem particularly prone to suffer from anxiety about the normality of their bodies and from consequent exaggerated fears of illness.

> Andrea, 13, came into a community clinic with a presenting complaint of "feeling bad all the time." The nursing history further identified the "feeling bad" as fatigue and depression. The history also yielded a passing remark from Andrea that she thought she was going to die. During the physical examination, she expressed curiosity about her heart sounds. This cue was pursued later when the findings of her assessment, which were all normal, were discussed with her. She then revealed that she had been experiencing (or had first noticed) palpitations in her chest and had surmised that they indicated a serious heart problem from which she would die. Captive in her anxiety, she had not been able to identify the heart palpitations as her presenting complaint or even, evidently, to link them clearly in her mind to her feelings of impending doom. Sensitive interviewing enabled Andrea to express her feelings and resolve the unfounded fear she had felt.

Andrea was not unusual in being alarmed by a normal somatic occurrence that was unfamiliar to her. Adolescents have been known to "find" their pelvic bones or suprasternal notch and fear that their skeletal structure is abnormal. Numerous normal consequences of illness or injury can also arouse fear and anxiety. For example, the temporary atrophy of an extremity that has been in a cast, or hypertrophy of the muscles used to compensate for the immobilized extremity, can give rise to expressed or unspoken questions about deformity. Similarly, quite normal but unfamiliar thoughts and emotions may cause the young adolescent genuine concerns about his or her mental health or character.

Adolescents, especially young ones, also tend to be quite suggestible and to overidentify with ill persons. They may believe they have developed a disease or disorder that some relative or acquaintance has or used to have. For example, a boy whose father died from myocardial infarction may suppose that he himself has heart disease, and headaches may be reported with epidemic frequency in a school in which one student is known to have a brain tumor. Uncertainty about identity, which is another characteristic of adolescence, combines with anxiety about one's physical apparatus to make it rather easy to identify with someone who is ill; for those adolescents who are influenced by the glamour that daytime television and some adults and subcultures associate with illness, it is still easier.

Early adolescence is characterized by a drive to reduce one's reliance on parents, particularly for physical care and activities that entail parental touch or inspection of the body in ways that imply childish dependency, intimacy, or breach of privacy. The young teenager also wishes to place peers in the roles of confidant, companion, and advisor and, to a considerable extent, to displace parents from those roles. These movements away from parents and toward age-mates are inevitable and necessary parts of the movement from childhood toward adulthood. When illness or disability either forces dependence on parents or isolates peers, the adolescent's developmental progress is endangered.

The developmental drives are strong, and most young adolescents who are stricken with even serious health problems are not easily diverted from seeking independence and peer alliances. In their fervor to be "normal," they may use defensive maneuvers such as denial of their illness.

James's first experience with a serious health problem came when he developed juvenile diabetes at the age of 14. His diabetes was initially not difficult to control but, unfortunately, this good control was primarily due to the fact that his mother managed his care for him. When, after about six months, James entered a "honeymoon" phase (temporary asymptomatic period common in new diabetes), he became ecstatic over the prospect of his cure. Although his physician told James that his symptoms and insulin dependence would return, the boy chose to believe otherwise and was devastated, when, a few months later, the remission ended. He sabotaged his maintenance program by overeating and faking his sugar and acetone records. After several bouts of severe ketoacidosis, James was given remedial counseling to help him deal with his feelings of helplessness and the disturbance of his sense of normality. As far as he was concerned, his body had betrayed him and the return of the disease threatened the physical integrity he was striving for.

As James demonstrates, refusal to participate cooperatively in one's health care regimen can be a dangerous by-product of the adolescent push for independence and self-esteem. But other manifestations of denial can be quite functional, as in situations in which a prognosis for dismal, unavoidable, long-range outcome is denied with the result that current function is not impaired by depression over future events about which nothing can presently be done.[2]

When health problems are present in early adolescence, the young person may, instead of struggling to achieve the developmental attainments of adolescence, revert to (or continue) the more dependent parent-child relationship of the school-age period. That is, when illness is superimposed on the ambivalence that many young people experience about having to give up things of childhood in order to achieve postchildhood prerogatives, the ambivalence may be resolved by opting for childhood patterns rather than striving for more mature ones. If the health problem truly is incapacitating and the adolescent objectively *is* reliant on parents for care and decision making, such so-called regression is not only necessary but also appropriate. If or when the health problem is not disabling enough to make reliance on parents necessary, the adolescent and the parents should relinquish unnecessary dependency patterns so that the youngster (and the parents as well) can progress toward age-appropriate behavior and developmental task mastery. Hofmann and her colleagues state that failure to work toward independence when recovery permits it is generally indicative of preexisting problems in the parent-child relationship, including either overprotectiveness or such a degree of deprivation that the child perpetuates the sick role in order to obtain nurturant attention that has previously been lacking.[3]

Health problems can interfere in several ways with peer relationships and hence with attainment of developmental tasks. The young adolescent who feels "different" may withdraw from peers because comparisons are painful or because of perceived or actual inability to participate as an equal in their activities. Some young people who feel that they are out of the mainstream of age-mates' activities become genuinely uninterested in those matters and in the people they involve, and their withdrawal and separateness intensify. Some develop a compensatory attitude of superiority to "ordinary people," although this defense is more common in middle or late adolescence than early. Whenever it arises, this attitude itself disinclines the adolescent to attempt peer involvement and also discourages approaches by peers.

On the other hand, an ill or handicapped young adolescent who does seek peer alliances may be rejected by age-mates who, as is typical of adolescents, repudiate persons whose qualities threaten their own unstable sense of identity and self-regard. Deviant appearance, impaired function, and retained dependency on parents may lead the peer group not only to exclude the adolescent from their activities and friendship but also in some instances to ridicule or otherwise attack. Such rejection, of course, very often produces withdrawal, self-absorption, depression, hostility, and poor self-esteem.

Middle Adolescence—Who Am I?

While early adolescents' major concern is about their normality, middle adolescents search for a more comprehensive sense of self, which goes beyond "Am I normal?" and includes such concerns as: What do I believe? What would I do if . . . ? Am I a good person? What do people think

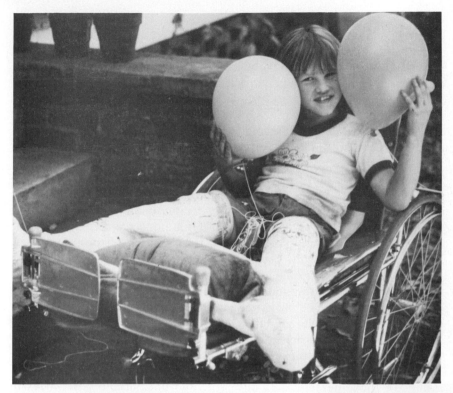

Young adolescents with health impairments may retain or resume some childhood behavior patterns and defer more age-typical behavior until they are able. Many illnesses simply do not permit increasing independence and extensive participation in well peers' interests and activities. (*Copyright © 1980 by Anne Campbell.*)

about me? Who would I like to be like? What can I become? What do I want? What do I like?

Middle adolescents involve people, especially other young people, to a great extent in the process of answering their questions about themselves. Personal sense of self is to a great extent a product of social interaction: One assesses oneself according to other persons' assessments. Adolescents, particularly in middle adolescence, are remarkably active in viewing themselves in the social "mirror" and sizing up the image that is reflected. Favorable evaluations by others build self-esteem, while unfavorable ones tend to lower it; in either case, however, one's sense of who one is (i.e., identity) becomes clearer.

A second way of using others to form one's identity, also heavily employed by adolescents, is to observe people and emulate those who seem appealing and successful. In early and middle adolescence, because personal identity is unformed, "understudying" in the theatrical sense of the word is common. Teenagers "try on" behaviors, mannerisms, attitudes, points of view, and roles or parts of roles they have observed in order to experience them temporarily as their own and see whether or not they "fit." This mimicking or borrowing of others' behavior may be evident in seemingly rather extreme or rapid changes of opinion, aspiration, style of dress, and so forth as the adolescent adopts and modifies or discards attributes of various public figures or personal acquaintances.

Health disorders can affect an adolescent's social experience in ways that interfere with the formulation of identity. Illness or disability can limit contact with others and hence restrict the pool of potential responders whose reactions can be used for self-definition. The deprivation is particularly severe for adolescents isolated from other teenagers, as in the case of those confined to home or to an institutional setting. When social experience is limited, so is the range of both models and critics, and the identity that develops is prone to narrowness and to the disproportionately large influence of the few persons the adolescent does encounter. The extreme hypothetical example in which an adolescent is isolated in the company of parents for months or years may serve to point out the range and richness of influence and experience that come from normal movement among peers and nonparent adults.

Even if a health problem imposes little or no social isolation, it may elicit negative reactions from other persons, which may well contribute to poor self-concept. Adolescence is in general characterized by intolerance of those perceived as different, and undesirable differences in physical appearance and function are very likely to diminish acceptability among peers; physical qualities are important status determinants in adolescence. Peer acceptance is a precursor of self-acceptance and hence an influence on identity formation.

Another way illness or disability may threaten the development of positive identity is by damaging the aspect of self-concept known as *body image*. Body image is most easily understood as the mental picture one has of one's own body. Body image is built up from a combination of experiences, including physical sensations (movement, pain, touch, comfort, etc.), familiarity with one's body from seeing it, and value judgments that incorporate the perceived attitudes of parents, peers, and other persons. The developmental egocentrism which is normal in adolescence and the idealism which can make imperfections seem intolerable (discussed in Chapter 1) make adolescents tend to exaggerate the flaws they perceive in themselves. Persons with defects of body form or function can, of course, suffer low self-esteem even without inaccuracies of body image.

When significant illness or injury arises, body image insult occurs and the body image must be revised to incorporate the change that has occurred in form or function. Body image can be damaged by ailments that are not

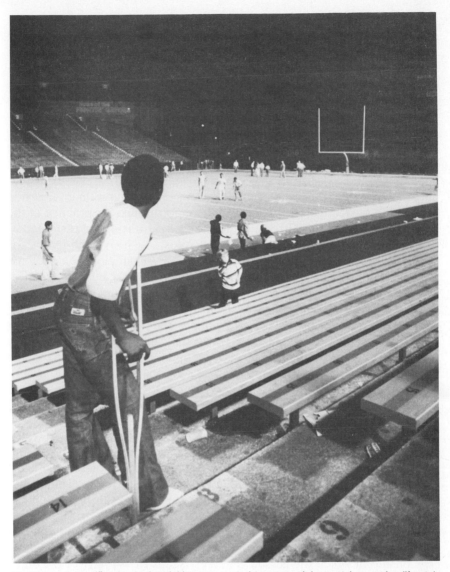

Mobility and specific physical activities are central to most adolescents' everyday life-style, self-expression, social contacts, and coping. Curtailment of function for even a few days can create severe stress. (*Copyright © 1980 by Anne Campbell.*)

outwardly detectable (e.g., heart disease, diabetes, or colitis) and also by emotional or cognitive impairments as well as by overt changes such as scoliosis, fracture, or hair loss. Body image insult can be crushing to adolescents, who are highly invested in "the body beautiful," and revising the body image to incorporate the deviation is likely to be a painful process.

Limited social experience, in addition to affecting identity development, can also impoverish the adolescent's repertoire of social skills. In other words, a teenager whose health prevents mobility in a heterogeneous social environment is prevented from obtaining the social experience necessary for developing versatility in relating to people. Social experience is an important part of becoming ready to assume late adolescent and adult roles.

Illness or handicap may compromise one's ability to participate in and effectively compete for dating activities. Adolescents tend to select dating partners in accordance with the teenage prestige criteria of physical appearance and physical function, such as athletic skill. Ill, handicapped, and disfigured young people, who rank low on these hierarchies, are often not chosen as dating companions. Their opportunities for practice in the social roles associated with dating are hence restricted, and they tend to feel insecure and inadequate in their sex roles.

Social experience is a major vehicle for the formation of a personal value system, which is part of identity. Moral standards, ethics, esthetics, and personal preferences about a wide variety of things are normally conceived, tested, and refined in social interaction. Adolescents whose social immobility or nonacceptance isolates them from a range of other persons may remain immature and narrow in their values. Trying one's values out on peers is an important part of updating and refining standards as well as a source of validating them so that one feels relatively secure with and affirmed in one's system of values.

Late Adolescence—Who Will Love Me and What Work Will I Do?

Late adolescence ideally is characterized by accomplishment of the developmental tasks that will enable the young person to assume an adult life-style. The sense of self (i.e., identity) should acquire a stability that gives the adolescent a sense of inner consistency and self-predictability. "Criteria" or developmental characteristics frequently considered to be indicative of healthy late adolescence and transition to adulthood are economic self-sufficiency, residence outside the parental home, and a love relationship in which the person genuinely seeks the welfare of the other person rather than (as is the case with less mature adolescents' love) using the other and the relationship as means toward self-definition. These "milestones" are clearly somewhat arbitrary, because some adolescents attain some of them early and some people who cannot reasonably be considered adolescents may never attain all of them. Nevertheless, as a general rule, independence from parents in housing and in finances and a mature love relationship seem acceptable as indicators that adolescence is at a close and adulthood has begun, and most adolescents view them as such. In addition, the process of selecting, preparing for, and commencing a work role is important as a means of attaining financial independence and as a personally meaningful, self-actualizing life experience.

Substantial health problems in late adolescence may impede the young person's passage into adulthood. An illness or handicap that interferes with attaining independence from parental care is obviously a serious obstacle. Educational and vocational opportunities are often limited for young people with health problems. Colleges, training programs, and employers may be reluctant to accept persons who are believed to be prone to accident or absenteeism or unable to perform and produce as required. The ill, and particularly the physically handicapped, may encounter many barriers to being able to function as independent adults, including resistive public attitudes, poor accessibility of public transportation, and architectural features that limit their mobility.

To love and accept love in an intimate, adult manner requires self-esteem and self-confidence, which, as discussed earlier, are predicated on successful social experience during earlier adolescence (as well as childhood). A secure sense of identity is a prerequisite to being able to enter into a self-disclosing, mutual, mature love without holding back for fear of diluting or losing one's own identity. Ways in which illness and disability may create difficulties in the development of identity have been discussed previously.

OTHER FACTORS AFFECTING RESPONSE TO ILLNESS OR DISABILITY

Type of Health Problem

The nature of the affliction is, of course, a major determinant of the adolescent's responses to illness, injury, or disability. A mild disorder can be expected to produce different reactions than a severe one; disfigurement has different effects than motor limitation; and chronic conditions evoke different responses than short-term ones. The various health problems carry quite dissimilar emotional connotations both for the ill person and for those in the social milieu. For example, note the variations in stigma among the following: femoral fracture, mental retardation, gonorrhea, infectious mononucleosis, cleft lip, scoliosis, elective abortion, alcoholism, and acne. The circumstances under which the health problem arises influence the way people, including the afflicted person, feel about it. Fracture due to football injury is likely to be viewed differently from a similar fracture incurred during criminal activity. Furthermore, the meanings attached to health disorders and to the circumstances surrounding them vary greatly among subcultures: An affliction that is looked upon as shameful in one adolescent subgroup may have quite a different value in another. Prognosis, of course, strongly colors responses to health disorders. Finally, as has so often been pointed out in the pediatric literature, reactions to illness are determined by the feelings, fears, fantasies, perceptions, and misperceptions the child or adolescent holds about his or her situation rather than by the "realities" as perceived by the health provider or parent.

Chronicity   Generally speaking, a congenital illness or disability or one that began early in childhood is more likely to be integrated into an adolescent's self-concept without great crisis than is one that arises during adolescence. A teenager who has been adapting to the effects of a health problem throughout the childhood developmental stages is likely to have an easier time attaining an adequate self-concept for adolescence and adulthood than is a person who must adjust to a new illness or disability at the same time the adolescent developmental tasks must be undertaken.

However, even those who adjusted well during childhood to their chronic illness or disability often experience crises in adolescence. The new social environment and expectations of adolescence lead the young person to a new awareness of the limitations and deviance accompanying the health condition. With the cognitive changes of adolescence comes a new appraisal of the impact the health disorder may have on one's present and future. As has been elaborated earlier, the developmental tasks can readily conflict with the exigencies of illness or handicap. Adolescents with limitations of physical function may have particular problems attaining independence. Those with chronic conditions may find it especially difficult to achieve an identity that is not disproportionately taken up by the disorder, whether or not the health problem is visible to themselves or others. Adolescents who have chronic illness that is not readily detectable to others may not suffer greatly from fear of peer rejection, but confusion, grief, and fantasy may make them withdraw from peer contact.

Adolescents who experience sudden acute illness are in crisis. The disruption in daily life, at a time when the emotional investment in carrying out day-to-day activities is enormous, creates a severe hardship. Increasing independence, spontaneity, mobility, and continual contact with friends typify the adolescent life-style, and interruption of that life-style for even a few days places great stress on a teenager's ability to cope. In addition, adolescents are typically highly anxious about their bodies, so even "minor" pain and "simple" procedures such as venipuncture are often tolerated less well than during the school-age period. Sedatives intended to ameliorate acute distress create for some teenagers additional anxious feelings of loss of control and fantasies of death.

Sexual Connotations of Illness and Disability   Any illness provokes apprehension regarding body functioning, but illness or other impairment during adolescence especially generates anxiety about one's sexual identity. The health problem need not have any overt effects on the sexual organs or sexual attributes in order to produce this apprehension. Adolescents may experience profound anxiety that *any* impairment will decrease their attractiveness as males or females. If an illness does involve a body part associated with sexual identity or function, the fear may be even more intense. In Western culture, high sexual value is attached to the breasts, hair, and genitals; pathology involving these areas can always be expected to engender strong response.

Hospitalization creates a set of special conditions that, along with the presence of illness, serve to magnify any insecurities about sexual identity. Dependency on others not only may signify loss of control but also may threaten one's sense of self as a person whose qualities include sexual identity. Young people who feel that others regard them as asexual or sexually inadequate sometimes resort to seductive or suggestive language and actions in order to assert their masculinity or femininity. Staff responses to this kind of behavior need to be tempered to protect all persons from infringement without further damaging the adolescent's self-concept. When nurses and others indeed consider adolescent patients asexual, any sexual behavior is likely to be condemned unduly, and needed information, counseling, and reassurance about current and future capabilities to fulfill sex roles and to function sexually and reproductively may be withheld. Peer encounters, especially heterosexual ones, are an important part of testing one's attractiveness and sex role functioning. Peer visiting in hospitals and social interactions among patients are useful adjuncts and can be arranged so that overt sexual activity is not encouraged.

Previous Patterns of Adjustment

Although adolescence is regarded as a unique developmental phase, most developmentalists also believe that there are many continuities, coming from childhood and extending into adulthood, in each person's overall patterns of coping and adjusting. Hence the style and adequacy of any adolescent's coping methods before the onset of illness or disability are widely presumed to have considerable impact on that person's responses to the health problem.[4] There is some rather conflicting evidence, however. Most discussions, like the present one, approach the relationship between illness and adjustment from the viewpoint that health status affects development and behavior (or personality); but there is a small body of literature that suggests the reverse order of events. Barton and Cattell,[5] for example, report the serendipitous discovery that their sample of ad-

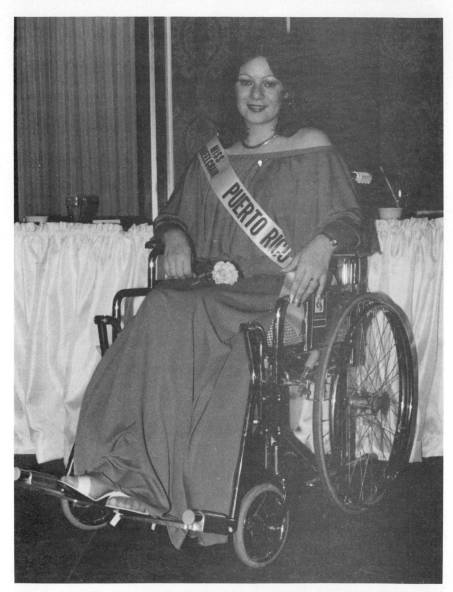

Adolescents with chronic health problems often have difficulty achieving an identity that is not disproportionately taken up by the disorder. *Compensation*, however—the substitution of constructive new activities or modes of expressing one's identity in place of activities that the health problem has made impossible—is an excellent way of coping. (*Copyright © 1980 by Anne Campbell*.)

olescents who developed chronic illness had different personality types (from peers who remained healthy) *before* they became ill. Their research also found that personality is altered by illness. Hence, regardless of certain methodological peculiarities of the Barton and Cattell study, it is valuable in that it calls into question two common assumptions: (1) that pre-illness personality patterns, including coping, will be retained after illness strikes and that therefore pre-illness adjustment somehow predicts adjustment to illness; and (2) that behavior patterns (dependency, emotional immaturity, depression, etc.) reported in persons with chronic illness are results of their illness experience rather than preexisting traits.[6]

Social Support Systems

Peers, family members, and health care professionals constitute a highly influential social support matrix within which the ill or handicapped adolescent responds to the health problem. The peer group ordinarily includes acquaintances from school, the neighborhood, and other social settings not particularly related to the health problem itself. For many ill and handicapped young people, the peer group, in addition, includes adolescents who are fellow patients from their clinic, hospital, or other treatment facility. This second group is often uniquely supportive to the young person grappling with illness or disability and, at the same time, with the developmental tasks that have been discussed earlier. Both techniques and attitudes to facilitate coping and promote task mastery can be obtained from fellow patients who have firsthand experience in being an adolescent with a health problem—especially if it is the same problem—and adolescents often identify with and trust peers in ways they are unable to do with adults, including health professionals. For adolescents whose disorder is detectable to others, the peer group of ill or handicapped young people also often provides an encouraging, accepting arena for social practice that eases the transition into the world of well peers.

Family members' reactions to an adolescent's illness or disability influence the teenager's own responses to it.[7] Parents, siblings, and members of the extended family network may promote or impede the adolescent's adjustment in myriad ways. Parents appear to be especially important. Their responses to the adolescent's health problem, of course, can be highly variable and are affected by many of the same factors that color the adolescent's own reactions: chronicity, severity, prognosis, functional impairment, social stigma, effects on appearance, and so forth. Parents also (like the adolescent) respond in accordance with the benefits and disadvantages that accrue to them because of the situation created by the health problem.

If serious illness or disability is of sudden onset during adolescence, most parents experience shock, guilt, depression, anger, anxiety, fear, and disruption of their life-style. Their relationship with the adolescent is likely to undergo marked change. Instead of a healthy and active teenager, they must now relate to a sick one who is also depressed, angry, anxious, fearful, and cut off from the usual daily activities and contacts which support coping. If, instead, the health disorder is a chronic one carried over from childhood, the parent-child interaction pattern is disrupted by the developmental changes of adolescence. In either sudden or ongoing illness, parental attitudes and actions about dependence and independence, guilt and blame-setting, acceptability of the illness, the adolescent's social relationships, the prospects for the future, and so on substantially affect the adolescent's own attitudes, behavior, and adjustment.

Because the purpose of this chapter is to examine *adolescents'* responses to illness and disability rather than the responses of significant others, parents' problems and adjustments will not be discussed in detail. However, two things should be made apparent here. One is that the adjustments required of parents are sizable both in terms of their interactions with the teenager (e.g., limit setting) and at a more personal level, as, for example, when parental aspirations for their child's future must be revised. The second point is that health professionals must view family members as candidates for professional intervention. Parents and siblings often need services provided by nurses or others (crisis intervention, support during grieving, and other types of professional care) both to maximize their own well-being and also to ensure that they in turn can facilitate the teenager's optimal adjustment.

INTERVENTIONS TO PROMOTE OPTIMAL
ADJUSTMENT AND DEVELOPMENT

There is much that nurses can do to facilitate healthy responses to illness or disability and to optimize the immediate and long-term outcomes of the adolescent's experience with a health problem. The remainder of this chapter discusses interventions for adolescents, that is, interventions based primarily on developmental characteristics. Some of the approaches also included are more general: For example, all health care consumers, regardless of developmental stage, need support from their significant others.

It should be said at the outset that one class of interventions of the utmost importance will not be addressed here. Physical care is neither secondary to nor isolated from the nursing care to be discussed. Because of its specificity, however, its inclusion in this material about adolescents in general is not feasible.

The reason that human development is useful as a basis for designing nursing care is that it allows nurses to minimize the extent to which health problems interfere with the client as a person. The objective of development-oriented nursing care is to enable persons to operate as near the top of their capacity as possible. The science of human development in a sense describes capacity and, in addition, identifies people's major methods of functioning (learning, coping, interacting, etc.) and the major hazards (social isolation, body image distortion, etc.) to reaching capacity.

Supporting Independence

The preceding pages have identified the drive for independence as a developmental earmark of adolescence. Health care for adolescents must provide for self-determination and self-reliance wherever possible. Adjustment to illness or disability, self-concept, and cooperation with the care regimen are all greatly improved when adolescent patients are partners in their care, from identifying problems and establishing care objectives right through providing interventions and evaluating their effectiveness.

A predicament that should be anticipated by health care professionals is that their objectives for the adolescent may be different from the objectives the adolescent has in mind. For example, teenagers generally take a short-term view of their situation and are far more interested in immediate relief of symptoms than in the long-range outcomes, which may hold a higher priority in the professional's view. An impasse can usually be avoided if the professional accurately understands what the patient hopes to accomplish from their interaction and advises the patient about the goals and interventions the professional considers desirable and feasible. Most adolescents react responsibly to a rational explanation about the various courses of action that are open to them and the outcomes that can be expected from each approach. One of the advantages of a written contract between client and professional (described in Chapters 3 and 11) is that it can be used to specify compromises or counteragreements that enable both adolescent and nurse to proceed with their care plan with the expectation that each will be satisfied with the outcomes of their work together.

Very often, adolescents who feel their self-determination being stifled respond by pushing harder to assert their independence. Conflict ensues with parents and health care professionals who view independence-asserting behavior as rebellion or resistance, ingratitude, self-destruction, or failure to understand the importance of complying with the care program the adults have formulated. More positive labels such as *testing* or *learning control* are rarely used. Adults normally experience some uneasiness about the awkward or abrupt processes by which adolescents achieve adult levels of independence and self-determination; when an adolescent is ill or handicapped, adult resistance to the teenager's efforts toward emancipation may readily become greater. One reason adults tend to be particularly restrictive with teenagers who have a health problem is that these young people are often considered less able than others to function independently and more vulnerable to physical or psychosocial injury from the "hard knocks" and mistakes that inevitably accompany the trial and error of assuming increasing responsibility for themselves. In addition, adults who have cared for the youngster during periods of necessary dependence sometimes have difficulty giving up that role.

The normal obstacles to self-reliance are enlarged by severe health problems. In the presence of physical disability, social deprivation, or overprotection, a young person's independence-seeking may be sporadic or may be expressed in ways that seem intolerable in the home or health care setting. In the search for a balance between dependency and independence, the adolescent may vacillate between extremes and may need sensitive responses from adults to prevent getting stranded at either extreme. New situations cause insecurity and a temporary need for increased dependency until self-assurance is sufficiently regained that the teenager feels able to step out more independently again. "Trial runs" from relative dependence to relative independence (and back again when the going gets tough) are the experiential basis on which an adult level of self-assertion and self-reliance is gradually attained. The environment that adults set up is an extremely important determinant of success in learning appropriate independence: It needs to foster the necessary trial runs rather than deter the adolescent in this critical task. Accepting retreats and at the same time supporting the teenager's forays into self-assertion are an important part of nursing care.

> Vicki, age 16, was hospitalized after an automobile accident. She had severe abrasions of the right arm and a fracture of the right tibia and fibula. She was in a semiprivate room on an adult orthopedic wing and had as a roommate a 72-year-old woman with a hip fracture.
>
> As soon as Vicki was over the initial shock of being injured, she began to make herself quite well known. Whenever her arm was dressed, she screamed that the nurses did not know what they were doing and that she would rather do it herself. She spent some days pulling her light all day for the nurses to move her, get her a telephone, hand her things, and pick up after her. She vacillated from this extreme of demanding care for a few days to refusing to allow anyone to do anything for her for several days. Vicki swung from whining to obstinacy without much between.
>
> A pediatric nurse clinician was called in by the orthopedic nurses. When she approached Vicki to explore with her what was happening, Vicki expressed surprise that anyone was interested. Vicki then became quite vocal about how no one would tell her what was going on and how long she would *really* have to stay in the hospital. She did not like the "old people" around,

and she did not like to have to ask for "every little thing." At times she felt that no one would respond to her requests anyway unless she made a commotion: She laughingly told of the time she had driven the nurses frantic by breaking the traction apparatus while stretching for an out-of-reach magazine. She complained that when she wanted to bathe herself, a nursing student would come in and want to "practice" bathing on her. But when she was really too tired to do some of these chores for herself, she said, an aide would generally leave the basin for her and she felt "dumb" if she asked for help.

The nurse clinician responded to this information by helping Vicki to set up a relationship with the staff in which Vicki would feel "safe" in asking for help when she needed it but also confident when she wished to do things for herself. When the nurses better understood Vicki's inconsistent and frustrating behavior as indications of a healthful struggle to maintain some degree of age-appropriate self-reliance, they modified her environment so that she received assistance when she wanted it and also planned and carried out her own activities to a greater extent without having to rely on others. Vicki's image as a problem patient changed to that of a patient with a problem: having experienced a topsy-turvy shake-up of her dependency-independency patterns during a time in her life when she was particularly unable to tolerate that.

Providing for Social Experience

Earlier passages of this chapter have emphasized the importance of the adolescent's peer affiliations and of social experience in general. Relationships with friends and family members and encounters with persons outside the family and health care staff must be permitted to continue with as little disturbance as possible through the course of an illness. In instances in which preexisting social affiliations and patterns are disrupted by the health problem, as when an adolescent is sent to a distant city for treatment, the young person's resumption of social exposure and opportunity to form new relationships needs to be a nursing care priority as soon as the patient's condition reasonably permits. Many adolescents benefit enormously from meeting others who share their particular health problem. The *camaraderie* common in rehabilitation hospitals demonstrates the support adolescents provide one another for self-confidence, self-acceptance, social acceptance, independent function, and coping. Other peer group experiences, such as summer camps for youngsters with diabetes, are valuable in much the same way as well as, of course, for their instruction in self-care. Individuals of any age who function well with a similar handicap can be inspiring models.

The adolescent's negative reactions to being different from healthy peers are seldom quickly resolved. It takes time to grieve over the differences and to develop an accepted self-concept, including body image. Social experiences are a necessary part of this process, since adolescents

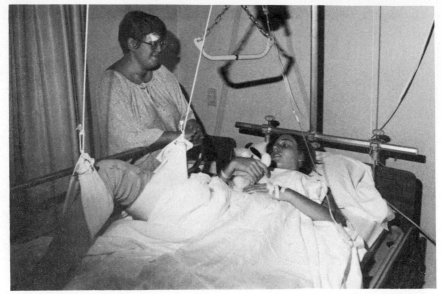

Ill adolescents, like well ones, seek to share their experiences and points of view with other adolescents. Peer sharing can greatly enhance adjustment and even recovery. (*Copyright © 1980 by Anne Campbell*.)

use others' reactions to them as an important part of the data with which they conduct their continual self-assessments. If the health problem is severe and differences from average adolescents are pronounced, some of the adolescent's social experiences are likely to be psychologically painful. Nurses can often considerably help the young person to weather the distresses of peer critique by, for example, helping the adolescent to identify personal qualities that enhance self-esteem, to understand others' reactions and place them in perspective, and to view the health disorder as but one of many personal characteristics. These kinds of ego supports are frequently better accepted from a professional or other non-family member than from parents, whom the teenager suspects of bias.

Information Sharing

Honesty is an indispensable part of the interventions used to assist an adolescent with adjusting to illness or disability. It is important to remember that adolescents, because of their age-typical idealism and tendency to view things as either all one way or all another, may feel that an adult who hedges about truth in even some minor matter is a liar and subsequently not a reliable source of help. To adolescents, honesty and trustworthiness include supplying pertinent information. Explanations about the treatment plan and expected outcomes must be provided. Being informed about one's situation opens the way for (1) participating in the care regimen as coplanner and partner in conducting and evaluating interventions; (2) developing a sense of responsibility for self that will help ensure responsible self-care in the future; (3) developing self-esteem based on knowing one has the confidence and respect of one's health care professionals; and (4) avoiding unnecessary mistakes that can easily occur when the naturally self-asserting adolescent takes action that is not based on sufficient information.

Recent nursing research demonstrated that an explicit description of the *sensory* aspects of a stressful procedure was a critical anxiety-reducing factor for children who subsequently underwent the procedure.[8] Because adolescents, particularly young ones, are so body-conscious, careful forewarnings about the sensations that accompany the various aspects of their health care presumably would be very helpful. Knowing what to expect to see, hear, smell, feel, and taste reduces anxiety about what is happening to that which is so highly important—one's body.

Adolescents who are experiencing very acute or emergency situations are, of course, not suitable candidates for teaching beyond the most basic explanations of what is being done to and for them. They are concerned only about the immediate issues of survival and body integrity. As soon as the emergency has subsided, these patients can absorb (and utilize for coping) more information about what has happened and what is expected to happen. They also should know that as soon as there are some decisions they can make to affect their situation, they will be notified.

Abruptness or cruelty in conveying to adolescents information about themselves is unconscionable. Potentially high-impact information should be given at a time and in a place in which the young person's access to support systems is assured and his or her privacy is protected. For example, distressing information should not be divulged at the end of an appointment, or as an inpatient goes out the door for a weekend pass, or in the hearing of persons whose awareness of the information might be distressing to the patient. The professional staff also is responsible for seeing that the adolescent receives follow-up support as needed to get through an experience with upsetting information.

As part of their need to be aware of their situation, adolescents require short-interval nursing reevaluations. "Come back in a month," which might be suitable if the patient were middle-aged, is not sufficient for adolescents, to whom a month seems a very long time to wait to see what progress is being made. The nurse and teenager need to talk frequently together to determine how well the care plan they have devised is working. The appropriate interval between follow-up evaluations, of course, varies with the circumstances, but the adolescent should help decide when they should meet or confer by telephone. Adolescents tend to be highly present-oriented and need to see quick results for their efforts. Positive changes that are discovered at reevaluation should be pointed out; where progress is slow, the patient should have an honest appraisal of the professional's interpretation of the situation and expectations for the future.

Understanding the Adolescent's Viewpoint

Adolescents do not always understand or share their parents' and health professionals' attitudes about the health problem and expectations for the plan of care. Professionals need to be aware that even adolescents who seem "old enough to know better" may hold views quite divergent from adults' and that those differences in viewpoint can impede the adolescents' physical or psychosocial well-being. James, Vicki, and Andrea, previously mentioned, all held points of view which were disturbing or dangerous to themselves and which could be effectively dealt with only after their health professionals became aware of them.

Adolescent behavior, sometimes described as unpredictable, is no more so than anybody else's if it is taken in context of teenagers' perceptions of their circumstances. Nurses increase their effectiveness in planning and providing nursing interventions for ill or handicapped adolescents by developing their ability to understand how teenagers look at things. The descriptions of adolescent behavior presented in the preceding pages and throughout this book are intended to increase the reader's understanding and facilitate empathy so that professional services may be well designed not only to fit the patients' health needs but also to win patients' collaboration and enhance their overall adjustment and development.

Besides using normative descriptions to anticipate how any particular adolescent may respond to illness or disability, nurses can very often learn more precisely how adolescents view their situations, what they think is going on and why, what they expect to happen, what they think will help, what they worry about, and so forth just by observing their behavior and conversing with them. Vicki's anger, frustration, and acting out became both understandable and remediable when she was asked about them. It was the nurse's observation of Andrea's examining room behavior and her talking with her, along with her awareness that young adolescents tend to fear that they are ill, that got to the bottom of the girl's belief that she was dying of heart disease. In light of James's noninvolvement in managing his diabetes and his joy over the honeymoon remission, his response to the return of his symptoms was not at all unpredictable: His therapeutic management assured his differentness from peers and promoted dependency on his mother. He was not in contact with other young people who had diabetes. His own strengths for managing his daily care were not utilized by his health care professionals or his mother. In short, James's health professionals failed to observe and interview for the conflicts that existed between his developmental characteristics and his care regimen and did not employ interventions to promote his acceptance of his chronic disease.

Role Maintenance

A fundamental way of promoting successful adaptation to a health disorder is to minimize the extent to which it interferes with the individual's customary patterns of living. Every feasible arrangement should be made to enable an ill or injured adolescent to continue the healthy, identity-supporting social roles he or she has performed in the past. Well-role behaviors rather than sick-role behaviors should be reinforced as the patient's condition permits. Even when the health problem unavoidably disrupts the former life-style, some old roles can be modified and retained.

> Cedric, age 16, became quite depressed and repeatedly expressed feelings of worthlessness while he was hospitalized for end-stage renal disease. As his disease had progressed over the past several years, he had relinquished most of his former activities and relationships outside his home. However, discussions with the nurses revealed that he was the family clown and spent much of his time entertaining and helping to supervise several younger adolescent and school-age siblings, to whom he was somewhat a hero. Cedric was invited by the nurse clinician to help her put together and manage a teaching group of a few younger renal patients. He functioned well in this role, effectively showing the other patients the ropes about dialysis and other aspects of their care and brightening both their outlook and his own in this semblance of a "big brother" role.

Old roles which were important to self-esteem and identity sometimes become impossible to maintain because of the health condition. Other roles are outgrown as the ill or handicapped adolescent either gets too old for them or becomes well enough rehabilitated that they are no longer appropriate. When important roles must be relinquished, they generally should, if possible, be replaced by others. Educational and vocational rehabilitation are often essential parts of an adolescent's preparation for resuming modified roles or taking on new ones.

Family Interventions

It has been said earlier that siblings and parents should be a focus of nursing attention because (1) they frequently need help to make their own adjustments to the ways the adolescent's health disorder impinges on their own lives, and (2) they constitute a significant part of the therapeutic environment for the patient and hence affect the patient's recovery.

Coherently functioning family members, especially parents, are among the priority needs of seriously ill or handicapped adolescents. The teenager whose family is a strong support system has a head start in the resolution of the crisis brought on by the health problem. The fostering of the intrafamily relationships through the provision of liberal visiting and rooming-in where appropriate is a basic nursing responsibility. So that family members can understand what they see—traction, altered consciousness, respirator, and so on—they must be given the explanations they need about the adolescent's condition and therapy. Also, they must be taught how they may safely maneuver equipment, touch the patient, perform appropriate parts of care, and so forth. More specific to the young person's developmental stage, the family members may need help to understand and cope with the behavioral manifestations that accompany loss of independence, loss of body integrity, and other problems that have been discussed earlier in this chapter.

Resumption of physical care-taking and acceptance of the adolescent's increased dependence can be quite taxing for some parents who thought they had gotten this child beyond that stage. Other parents may find their child's dependency gratifying in unhealthful ways.

Financial cost of major illness presents a problem for most families in spite of insurance or other resources. Parents may take second jobs, and the family's usual patterns of operating with regard to meals, care of other children, family communication, and so forth may be severely compromised. The ill adolescent may be blamed, particularly by siblings, as the cause of all the trouble, and ill teenagers can be very self-condemning. Role realignment within the household is usually difficult for all family members as functions that previously were performed by one person must now be assumed by someone else or done without.

Parents and sometimes siblings carry heavy burdens of guilt for the adolescent's illness or injury. Parents of adolescents almost daily weigh the risks of extending privileges that are dangerous in some ways, and siblings commonly initiate or participate in some hazardous activity and then blame themselves because someone else must pay the consequences. Parents may feel guilty for not recognizing disease symptoms earlier, although many teenagers, because of doubt, fear, denial, or a heightened sense of privacy, conceal their symptoms.

In summary, parents and sometimes other family members need information about the ill teenager's developmentally determined responses to illness, instruction in relating to the patient and caring for him or her in ways that promote optimal adjustment, and supportive interventions as necessary to resolve particular needs of their own. These latter interventions vary widely but include both direct nursing services (teaching and counseling) and referral to appropriate sources (crippled children's agencies, parent groups, etc.).

Therapeutic Milieu

Physical facilities, staff characteristics, and therapeutic programs for adolescents vary broadly in accordance with the adolescent's particular health problem. Treatment settings and their effective design and management for providing health services to adolescents are discussed more thoroughly in Chapters 13 through 21.

POSITIVE EFFECTS OF ILLNESS OR DISABILITY IN ADOLESCENCE

It is often overlooked that illness or disability can foster development as well as threaten it. It is not trite optimism to note that stress often produces strength rather than breakdown and that the potential for personal growth is inherent in crisis.

Many adolescents who have adequate support systems, including nursing intervention, develop strengths that enhance their preparation for adulthood. Their personal values may become quite mature and add to their ability to cope with future crises. They may learn tolerance for differences among people and may have a special benevolence for those who are different, including themselves. Many whose health problems last for any length of time develop compensatory skills or attitudes that serve them well, and they may acquire special abilities that facilitate their social relationships, vocations, and other aspects of living.

With the cooperation of family and health professionals, adolescents can play a major role in designing and carrying out their health care program. This role results in a degree of control over oneself and one's environment that can be very enhancing to self-esteem. Self-concept is also fostered by the supportiveness of friends, family, and health care workers who rally to assist and encourage the young person. Friendships and family love and cohesiveness may emerge out of the hardships engendered by the illness, and the special "togetherness" of similarly afflicted people can be intensely rewarding and supportive of self-esteem. Courage, determination, and many pragmatic skills for living can result from encountering the difficulties that accompany adolescent health disorders.

REFERENCES

1 A. D. Hofmann, R. D. Becker, and H. P. Gabriel, *The Hospitalized Adolescent: A Guide to Managing the Ill and Injured Youth*. New York: The Free Press, 1976.
2 Ibid.

3 Ibid.
4 Ibid., pp. 22, 151.
5 K. Barton and R. Cattell, "Personality Before and After a Chronic Illness," *Journal of Clinical Psychology*, **28**:464–467, 1972.
6 J. W. McDaniel, *Physical Disability and Human Behavior*, 2d ed. New York: Pergamon Press, 1976.
7 Ibid., p. 24.
8 J. E. Johnson, K. T. Kirchhoff, and M. P. Endress, "Altering Children's Distress During Cast Removal," *Nursing Research*, **24**(6):404–410, 1975.

BIBLIOGRAPHY

Conway, B.: "Effect of Hospitalization on Adolescents," *Adolescence*, 6:77–92, 1971.
Dempsey, M. O.: "The Development of Body Image in the Adolescent," *Nursing Clinics of North America*, 7(4):608–615, December 1972.
Dreikurs, R.: "The Socio-Psychological Dynamics of Physical Disability: A Review of the Adlerian Concept," *Journal of Social Issues*, 4(4):39–54, 1948.
Erikson, E.: *Identity, Youth and Crisis*. New York: W. W. Norton and Co., 1966.
Goffman, E.: *Stigma: Notes on the Management of Spoiled Identity*. Englewood Cliffs, N.J.: Prentice-Hall, 1963.
Matteson, D. R.: *Adolescence Today*. Homewood, Ill.: The Dorsey Press, 1975.
Parsons, T. and R. Fox: "Illness, Therapy, and the Modern Urban American Family," *Journal of Social Issues*, 8:31–44, 1952.
Riddle, I.: "Nursing Intervention to Promote Body Image Integrity," *Nursing Clinics of North America*, 7(4):651–661, December 1972.
Schowalter, J. E. and W. R. Anyan: "Experience on an Adolescent Inpatient Unit," *American Journal of Diseases of Children*, 125(2):212–215, February 1973.
Wright, B. A.: *Physical Disability—A Psychological Approach*. New York: Harper and Brothers, 1960.

Chapter 5

Nutrition

Jane Wentworth

Except for infants, adolescents have greater food requirements per unit
of body weight than persons in any other age group. Because of this and
other developmental characteristics that affect their diet and food utilization, adolescents are a high-risk group for nutritional inadequacy. Nutrition has often been identified by professionals as a major area in which
adolescents particularly need assessment and intervention (including
teaching for self-care). It is widely accepted, for example, that faulty
eating practices in adolescence are associated with major complications
of pregnancy and with obesity and heart disease in later life. Adolescents
themselves do not usually include nutritional adequacy among their principal health concerns, but they do identify numerous problems that have
direct or indirect implications for nutrition: dental health, nervousness,
obesity, acne, menstrual difficulties, and venereal disease.[1] Adolescents
are infamous for their concerns over body weight[2] and may take weight-
control measures that run counter to their overall present and future health
and well-being. Other health-related phenomena of adolescence that affect
nutrition are tobacco use by about one-fourth of young people 12 to 19

years of age and use of beverage alcohol by about one-third of this age group.[3]

This chapter describes methods for assessing the nutritional status of adolescents; discusses the nutrient requirements of young people; reports findings of national studies of adolescents' nutritional status; discusses pregnancy, athletics, obesity, and drug use as they pertain to nutrition; and makes recommendations for approaches to nutrition education.

NUTRITIONAL ASSESSMENT

Nutritional assessment, as part of the total health assessment, is a means for identifying nutritional status and nutritional needs; it also frequently reveals problems that are not primarily nutritional. Obviously, a sound assessment must precede dietary counseling and is the basis for nutrition intervention and evaluation activities. Nutritional assessment consists of physical, biochemical, clinical, and dietary studies made in conjunction with health and socioeconomic histories. Three levels of intensity of nutritional assessment for teenagers have been delineated (see Table 5-1). Table 5-2 presents criteria that were distributed in 1976 to health professionals throughout the United States by which to select individuals for further assessment. The information in Table 5-2 can be used to establish priorities and policies when planning and providing services for improving nutritional care of groups as well as individuals. The hematologic criteria apply to adolescents who are pregnant as well as to those who are not.

Diet History

Determining the client's dietary practices is a basic part of the nutritional assessment. *Twenty-four-hour recall*, in which the adolescent recounts what he or she has eaten in the past day, is not an effective way of evaluating food intake, because any single day's intake may be unrepresentative of day-to-day eating patterns and hence provides an unreliable data base for individual dietary counseling. A *diet history* provides a better picture of food intake patterns and the amounts of the foods most commonly eaten. However, a diet history takes 30 to 45 minutes to complete, and time is often in short supply in practice settings. In addition, the analysis of the diet history findings is lengthy unless computer assistance is available. The Public Health Service has provided a questionnaire (see Table 5-3) for school-age children and adolescents. This form helps identify major food intake weaknesses. It does not provide adequate information from which to assess the kilocalorie, protein, vitamin, and mineral content of a diet, but it does identify bizarre diets and those devoid of

Table 5-1 Levels of Nutritional Assessment for Adolescents

| Levels of approach | History | | Clinical evaluation | Laboratory evaluation |
	Dietary	Medical and socioeconomic		
Minimal level	1. Frequency of use of food groups 2. Habits, patterns 3. Snacks 4. Socioeconomic status	1. Previous diseases and allergies 2. Abbreviated system review 3. Family history	1. Height 2. Weight	1. Urine: protein and sugar 2. Hemoglobin
Mid-level	1. Above 2. Qualitative estimate 3. 24-hour recall	1. Above in more detail	1. Above 2. Arm circumference 3. Skinfold thickness 4. External appearance	1. Above 2. Blood taken by vein for albumin (serum), serum iron and TIBC; vitamins A and beta carotene; RBC indices; blood urea nitrogen (BUN); cholesterol; zinc
In-depth level	1. Above 2. Quantitative estimate by recall (3–7 days)	1. Above	1. Above 2. Per ICNND Manual 3. X-ray of wrist and bone density	1. Above 2. Blood tests: folate and vitamin C; alkaline phosphatase; RBC transketolase; RBC glutathione; lipids 3. Urine: creatinine; nitrogen; zinc; thiamine; riboflavin; loading tests (xanthurenic acid/FIGLU) 4. Hair root: DNA; protein; zinc; other metals

Source: G. Christakis, ed., "Nutritional Assessment in Health Programs," *American Journal of Public Health*, **63**(supplement):1–82, November 1973.

**Table 5-2   Criteria for Selecting Persons for Further
Nutritional Assessment**

For all individuals:	Serum cholesterol concentrations greater than 230 mg/100 ml.
	Dental caries.
	Low hemoglobin concentrations—less than 11 g/100 ml for persons under 10 years of age, less than 12 g/100 ml for persons over 10 years of age, or less than 13 g/100 ml for males over 14 years of age.
	Diseases or conditions in which nutrition plays a key role— cardiovascular disease, hyperlipidemia, diabetes, gastrointestinal disorders, hypertension, metabolic disorders, physical or mental handicaps affecting feeding, allergies, surgery, burns.
	Weight for height below the 5th percentile or above the 95th, or height for age below the 5th percentile.
	Inadequate income, food supply, or facilities for food preparation.
	Substance abuse—alcohol, tobacco, other drugs.
	Pica.
	Use of oral contraceptives, dilantin, or other drugs or medication affecting nutritional requirements.
For pregnant and lactating women:	Any of the items listed for all individuals.
	Under 15 years of age or over 35.
	Unfavorable outcome of previous pregnancy.
	Short interval between pregnancies.
	Preexisting complications such as cardiovascular disease, renal disease, or diabetes.
	Significant deviation in weight gain.
For infants and children to 18 years of age:	Any of the items listed for all individuals.
	Low birth weight.
	Failure to thrive.

Source: Adapted from *Guide for Developing Nutrition Services in Health Care Programs*. Rockville, Md.: USDHEW, Pub. No. (HSA)78-5103, 1978.

Table 5-3 A Sample Dietary Questionnaire

	Yes	No
Do you drink milk?	☐	☐

If yes:
Whole milk ☐
2% milk ☐
Skim milk ☐
Other ☐
Specify _____

Please indicate which of the following foods you eat and how often.

	Never or hardly ever (less than once a week)	Sometimes (not daily but at least once a week)	Every day or nearly every day
Cheese, yogurt, ice cream	☐	☐	☐
Eggs	☐	☐	☐
Dried beans, peas, peanut butter	☐	☐	☐
Meat, fish, poultry	☐	☐	☐
Bread, rice, pasta, grits, cereal, tortillas, potatoes	☐	☐	☐
Fruits or fruit juices	☐	☐	☐
Vegetables	☐	☐	☐

If you eat fruits or drink fruit juices every day or nearly every day, which ones do you eat or drink most often? (Not more than three.)

_____

If you eat vegetables every day or nearly every day, which ones do you eat most often? (Not more than three.)

_____

	Yes	No
Do you usually eat anything between meals?	☐	☐

If yes, name the two or three snacks (including bedtime snacks) that you have most often.

_____

Do you or the person who prepares your meals have use of a

	Yes	No
Working stove	☐	☐
Refrigerator	☐	☐
Piped water	☐	☐
Do you take vitamins or iron?	☐	☐

If yes, how often? _____
What kind? _____

	Yes	No
Are you on a special diet?	☐	☐

If yes, what is the reason?
Allergy (specify type of diet)

_____

Weight reduction (specify type of diet)

_____

Other (specify reason for diet and type of diet)

_____

Table 5-3   A Sample Dietary Questionnaire (*Continued*)

Who recommended the diet?_____

	Yes	No
Do you eat clay, paint chips, or anything else not usually considered food?	☐	☐

  If yes, what?_____

  How often?_____

Source: S. J. Fomon, *Nutritional Disorders of Children—Prevention, Screening and Follow-up.* Rockville, Md.: USDHEW, Pub. No. (HSA) 76-5612, 1976.

certain food groups and is useful in selecting persons who may be at nutritional risk and in need of further assessment. It is recommended here that the form be used by health professionals as an interview schedule rather than by adolescents for self-completion; however, it is suitable as a self-report questionnaire for school classes or other literate groups when group information is needed. Several dietary interview forms have been published recently [4,5,6] and can be adapted if Table 5-3 is not suitable for local use. A recent article describing the role of the nurse in health assessment and promotion suggests that information be obtained about condition of the buccal cavity, ability to chew and swallow, appetite, ingestion and digestion of nutrients, weight, and elimination,[7] all helpful information with which to evaluate patient needs.

Height and Weight

The assessment of growth by measurements of height and weight is extremely important. Data collected must be accurate. A beam scale permitting readings to the nearest 20 g should be used and should be calibrated every three to four months. Specific details for measuring have been distributed by the Center for Disease Control.[8] Height is taken most accurately by using a measuring stick attached to a true vertical flat surface. A block, squared at right angles against the wall, is placed on the crown of the head, and the measurement on the stick is then read. Measuring rods attached to platform scales are not recommended. In a study carried out by the Center for Disease Control to determine sources of error in weighing and measuring children, several types of errors were found to occur. Inaccurate measuring, recording errors, or both were found, and inadequate weighing and measuring equipment also led to inaccurate data. These problems were categorized as being of three different kinds: equipment-related, skill- or knowledge-related, and motivation-related.[9] Since other types of assessments such as dietary histories, clinical examinations, and laboratory tests may have greater errors which are less easily detected or eliminated,[10] every effort should be made to adequately train and supervise personnel responsible for height and weight measurements.

Updated growth data have been compiled by the National Center for Health Statistics and are now available from the Public Health Service.[11] Information provided consists of smoothed growth curves of height and weight, expressed as percentile curves showing the 5th, 10th, 25th, 50th, 75th, 90th, and 95th percentiles. Growth curves for the adolescent group are available for both males and females through 18 years of age. Figures 5-1 through 5-4 present a reduced version of the larger graphs currently available. (Ross Laboratories and Mead Johnson have reproduced the PHS growth curves and distribute them for professional use.) Criteria for using height and weight assessments for identifying individuals with nutritional problems have been provided by the Center for Disease Control[12] and are consistent with those recommended by Fomon.[13] These criteria are:

1 *Low height for age*: Height for age less than the 5th percentile for persons of the same sex and age in the reference population.
2 *Low weight for age*: Weight for age less than the 5th percentile for persons of the same sex and age in the reference population.
3 *Low weight for height*: Weight for height less than the 5th percentile for persons of the same sex and height in the reference population.

A one-time measurement of height and weight is of little value in the assessment of growth: Patterns across time are far more meaningful. An

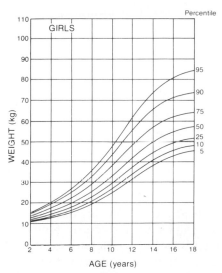

Figure 5-1 Weight for age of girls from 2 to 18 years. (*Source: P. Hamill et al., "NCHS Growth Charts, 1976,"* Monthly Vital Statistics Report, **25**[3] [*supplement*], *June 22, 1976.*)

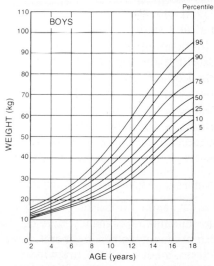

Figure 5-2 Weight for age of boys from 2 to 18 years. (*Source: P. Hamill et al., "NCHS Growth Charts, 1976,"* Monthly Vital Statistics Report, **25**[3] [*supplement*], *June 22, 1976.*)

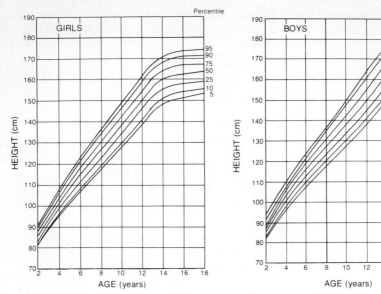

Figure 5-3 Height for age of girls from 2 to 18 years. (*Source: P. Hamill et al., "NCHS Growth Charts, 1976,"* Monthly Vital Statistics Report, **25**[3] [*supplement*], June 22, 1976.)

Figure 5-4 Height for age of boys from 2 to 18 years. (*Source: P. Hamill et al., "NCHS Growth Charts, 1976,"* Monthly Vital Statistics Report, **25**[3] [*supplement*], June 22, 1976.)

unexplained increment or decrement in the growth trend may be one of the first signs of a serious health problem, and movement from one percentile group to another should be investigated. Children and adolescents at either the top or bottom extreme of the curves need closer scrutiny than others. Mild or marginal nutritional abnormalities may be a cause of growth deviations. Dietary and biochemical assessment should be obtained for youngsters who are small or who drop to lower percentiles over time. At the other extreme, obesity may be prevented if counseling is begun with minimally overweight adolescents and those whose weight is increasing across percentile "channels."

Nutritional Assessment in Pregnancy

Anemia Because guidelines specifically for screening *adolescents* for anemia in pregnancy have not been established, the screening criteria for pregnant women in general, developed at the Conference on Nutritional Assessment[14] in 1972, are widely used. Hematologic tests used to screen for deficiencies are given in Table 5-4. Values less than those given in the table may indicate some form of anemia. Specific anemias are then identified by blood smear to ascertain types of erythrocytes present, and

Table 5-4   Criteria of Deficiency for Hematological Laboratory Tests in Adult Women*

Determination	Level
Hemoglobin	
Pregnant	< 11 g/100 ml
Nonpregnant	< 12 g/100 ml
Hematocrit	
Pregnant	< 33%
Nonpregnant	< 36%
Serum iron	< 50 μg%
% Saturation	< 15%
Serum folate	< 3 ng/ml†
Serum vitamin B_{12}	< 80 pg/ml‡

*Modified from W.H.O. Tech. Rep. Ser. No. 405, 1968.
†nanograms per ml
‡picograms per ml
   Source: G. Christakis, ed., "Nutritional Assessment in Health Programs," American Journal of Public Health, 63(supplement):1–82, November 1973.

additional blood studies such as mean corpuscular volume, mean corpuscular hemoglobin, serum folic acid and vitamin B_{12} levels, and others may be done.

Weight Gain   Weight gain during pregnancy can be monitored by using the chart presented in Figure 5-5. Weight increments should be gradual rather than characterized by the peaks and valleys so often typical of teenagers' weight gain. Body weight during pregnancy is further discussed in the later section of this chapter that focuses on nutrition in pregnancy.

Referral for Nutrition Counseling

When the nutritional assessment reveals a need for intensive or specialized dietary counseling, referral to a dietitian or public health nutritionist may be desirable. A sample referral form developed by the Public Health Service is given in Table 5-5.

NUTRIENT REQUIREMENTS

The actual human requirements for many of the nutrients essential for growth, reproduction, and maintenance are still unknown. The reasons for this are complex, but they include ethical constraints against experimentally inducing deficiencies, the enormous expense of the necessary biochemical measurements, and the difficulties involved in manipulating experimental subjects' diets over months or years. Since precise deter-

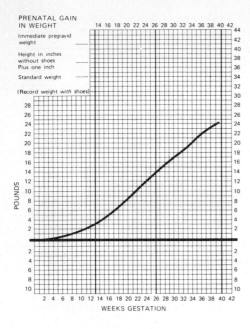

Figure 5-5 Prenatal gain in weight. (*Source: R. B. Howard and N. H. Herbold,* Nutrition in Clinical Care, *McGraw-Hill Book Company, New York, 1978, p. 247.*)

minations of requirements have not been feasible, dietary standards are used instead to define desirable intakes of nutrients. In the United States the Recommended Dietary Allowances (RDAs) have been developed by the Food and Nutrition Board of the National Research Council, National Academy of Sciences[15] as a guide for planning diets. RDAs do not represent specific individuals' requirements but are averages for different age groups. The values have been based on estimated requirements with a safety margin added to allow for individual variation. The RDAs for children, teenagers, and young adults are provided in Table 5-6. The revised edition of the RDAs will include provisional values for sodium, potassium, copper, molybdenum, selenium, manganese, fluorine, chromium, pantothenic acid, and biotin. These will be helpful not only in dietary assessment but also in dietary counseling. The Food and Agricultural Organization and the World Health Organization of the United Nations and numerous countries have also established standards for intake of energy, protein, and selected vitamins and minerals.[16]

To determine the dietary intake needs of a particular teenager, it is necessary to take into consideration influential factors such as physiological state, body size, sex, age, state of health, amount and kind of physical activity, and use of tobacco, alcohol, and other drugs. Because of the rapid rate of growth during adolescence, the effect of some of these

Table 5-5 Sample Nutrition Referral Form

Patient's name	Identifying number	Referral reason
Address	Phone	County
Sex Birth date Ht. Wt.	Physician	Diet order
Diagnosis	Physical and biochemical findings	
Personal— occupation and/or school, grade, etc.	Other personnel working with patient	
Summary of nutrition history		
Background—education, nationality, etc.		
Economic considerations—available funds, shopping facilities, commodity food, food stamps, etc.		
Food storage and cooking facilities		
Problems involved in following good habits or in carrying out diet plans		
Diet instructions given		
Follow-up plans		
Referral to: Person Title Referral from: Person Title Date		

Source: S. J. Fomon, *Nutritional Disorders of Children—Prevention, Screening and Follow-up*. Rockville, Md.: USDHEW, Pub. No. (HSA) 76-5612, 1976.

factors is intensified at this stage of life, and cell depletion can occur if diets are marginal or inadequate in some nutrients. The age of onset of rapid growth varies greatly among young people and is influenced by genetic programming, nutritional status, and environmental factors. Children with a more advanced biological age (indicated by bone age) attain puberty at an earlier chronological age than other children and require additional energy and nutrients to support their growth needs.[17] Puberty is delayed among the malnourished and in many low-income children.[18]

In the United States the average age at which girls begin the adolescent growth spurt is around 10.5 years, while the average for boys is about 13 years.[19] The RDAs reflect these sex differences (as shown in Table 5-6), with the higher need for kilocalories in females occurring during the years

Table 5-6   Recommended Daily Dietary Allowances

	Units	Children	Males				Females		
			11–14	15–18	19–22	11–14	15–18	19–22	
Age	years	7–10	11–14	15–18	19–22	11–14	15–18	19–22
Weight	kg	30	44	61	67	44	54	58
Height	cm	135	158	172	172	155	162	162
Energy	kcal	2400	2800	3000	3000	2400	2100	2100
Protein	g	36	44	54	54	44	48	46
Calcium	mg	800	1200	1200	800	1200	1200	800
Phosphorus	mg	800	1200	1200	800	1200	1200	800
Iodine	μg	110	130	150	140	115	115	100
Iron	mg	10	18*	18*	10	18*	18*	18*
Magnesium	mg	250	350	400	350	300	300	300
Zinc	mg	10	15	15	15	15	15	15
Vitamin A	IU	700	1000	1000	1000	800	800	800
Vitamin D	IU	400	400	400	400	400	400	400
Vitamin E	IU	10	12	15	15	12	12	12
Ascorbic acid	mg	40	45	45	45	45	45	45
Folacin	μg	300	400	400	400	400	400	400
Niacin	mg	16	18	20	20	16	14	14
Riboflavin	mg	1.2	1.5	1.8	1.8	1.3	1.4	1.4
Thiamine	mg	1.2	1.4	1.5	1.5	1.2	1.1	1.1
Vitamin B_6	mg	1.2	1.6	2.0	2.0	1.6	2.0	2.0
Vitamin B_{12}	μg	2.0	3.0	3.0	3.0	3.0	3.0	3.0

*This allowance cannot be met by ordinary diets; therefore the use of supplemental iron is recommended.
    Source: *Recommended Dietary Allowances* (8th rev.), Washington, D.C.: National Academy of Sciences, National Research Council, Food and Nutrition Board, 1974.

from 11 to 14, while for males the highest recommended allowance for kilocalories begins around age 15 to 18 years. The large appetite that accompanies this rapid growth phase also decreases at a much earlier age in females than in males.[20] Because of the fewer kilocalories females require, they must be more selective than males about their food intake in order to consume adequate amounts of nutrients such as iron, folic acid, and vitamin B_6 without exceeding their caloric needs. The figures in Table 5-7 for kilocalorie and protein allowances are calculated from averages provided by the National Academy of Sciences and should be used only as a guide to establish needs for groups and not for determining requirements of specific individuals. Munro[21] feels that the recommendation for protein is lower than the amount actually needed during the adolescent growth spurt. The next revision of the RDAs will no doubt reflect findings from current and continuing research and, it is hoped, will define more specifically the protein needs during this period of intensive growth.

Energy intake of healthy adolescents 11 to 18 years of age in the longitudinal study of the Denver Child Research Council ranged from 10

Table 5-7 Energy and Protein Allowances

	Age (years)	Energy (kcal/kg)	Energy* (total kcal)	Protein (g/kg)	Protein* (total g)
Children	7–10	80	2400	1.20	36
Males	11–14	64	2800	1.0	44
	15–18	49	3000	0.88	54
	19–22	45	3000	0.81	54
Females	11–14	55	2400	1.0	44
	15–18	39	2100	0.89	48
	19–22	36	2100	0.79	46

*Calculated values are based on the average weight for each age group.
Source: Recommended Dietary Allowances (8th rev.), Washington, D.C.: National Academy of Sciences, National Research Council, Food and Nutrition Board, 1974.

to 19 kcal/cm for females and from 13 to 23 kcal/cm for males.[22] These values compare favorably with the 16 kcal/cm mean intake of a group of female adolescents studied by Wait and Roberts.[23] In the dietary intake findings of the first Health and Nutrition Examination Survey carried out by the Public Health Service, a 24-hour recall of foods eaten revealed that adolescents aged 10 to 19 years had a mean kilocalorie intake below the Public Health Service's recommendation. That agency's standards for evaluating the daily intake of young people participating in the survey are given in Table 5-8. A comparison cannot be made at this time with the Denver and Wait and Roberts studies since data have not been published about energy intake in relation to height. The data showed that among all subjects 12 to 17 years old the average of kilocalories consumed by blacks

Table 5-8 Health and Nutrition Examination Survey (HANES) Standards for Evaluation of Daily Dietary Intake

	Males			Females		
	10–12 years	13–16 years	17–19 years	10–12 years	13–16 years	17–19 years
Calories (kcal/kg)	68	60	44	64	48	35
Protein (g/kg)	1.2	1.2	1.1	1.2	1.2	1.1
Calcium (mg)	650	650	550	650	650	550
Iron (mg)	10	18	18	18	18	18
Vitamin A (IU)	2500	3500	3500	2500	3500	3500
Vitamin C (mg)	40	50	55	40	50	50
Thiamine	0.4 mg/1000 kcal for all ages					
Riboflavin	0.55 mg/1000 kcal for all ages					
Niacin	6.6 mg/1000 kcal for all ages					

Source: "Dietary Intake of Persons 1–74 Years of Age in the United States." National Center for Health Statistics, Advance Data, No. 6, March 1977, p. 3.

was about 300 lower than the intake of white participants. The greatest deficits were among the low-income blacks.[24]

Health professionals are confronted with the task of choosing a standard by which to estimate dietary needs. Most nutritionists continue to use the most current revision of the National Research Council RDAs. It is based on current and past research literature as interpreted by a group of scientists trained in physiology, biochemistry, medicine, and nutrition and remains the single most authoritative document about the nutritional needs of healthy persons in the United States. However, a personalized approach must be taken in the evaluation of the nutritive needs of adolescents, since considerable variation in requirements has been found.[25-28]

The U.S. Recommended Daily Allowances (U.S.RDAs), not to be confused with the National Research Council RDA, were developed by the Food and Drug Administration to be used to provide nutritional content information on food labels in instances in which the food processor desires to display this information or makes some claim for the food product.[29] The U.S.RDA was derived partially from the 1968 revision of the RDA and replaced the Minimum Daily Requirement (MDR). There are actually four different allowances: for adults and for children 4 or more years old, for infants, for children under 4 years of age, and for pregnant or lactating women. The last two categories are used with "special dietary foods."[30] Values for adults and for children over 4 years of age are given in Table 5-9. Some assessment of nutrient intakes can be made by observing the percent of the U.S.RDA met as expressed on the labels of foods. Recommendations for protein intake for males from 15 to 22 years of age vary substantially (45 g per day in the U.S.RDA and 54 g per day in the RDA). A comparison of Table 5-6 with Table 5-9 reveals differences in other nutrients such as vitamin E, ascorbic acid (vitamin C), and vitamin B_{12}, but the differences probably are not large enough to warrant revision of the U.S.RDA at this time.

In the United States, where there are two problems related to long-time dietary practices—atherosclerosis and obesity—the question of maximum recommended dietary allowances for some nutrients arises. Serum cholesterol levels begin to rise sharply after age 17 in both males and females, as recently reported.[31] Research is needed to further clarify the relationship between dietary practices during adolescence and health during adulthood. The effects that alcohol, steroid contraceptives, and other drugs have on the intake and utilization of nutrients need to be studied, as do the results of fad diets for rapid weight loss or gain.[32]

Nutrional needs, of course, vary with state of health. For example, all infections increase the body's need for protein, calories, vitamins, and some minerals, especially when fever is present. The severity and duration of infection determine whether or not therapeutic vitamin supplements are indicated in addition to an adequate diet. Young people, as well as their health care professionals, need to be aware of this effect of infectious processes (including sexually transmitted diseases). Nutrition problems generated by health disorders such as cardiac disease and renal disease are beyond the scope of this book, but excellent resources are available elsewhere.[33]

NUTRITIONAL STATUS

Nutrition is here defined as "the science that interprets the relationship of food to the functioning of the living organism,"[34] and *nutritional status* as "the condition of health of an individual as influenced by the intake and utilization of nutrients, determined from the correlation of information obtained from physical, biochemical, clinical, and dietary studies."[35] For easily understandable reasons, few studies have been comprehensive enough to provide physical, biochemical, clinical, and dietary data. Most research and many clinical practitioners look at the relative presence or absence of particular nutrients, such as riboflavin or iron, as opposed to the nutritional status of individuals. In the United States, the two national studies that have carried out in-depth nutritional assessments are the Ten-State Nutrition Survey[36] and the first Health and Nutrition Examination Survey (HANES).[37] The ten-state study unfortunately involved a population sample that was not representative of the people of the United States. Another drawback of these two studies is that the criteria used to evaluate dietary adequacy (see Table 5-8) were different from the RDAs, which are the standards commonly used for assessing diets of groups.

Table 5-9 U.S. Recommended Daily Allowances (U.S.RDAs) for Adults and Children Four or More Years of Age

Vitamin A	5000 IU	Biotin	0.3 mg
Vitamin D	400 IU*	Pantothenic acid	10 mg
Vitamin E	30 IU	Calcium	1.0 g
Vitamin C	60 mg	Phosphorus	1.0 g
Folic acid	0.4 mg	Iodine	150 μg
Thiamine	1.5 mg	Iron	18 mg
Riboflavin	1.7 mg	Magnesium	400 mg
Niacin	20 mg	Copper	2.0 mg
Vitamin B_6	2.0 mg	Zinc	15 mg
Vitamin B_{12}	6.0 μg	Protein	45 g†

*Optional.
†If protein efficiency ratio of protein is equal to or better than that of casein.
Source: U.S. Department of Health, Education, and Welfare, FDA, PHS, Rockville, Md., HEW Pub. No. (FDA) 76-2042, 1976.

(The margin of safety used to cover individual variations was narrower than in the RDAs.)

More than half of the adolescents in the Ten-State Nutritional Survey had kilocalorie intakes lower than the standard considered adequate. With the exception of the Spanish-American females, adolescents in the low-income-ratio states had lower intakes than teenagers in the high-income-ratio states. In the HANES study, girls 15 to 17 years old had the lowest kilocalorie intake (66 to 71 percent of the standard), and persons from ages 10 to 19 failed to meet the recommended energy level in each age subgroup. Mean iron intake was low in all groups of adolescents in the ten-state study. Over 80 percent of the females had intakes below 18 mg and about three-fourths of the males in the 12 to 14 and 15 to 16 year groups had intakes below the 18 mg standard. One-third of the younger males (10 and 11 years old) failed to meet their standard of 10 mg. Iron was the nutrient most often found low in the total population of the HANES study, but adolescent females were 35 to 55 percent below the standard of 18 mg, while white males 15 to 19 years old averaged 17 percent below the standard of 18 mg. Thirty percent of the low-income black males 15 to 17 years old had mean iron intakes below the standard, and 26 percent of upper-income black males 15 to 19 years of age failed to meet the standard.

Among the lower-income groups, 3.7 percent of whites between 12 and 17 years old had low hemoglobin values, while 20.4 percent of the blacks had low levels. In the upper-income group, blacks (15 percent) again outnumbered whites (2.5 percent) among adolescents with low hemoglobin. Of interest is the surprising finding that 7.4 percent of all males in this age group had low hemoglobin levels, but only 1.9 percent of the females were low. Serum iron was found to be low in some of these young people with reduced hemoglobin, but the highest prevalence was among black males 12 to 17 years of age (6 percent). Serum transferrin saturation values were lowest among low-income blacks in the population from 12 to 17 years old, of whom 12.5 percent had levels below the standard.

The appearance of anemia during pubescence among males in the low-income groups parallels the increased demand for iron to synthesize red blood cells and to increase muscle mass.[38] Marginal iron intake probably delays the growth spurt and causes smaller body size than the potential, as data collected in developing countries tend to support. It is not known whether it is malnutrition during infancy or during pubescence that affects the growth spurt, but a large number of children in developing countries have little or no growth spurt during adolescence.[39]

The ten-state and HANES studies showed considerable variation in the intake of vitamins A and C but revealed a large number of adolescents with intakes both below and above the standard. Spanish-Americans had

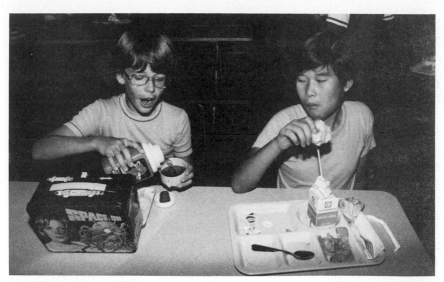

After children become adolescents, their dietary preferences and practices are influenced increasingly by current social experiences and peers and decreasingly by family and cultural background. (*Copyright © 1980 by Anne Campbell*.)

lower intakes of vitamin A than black or white adolescents. Only the adolescents 12 to 14 years old met the recommended intake of 3500 IU. Biochemical and dietary data were consistent in showing a high prevalence of ''deficient'' and ''low'' vitamin A values in the low-income-ratio states. In the HANES survey, all groups of males had mean intakes above the standard, but black females 12 to 14 years old in the upper-income group and 15 to 17 years old in the lower-income group had mean intakes 15 and 27 percent, respectively, below the standard.

The same pattern appeared in the ten-state survey with regard to vitamin C. Despite the high mean intake value, the data for individuals showed that almost half of the adolescents aged 10 to 16 years had intakes below the recommended 30 mg. However, the HANES study found that adolescents had mean intakes well above the standard. There was a tendency to increase vitamin C intake with age, but when intake was measured in relation to body weight, it decreased with age.

Protein intake was found to be less than 50 g in about one-third of the females in the ten-state study; however, the mean protein intake for the adolescent population was above the dietary standard for each age subgroup. Except for girls 15 to 17 years old, adolescents approached or exceeded the protein intake recommended in the HANES study. Girls 15 to 17 years old had mean values that averaged around 16 percent below the standard. There was little biochemical evidence that protein deficiency existed among the adolescent group 12 to 17 years old. Less than 3 percent for both sexes had low serum protein levels.

Earlier studies have reported that diets of boys have been more adequate in nutrients than those of girls,[40] but the more recent surveys highlight the lack of some nutrients in the diets of many low-income boys as well as girls. The failure of the biochemical studies on iron to correlate with dietary intake in women may indicate increased use of iron supplements by this group and needs further study.

NUTRITION FOR PREGNANT ADOLESCENTS

The incidence of pregnancy during adolescence has risen during the past two decades, and the increase has been accompanied by an increase in serious medical, psychological, educational, and social problems.[41] During this time contraceptives have become more available to adolescents; nevertheless, from 1968 to 1974 births to adolescents increased by 47,000 in the United States, making a total of 247,000.[42] In 1972 Hofmann[43] reported that 2 of every 100 unmarried 15- to 19-year-old females became pregnant, while McDonald[44] estimated that 1 of 10 young women became mothers before graduating from high school. Information about the number of abortions occurring is not available since this is not included in pregnancy statistics, and the magnitude of the situation is unclear because not all pregnancies are reported. The birth rate in 1975 was reported as 36.6 mothers 15 to 17 years old per 1,000 mothers of all ages. This is an increase of 21.7 percent over the 1966 rate, while the rate for all other age groups except 25 to 29 years declined.[45]

The increase in abortions among adolescents creates concern for the health and nutritional care of this group. Mental health as well as physical health is often affected, and, of course, both can affect nutrition. A recent survey of women who became pregnant during adolescence revealed that subsequent unwanted pregnancy was a serious problem despite participation in comprehensive health service programs. The study indicated that some 40 percent of all mothers in the population studied who became pregnant during adolescence resorted to abortion or sterilization or both methods to control subsequent fertility.[46]

Despite renewed interest in maternal nutrition within this decade, many health professionals, while focusing on social or psychological well-being, overlook the need for adequate nutritional care during adolescent pregnancy. A comprehensive approach to total health care including nutrition has repeatedly demonstrated a beneficial effect on the outcome of pregnancy.[47-49]

Pregnancy in younger adolescents (under 15 years of age) is accompanied by higher perinatal mortality rates, more cases of toxemia, and a greater number of low birth weight infants than in adolescents 15 to 18 years old.[50] The specific causes of these complications are not yet known, but immaturity of maternal organs could contribute. Depletion of nutrient stores during the rapid pubescent growth spurt cannot be ruled out. Other factors contribute to the fact that, nutritionally, the teenager is not at the prime of her life for reproduction. Poor dietary habits, including crash dieting and skipping meals, can deplete tissue stores of nutrients. Undesirable health practices such as smoking and the use of alcohol and other drugs increase nutrient requirements and often directly interfere with adequate food intake. The use of "the pill" also increases nutrient needs for some vitamins and minerals. Brewer's review of the literature on nutrition in pregnancy indicates that there is sufficient evidence to implicate poor nutritional status as a major cause of toxemia of pregnancy.[51]

Contrary to popular belief, only a few teenage pregnancies might be complicated by the continued growth of the mother. If fertilization occurs before or soon after menarche, growth requirements of the mother could compete with the pregnancy; however, such cases are rare in the United States since for females the peak velocity of growth in height occurs around 12.5 years.[52] At the present time there is insufficient evidence to support the hypothesis that pregnancy in adolescents imposes greater nutritional requirements than does pregnancy in postadolescent women.[53] The RDAs for pregnancy during the years from 15 to 18 are either the same or slightly more than allowances for pregnancy during adult years. The RDAs and percent of increase recommended for pregnancy and lactation in the adolescent are provided in Table 5-10. More energy, protein, niacin, riboflavin, and thiamine are recommended for pregnant adolescents, but recommendations for vitamin D, calcium, and phosphorus are unchanged from those for nonpregnant adolescents. It is interesting that the recommended percent increase over the nonpregnant state for energy, protein, niacin, riboflavin, and iodine is actually less for the pregnant adolescent than for the pregnant postadolescent woman. If during pregnancy lean body mass continues to increase in the adolescent, additional protein intake over the current RDAs would be required to support this growth, but according to Thompson the amount is not yet known.[54]

To support tissue synthesis, the RDAs for protein intake for pregnant adolescents are 1.7 g/kg for 11- to 14-year-olds and 1.5 g/kg for those 15 to 18 years of age. Adequate energy must be provided to continue both maternal maturation and fetal development, and the quality of protein ingested should allow for 75 percent efficiency of utilization.[55] A steady increase in weight gain of 0.25 to 0.45 kg per week during the nine months is recommended in addition to weight increase comparable to that of nonpregnant females of the same maturity. Adequate weight gain in the pregnant adolescent is extremely important. Two of the nutritional factors

Table 5-10 Recommended Dietary Allowances during Pregnancy and Lactation in Adolescence

Energy and nutrients	Pregnancy		Lactation	
	Total	Percent increase over nonpregnant*	Total	Percent increase over nonpregnant*
Energy	2400 kcal	14	2600 kcal	24
Protein	78 g	62	68 g	42
Vitamin A	5000 IU	25	6000 IU	50
Vitamin D	400 IU	0	400 IU	0
Vitamin E	15 IU	25	15 IU	25
Ascorbic acid	60 mg	33	80 mg	33
Folacin	800 μg	100	600 μg	100
Niacin	16 mg	14	18 mg	29
Riboflavin	1.7 mg	21	1.9 mg	36
Thiamine	1.4 mg	30	1.4 mg	27
Vitamin B_6	2.5 mg	25	2.5 mg	25
Vitamin B_{12}	4.0 mg	33	4.0 mg	33
Calcium	1200 mg	0	1200 mg	0
Phosphorus	1200 mg	0	1200 mg	0
Iodine	125 μg	9	150 μg	30
Iron	18 mg†	suppl.	18 mg	0
Magnesium	450 mg	50	450 mg	50
Zinc	20 mg	33	25 mg	33

*Percent increase has been calculated from the RDA values for 15- to 18-year-old females.
†The use of 30–60 mg of supplemental iron is recommended.
Source: *Recommended Dietary Allowances* (8th rev.), Washington, D.C.: National Academy of Sciences, National Research Council, Food and Nutrition Board, 1974.

most strongly associated with the outcome of pregnancy are the mother's weight gain during pregnancy and her prepregnancy weight.[56] The recommended average weight gain for adult women is 11 kg (about 24 lb) with a range from approximately 9 to 13 kg; an adolescent would be expected then to gain an additional 1 to 2.5 kg, depending on her stage of maturity. The adolescent's need for this additional weight gain is often overlooked. The psychological effect of learning that she must gain this weight and accept a new body image is often distressing to the adolescent and must be considered in dietary counseling. The overweight pregnant adolescent also needs to gain, but probably only about the average 11 kg. Weight loss during pregnancy should be avoided, for it can present problems: ketone bodies formed during fat metabolism can cross the placenta and cause neurological damage to the fetus. Winick and Brasel[57] reported evidence that a greater number of low birth weight babies have learning disabilities. Insufficient nutrient intake during the period of organogenesis (first eight weeks of pregnancy) increases the chances of producing a defective or low birth weight infant.

**Table 5-11   Components of the Average Weight Gained
in Normal Pregnancy**

Component	Amount (g) gained at:			
	10 weeks	20 weeks	30 weeks	40 weeks
A. Total gain of body weight	650	4000	8500	12,500
Fetus	5	300	1500	3300
Placenta	20	170	430	650
Liquor amnii	30	250	600	800
Increase of:				
Uterus*	135	585	810	900
Mammary gland†	34	180	360	405
Maternal blood	100	600	1300	1250
B. Total (rounded)	320	2100	5000	7300
C. Weight not accounted for (A−B)	330	1900	3500	5200

*Blood-free uterus.
†Blood-free mammary glandular tissue.
Source: Maternal Nutrition and the Course of Pregnancy. Washington, D.C.: Pub. No. 1761, National Academy of Sciences, National Research Council, 1970.

Holey[58] has been successful in promoting adequate weight gain during pregnancy when the pregnant woman understands the relationship between the nutritional needs of her body and those of her developing fetus. During pregnancy, oxygen consumption is increased as the fetus and maternal tissues (including the placenta, uterine muscle, and breast tissue) grow. The cardiac and respiratory systems have an increased work load which also requires additional oxygen uptake.[59] This information and Table 5-11's figures on the average weight gain in both maternal and fetal tissue can be adapted for use in patient education. The prenatal weight gain grid (Figure 5-5) can also be used as an educational tool to help patients compare their weight gain with the expected gain as determined from their height and weight prior to pregnancy.[60,61]

A daily iron supplement of 30 to 60 mg is recommended, since anemia has been shown to be a common problem among pregnant teenagers.[62] Iron-rich foods are not widespread in our food supply, and some, such as cooked greens, are poorly accepted by many adolescents. The 30- to 60-mg supplement provides adequate maternal levels to overcome iron deficiency anemia and enables the fetus to store iron during the last trimester in preparation for the first few months of extrauterine life when the iron intake of infants is very low.

The 1970 report of the Committee on Maternal Nutrition of the National Academy of Sciences indicated that a daily supplement of 200 to 400 μg of folic acid "should easily prevent folic acid deficiency in practically all women."[63] This supplement would also eliminate some of the folic acid (folacin) deficiency seen in premature infants[64] and help in overcoming the depletion of folacin caused in some women by taking oral contraceptives prior to pregnancy.[65] Healthy adolescents whose diet is adequate may not need supplements of either iron or folacin.

Vitamin A nutriture in pregnant adolescents needs further research. Hodges[66] indicated that much lower levels of vitamin A are present in the livers of adolescents than of average adults, and that in animal studies inadequate vitamin A increases the incidence of birth defects. In 1970 Giroud presented evidence that the high rate of birth defects among infants of adolescents was of nutritional origin.[67] Current data about vitamin A appear to be inadequate to draw any firm conclusions.

One of the physiological adjustments of pregnancy is the retention of extracellular fluid, which in turn requires an increase in sodium for electrolytic balance. An average of 11.5 to 20.7 g (500 to 900 meq) is accumulated during the gestation period.[68] The old practice of restricting sodium in the diet has proved to be counterproductive, because an actual increase in sodium intake is needed. For adolescents, however, who are partial to potato chips, salted french fries, salted peanuts, vending machine crackers, and other high-sodium foods, a word of caution about overusing salt may help avoid excessive water retention. Diuretics cause excretion not only of sodium but also of potassium and should be avoided during pregnancy unless cardiac or renal problems necessitate their use. Salt substitutes such as lithium chloride may also be harmful during pregnancy and should also be eliminated from the diet.[69]

Edema in pregnancy is due in part to the dramatic change of total osmolality of the blood. The total concentration of plasma proteins decreases during the first trimester from 7 g/100 ml to 5.5 or 6 g/100 ml and remains at this lower level throughout the remainder of pregnancy. In toxemia of pregnancy, the excessive fluid retention which occurs is a direct result either of inadequate protein consumption[70] or of excessive loss of protein or amino acids through glomerular filtration, a very severe problem that requires nutritional and medical intervention.

Digestive problems are frequently among the discomforts experienced during pregnancy. Some women find relief from nausea and other gastrointestinal disturbances by eating smaller and more frequent meals. Also, eliminating erratic eating schedules and avoiding long periods between snacks or meals helps reduce nausea. Increasing fiber (bulk) content in the diet by adding more fruits, vegetables, whole grain cereals, and nuts (or any one of these) relieves constipation caused by a normal decrease in gastrointestinal motility during pregnancy. It has been observed that, among low-income Southerners, whose daily diet contains dry beans or peas, potatoes, and/or large amounts of bread, few pregnant women experience constipation.

Lactose intolerance is now known to be quite common among blacks and Orientals in the United States. This inability to digest milk and milk products is attributed to lack of synthesis of the enzyme lactase. Disaccharides subsequently accumulate in the bowel lumen, and diarrhea, nausea, flatulence, and a sense of fullness result. Symptom severity varies, depending on the amount of lactase present and the amount of the milk product consumed. Dietary counseling is important for lactose-intolerant pregnant women, since the elimination of some or all milk products from the diet places the woman and fetus at risk for calcium insufficiency unless other calcium sources are substituted. Luke,[71] in a recent review of the extent and implications of lactose intolerance during pregnancy, has developed a basic daily food plan to provide calcium for lactose-intolerant women during pregnancy and lactation. Leafy green vegetables can contribute substantially to the calcium content of the diet. Calcium is absorbed also from baking powder used in biscuits, cornbread, and home-prepared cakes and cookies. The bones in canned salmon and sardines provide a ready source of calcium. Some women for whom fluid milk creates problems can tolerate cottage cheese and other cheeses, yogurt, and ice cream. Liquid breakfast mixes have been recommended by Luke, but they should be used minimally by most women because they are extremely high in purified sugars.

Pica, the practice of eating substances not ordinarily considered foods, constitutes a nutritional danger to both the pregnant teenager and her unborn baby. The causes of this very old, culturally derived practice are unknown. Iron deficiency and other dietary inadequacies have variously been proposed as either causes or effects of pica. In some segments of the population of the United States, pica continues despite the unavailability of the nonfood substances traditionally used by earlier generations. Women today substitute such things as dry laundry starch, flour, baking soda, paraffin, coffee grounds, and ice for the clay (earth) that was most commonly used by their mothers and grandmothers. Pica is associated with anemia, although the cause-effect relationships have not been conclusively identified. The substances ingested may limit absorption of iron and other minerals and/or may displace essential nutrients from the diet.

Luke, in her review of pica during pregnancy,[72] suggests that eating patterns may be changed if the patient is helped to understand that her unborn baby is reliant upon her for good nutrition and that pica deprives the fetus. Those persons who eat nonfoods in an effort to decrease morning nausea may be amenable to dietary counseling about substituting dry foods such as crackers, and they may find it helpful to eat a small snack before retiring at night to reduce the time span between feedings. Including a greater variety of foods in the diet may satisfy cravings.

The diet of the pregnant teenager can be individualized to her tastes and still be nutritionally sound. Table 5-12 presents a daily pattern to help build an adequate diet. Table 5-13 identifies foods containing selected nutrients and indicates the proportion of the Recommended Dietary Allowances they provide.

NUTRITION FOR ADOLESCENT ATHLETES

The energy requirements of any person are based on three major factors: basal metabolism, activity, and the calorigenic effect of food (also called the specific dynamic effect). During puberty there may be a slight increase in the basal metabolic rate (BMR), which declines later in adolescence and following completion of growth. There are conflicting reports on BMR,[73] but in females it declines gradually from the time of menarche. Energy is used for both internal (physiologic) and external activities, the latter being the most variable factor influencing energy requirements and, for athletes, the cause of extreme increases in energy needs. Trained athletes appear to have a slightly higher BMR than nontrained athletes. This increase is probably caused by the presence of a greater amount of lean body mass (LBM);[74] however, these differences are negligible, and only a very small increment of protein would be needed to maintain this slightly larger LBM.

Extensive review of the research on nutritional needs of athletes indicates that total energy intake is the principal requirement that is sig-

Table 5-12 Daily Food Intake

Food groups	Number of servings
Milk, cheese, etc.	3–4 servings
Meats, poultry, fish, dry beans, dry peas, eggs, nuts	2 servings
Fruits and vegetables	2 servings fruit
	3 servings vegetables
Use a dark green leafy vegetable daily	
Use a food high in vitamin C daily	
Bread, cereals, and pasta products	4–5 servings of whole grain or enriched
Margarine, butter, salad dressing, mayonnaise, vegetable oil	2 tablespoons

Additional foods to provide calories should be chosen from breads and cereals and the more concentrated vegetables such as potatoes (baked or boiled), sweet potatoes, corn, peas, carrots, etc. Only occasionally use foods concentrated in sugars and fats such as pastries, candies, potato chips, salted crackers, soft drinks.

Source: Adapted from *Essentials of an Adequate Diet* (rev.). Washington, D.C.: U.S. Dept. of Agriculture, 1971.

nificantly increased for athletes as compared to other people of their age and sex. It should be pointed out, however, that with an increase in oxygen intake and carbon dioxide excretion there is an increased requirement for ascorbic acid. Also, as energy intake increases, so do the RDAs for some nutrients.[75] Thiamine, riboflavin, and niacin needs are directly related to

Table 5-13 Food Sources of Nutrients in Relation to Recommended Dietary Allowances*

| Nutrient | Sources | | | |
	Excellent (75% RDA)	Good (50% RDA)	Significant (25% RDA)	Fair (10% RDA)
Ascorbic acid	Orange Strawberries Cauliflower Broccoli Br. sprouts Green pepper Tomato Grapefruit Honeydew melon Mustard greens	Cabbage Spinach Tangerine Asparagus	Banana Blueberries Lima beans Raspberries Green peas Radishes Sauerkraut	Apple Peach Corn
Vitamin A	Liver Carrot Pumpkin Sweet potatoes Spinach Winter squash Turnip greens Mustard greens Beet greens	Apricots Watermelon Broccoli	Honeydew melon Peaches Prunes Tomato Nectarines	Asparagus Green beans Br. sprouts Cheddar cheese Green peas Tomato juice
Thiamine	Pork	Dried peas Macaroni	Green peas Ham Peanuts	Orange Watermelon Dried beans Noodles Spaghetti Lamb liver Rice Cashew nuts
Riboflavin	Liver		Macaroni Cottage cheese Buttermilk Milk	Avocado Tangerine Prunes Asparagus

*Based on average serving size as follows:
  Meat—3 oz., edible portion
  Fruit—3 to 4 oz.
  Vegetables—3 to 4 oz.
  Cereals—1 oz.
  Milk—8 oz.

Table 5-13   Food Sources of Nutrients in Relation to Recommended Dietary Allowances (*Continued*)

| Nutrient | Sources | | | |
	Excellent (75% RDA)	Good (50% RDA)	Significant (25% RDA)	Fair (10% RDA)
Riboflavin (*cont'd*)			Yogurt	Broccoli Mushrooms Ice cream Beef Salmon Turkey
Vitamin B$_6$		Soybeans Beef liver Tuna	Lima beans Pork Beef Veal Halibut Salmon Chicken Bananas Avocado	Cauliflower Green pepper Potatoes Spinach Raisins Perch
Vitamin B$_{12}$	Beef liver Clams Salmon Trappist cheese Lamb Eggs		Veal Cheese Scallops Swordfish	
Magnesium	Molasses Peanuts	Beet greens	Spinach Lima beans Green peas	Raisins Sweet potatoes Br. sprouts Cod
Iron	Calves' and pork liver Clams	Beef liver	Asparagus Ham Veal Beef Chicken Macaroni Prunes Raisins Spinach	Banana Beans Br. sprouts Cod Green peas Noodles Rice Cashew nuts Peanuts
Calcium			Turnip greens Swiss cheese Buttermilk Milk Yogurt Salmon	Prunes Broccoli Beet greens Cottage cheese Ice cream Haddock Scallops

Source: Helen Andrews Guthrie, *Introductory Nutrition* (3d ed.). St. Louis: The C. V. Mosby Company, 1975.

kilocalorie intake; the RDAs for these are 0.5 mg of thiamine, 0.6 mg of riboflavin, and 6.6 mg of niacin per 1000 kcal.[76] (There are lower limits below which dietary intakes of each vitamin should not fall regardless of the level of kilocalories consumed, but athletes seldom restrict their caloric intake to the point that this becomes a concern.) Foods added to increase energy intake should be nutritious ones such as whole grain breads, cereals, pasta, potatoes, and fresh fruits. Highly refined foods should be avoided since they are deficient in both vitamins and minerals.

Complex carbohydrate foods are desirable to provide the extra energy, vitamins, and minerals athletes need. Even though energy can be derived from protein, protein causes a greater increase in the specific dynamic effect and leads to greater energy expenditures for metabolism than carbohydrate foods produce. The specific dynamic action of a mixed diet contributes about 10 percent to the total energy needs of a moderately active adolescent, while in a diet where most of the kilocalories are derived from protein an increase in metabolism as high as 30 percent can occur.[77] In addition, the excess nitrogenous end products of protein metabolism must be metabolized and excreted; hence, a high-protein diet puts a greater work load on the liver and kidneys. As compared to nontrained athletes, trained athletes have the ability to store greater amounts of glycogen as reserves for conversion to glucose during performance. One technique used to accomplish this is to eat a high-carbohydrate diet following extreme exercise, which depletes liver and muscle glycogen stores. As glycogen is taken up by these tissues, they store an increased amount over their normal resting level.[78]

To specify the energy requirements for adolescent athletes, who are also growing, is a very complex undertaking and, because of rapid changes in the biological system from day to day, is probably not feasible. But estimates can be made, and one method is to use the RDA for sex and age as a baseline and then adjust for stage of puberty, growth status (height, weight, and skinfold thickness), and physical activity. Appetite in the healthy adolescent is usually the best controlling factor in energy balance. Several excellent guides are available to help young people select adequate diets for increased physical activities.[79,80] The guidelines in Table 5-14, which can be used as a starting point, provide around 1850 kcal and allow the athlete to add foods from any of the food groups to increase his or her energy intake. Snacks to increase kilocalories should consist of fresh and dry fruits, fruit juices, vegetable juices, raw vegetable strips, nuts, seeds, and a variety of sandwiches. Home preparation of "pocket snack" is becoming popular among young adolescents and college students.* Pocket snack is a rich source of calories and nutrients.

*Pocket snack is made by mixing 2 cups of nuts, 2 cups of raisins or other dried fruit, 1 cup of sunflower seeds, and 1 cup of pumpkin seeds. It should be refrigerated until used.

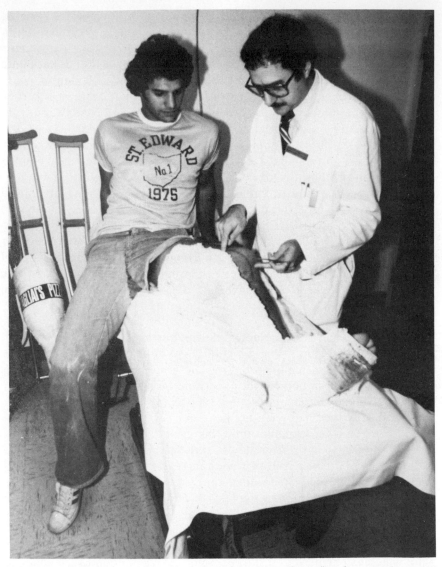

Nutrient needs fluctuate considerably during adolescence, depending, for example, on rate of growth, medicine or other drugs used, sex, state of health, and—as in the case of this young athlete whose ball playing has been curtailed by injury and surgery—activity level. *(Copyright © 1980 by Anne Campbell.)*

Water, an essential nutrient, is very important for athletes. Around one quart per 1000 kcal should be consumed.[81] Milk, fruit drinks, and soft drinks do not substitute for water. Mullis and Thye[82] have developed *The Nutritionist's Game Plan* to provide nutrition information for coaches of young athletes. They promote the drinking of water. Water intake should be increased on the day of the athletic event, since performance is diminished when water loss is great. The use of salt tablets during strenuous exercise periods is discouraged, but some coaches have found that dilute saline solutions are helpful. One tablespoon of salt per gallon of water aids in replacing sodium without disturbing water balance. During practice or game time, one to three glasses of this saline solution should be consumed hourly. The pregame meal should be made up primarily of carbohydrate foods that are easy to digest. This meal does not supply the energy required in the upcoming athletic event, but it "may serve a physiological function."[83]

There are a great number of high protein and "super" foods and unreliable books about special foods for athletes. A well-balanced diet of foods from the five groups in Table 5-14 provides plenty of energy and is much to be preferred. Darden[84] has recently revised his book, *Nutrition and Athletic Performance*, which can be recommended for high school and college athletes. Coaches may wish to obtain *Nutrition for Athletes: A Handbook for Coaches*,[85] also a helpful and reliable text.

Table 5-14   Basic Food Guide for Athletes

Food group	Servings
Milk or milk products	2 or more cups, or 2 $2/3$ cups cottage cheese, or 2 $2/3$ ounces natural cheese or the equivalent.
Lean meat, poultry, fish, dry beans, dry peas, lentils, nuts, eggs, cheese	2 or more servings providing a total of 6 ounces. Use of a combination of these foods to obtain the 6 ounces is recommended.
Vegetables and fruits and their juices	3 servings vegetables, including a dark green or yellow one daily.
	3 servings fruit.
	1 serving of potatoes, carrots, beets, lima beans, peas, or onions (or substitute a whole grain bread or cereal or enriched or brown rice).
	A food rich in ascorbic acid should be included daily.
Bread, cereal, and pasta products	6 servings of whole grain or enriched breads or cereals.
Butter, margarine, salad dressing, mayonnaise, vegetable oil	1 tablespoon (use to season food if desired).

Source: Adapted from *Essentials of an Adequate Diet (rev.)*. Washington, D.C.: U.S. Dept. of Agriculture, 1971.

OBESITY

Incidence and Causes of Adolescent Obesity

During the adolescent years, obesity is a common form of malnutrition and constitutes a substantial threat to health and development. One-tenth to one-fourth of the adolescents in the United States are obese (the incidence varies among demographic subgroups).[86] Significant numbers of these overweight teenagers will become obese adults with increased chances of developing degenerative diseases at an early age and, ultimately, of shortening their lives. Obesity also places an adolescent at risk for low self-esteem, poor peer acceptance, and the many distortions of psychosocial adjustment that accompany them. The obese adolescent who avoids social interactions or who is excluded from them by other persons is handicapped in attaining the developmental tasks of this stage of life. Physical health may be compromised by long-term adherence to nutritionally inadequate fad diets that many overweight teenagers, particularly young women, adopt in their effort to conform to the "slim youth" stereotype.

The causes of obesity are multiple and complex and, even after many decades of study, poorly understood. Current research on human appetite and eating behavior focuses on central nervous system influences, hormonal and peripheral (not found in the brain) mechanisms, and psychological aspects.[87] Childhood obesity is so widespread that it has been declared a world health problem,[88] and about four out of five fat children continue to be overweight as teenagers. The "fat cell hypothesis" posits that infancy is the critical period for proliferation of adipose tissue and that overfeeding at that time develops an excessive number of permanent fat cells, which predispose to obesity throughout life. Controversy continues over this hypothesis; lack of standardization among methods used to assess obesity in infancy has contributed to the uncertainty, as has a dearth of longitudinal studies to determine the percentage of obese infants who are obese as adults. Poskitt and Cole recently reported that only one of nine overweight babies was still obese at five years of age.[89] Heald[90] agrees that adipose hyperplasia (increased numbers of adipose cells) arising during early childhood contributes to juvenile obesity and is more resistant to treatment than is obesity that begins during the adult years. He indicates that some of the factors that lead to hyperplasia of adipose tissue are unknown but that caloric intake in excess of energy needs contributes to the problem.

One excellent study investigated the influence of early caloric deprivation on the subsequent development of obesity by age 19 in males.[91] During the Dutch famine of 1944–45, women who experienced low caloric intakes for one to three months during the last trimester of pregnancy and whose infants were underfed for the first three to five months of postuterine life had significantly fewer sons who were obese at age 19 than did a control group of women. This difference supports the hypothesis derived from animal experiments that the last trimester of pregnancy and the first year of the infant's life is the critical period for development of the adipose tissue. It has also been reported by Knittle[92] that an increased number of fat cells are present in humans whose obesity begins early in life, while obesity arising during adulthood results in increased cell size rather than cell numbers.

The three periods during childhood when obesity is most likely to occur are late infancy, early childhood or around age six, and adolescence.[93] The reasons for this timing are not known, but both physiologic factors and psychologic or interpersonal relationships have been found to play a role.

Although the causes of obesity remain elusive, it is evident from the hazards of being overweight and the great difficulty in regaining and retaining normal weight after obesity has occurred that prevention of obesity is of utmost importance. Obviously, adolescence is too late a time to prevent obesity in the already obese teenager, but health professionals and health educators can and must provide the very substantial service of helping these adolescents learn of the importance and methods of preventing overweight in their own children and other children who may come under their care.

Assessment of Obesity

A large weight gain during adolescence is, of course, normal and desirable. Between 10 and 18 years of age, males typically at least double their weight and females increase their weight by about 60 to 80 percent. It is the kind of tissue gained that is important: Is it lean body mass or fat? It is quite possible to be overweight but not obese, as many athletes demonstrate. Similarly, very sedentary persons may be obese but not markedly overweight. Seltzer and Mayer[94] have published standards for assessing obesity by using skinfold thickness measurements rather than weight. Calipers are used to determine the minimum triceps skinfold thickness, and findings are compared to the standard in Table 5-15. The measurement should be taken at exactly one-half the distance between the shoulder and the elbow while the subcutaneous tissue is held between the thumb and forefinger 1 cm above the site where the calipers are placed. The skin is pulled gently away from the muscle and held during the measurements. The dial should be read to the nearest 0.5 mm for three stable readings. For the very thick skinfolds of obese individuals, readings should be obtained three seconds after the calipers handle is released. Figure 5-6 shows the proper position for skinfold measurements.

Normative height and weight charts are helpful in the assessment of obesity during adolescence. These, as well as skinfold thickness mea-

Table 5-15 Triceps Skinfold Thickness (in Millimeters) Indicative of Obesity*

	Skinfold thickness	
Age	Male	Female
10	16	20
11	17	21
12	18	22
13	18	23
14	17	23
15	16	24
16	15	25
17	14	26
18	15	27
19	15	27
20	16	28
21	17	28
22	18	28
23	18	28
24	19	28
25	20	29

*Adapted from data standardized on United States Caucasians.
Source: C. C. Seltzer and J. Mayer, "A Simple Criterion of Obesity," Postgraduate Medicine, 38:A101–107, 1965 (© McGraw-Hill, Inc.).

surements, are of interest to adolescents as they assess their own physical development and can be useful aids in nutrition awareness sessions.

Treatment of Obesity

In the treatment of obesity in adolescence, care must be taken to avoid interfering with growth. During the rapid growth spurt, teenagers are extraordinarily sensitive to caloric restriction: If weight loss exceeds 1 percent of the total body mass per unit of time, marked decreases in growth result.[95] Hence, the objective of weight control programs for teenagers who are still growing rapidly should be to halt or retard the *rate* of weight *gain* for a period of time rather than to induce weight loss. Older adolescents whose growth is complete can tolerate loss of weight. The key to weight control in adolescence, as in other stages of life, is to adjust diet or activity level (usually both) so that energy intake is aligned with energy expenditure.

Most normal adolescents are able to adjust their diet and exercise to control their weight if they feel they are "too fat," but they need sound information about meeting nutrient requirements and avoiding the seductions of radical diets or dangerous extremes of physical activity. Coun-

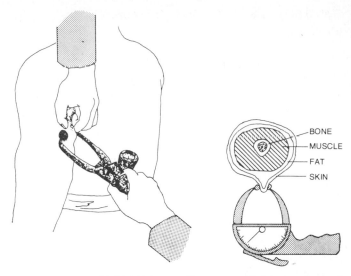

Figure 5-6 Calipers measurement of skinfold thickness. Measurement is taken on the back of the upper arm, exactly midway between the shoulder tip and the point of the elbow.

seling must be skillfully offered lest it engender the so-called adolescent rebelliousness and counteract its purpose. (See Chapter 11 for information about health counseling approaches.) Young people with emotional and personality disturbances may become so upset by even a small excess in weight that they become overly rigid in their eating behavior and develop eating disorders such as anorexia nervosa, overingestion followed by self-induced vomiting, depression anorexia, food faddism, or other eating problems.[96] These adolescents need professional psychologic intervention.

Obesity is a multifaceted problem involving highly complex physiologic and psychologic phenomena, and a treatment approach that works for one teenager often fails for another. Behavior modification programs have enabled many persons to correct their obesity: Self-help groups, programs for individuals, and groups assisted by psychologists and nutritionists have all been described.[97,98] The basis of the behavior modification approach is to determine what cues elicit the desire to eat and then to modify the environment to reduce those cues. The obese are influenced more than nonobese persons by external factors such as food palatability, time of day, and availability of food than by internal factors such as hunger. Behavior modification programs attempt to make the obese person aware of these factors[99,100] and induce the realization that undesirable eating behavior can be unlearned and new behavior substituted.[101,102] Self-reward mechanisms have also been useful in the treatment of obesity in adolescence.[103]

DRUG-INDUCED NUTRITIONAL DEFICIENCIES

Oral Contraceptives

When oral contraceptives became available in the 1960s, they were not suspected of having adverse effects on nutrition. With long-term use came reports of the various side effects, one of which is the possible alteration of the body's need for a number of minerals and vitamins. Table 5-16 provides a summary of these effects. The changes in requirements for some nutrients vary with the type of oral contraceptive taken. In 1975 the Committee on Nutrition of the Mother and Preschool Child of the Food and Nutrition Board indicated that, until further information was available about the clinical consequences of using oral contraception, "no definitive recommendation regarding use of nutritional supplements can be made."[104] However, dietary assessment and nutritional counseling should be an essential component of family planning services. Some authorities advocate the use of supplements such as vitamin B_6 as a prophylactic measure to prevent depression, even though data to confirm the effectiveness of this treatment are lacking.[105] A wise practice is to assess the adequacy of the adolescent patient's diet and, if she uses an oral contraceptive, encourage her to add foods that are rich in folic acid, vitamin B_6, vitamin B_{12}, vitamin C, and riboflavin. Helping her to balance her diet now will support her nutritional well-being if she later becomes pregnant.

Other Drugs

Antineoplastics Folic acid is one of the vitamins required for synthesis of deoxyribonucleic acid (DNA) and ribonucleic acid (RNA). The folic acid antagonists aminopterin and methotrexate are sometimes used to interrupt cellular proliferation in neoplastic disease. Because of folic acid's role in DNA and RNA formation, it is essential during embryogenesis and again during the last trimester of pregnancy, when the brain of the fetus is growing at a rapid rate. In animals, severe folic acid deficiency during organogenesis has been shown to promote fetal malformations.[106] There have been several reports of malformed infants born to women who had received folic acid antagonists early in pregnancy.[107]

Antituberculosis Drugs Adequate intake of vitamin B_6 (pyridoxine) during the last trimester of pregnancy is critical, since this vitamin is essential in the synthesis of proteins and in the production of neuro-transmitters in the nervous system. The antituberculosis drugs isoniazid (INH) and cycloserine are vitamin B_6 antagonists. Para-aminosalicylic acid (PAS) interferes with the absorption of vitamin B_{12} and in time can

Table 5-16 The Effects of Oral Contraceptives on Nutritional Status

Nutrient	Effect	Mechanism
Folic acid (folacin)	Reduction in serum and/or erythrocyte folate levels; alterations in urinary formiminoglutamic acid excretion (these effects not found in all users); megaloblastic anemia in some.	Interferes with absorption or contributes to an increased rate of folate clearance from plasma to tissues.
Vitamin B_6 (pyridoxine)	Subclinical deficiency of vitamin B_6; evidence of depression in some women.	Increased excretion of the tryptophan metabolites 3-hydroxykynurenine and xanthurenic acid; may be caused by a block in the activity of the enzyme kynureninase (more research is necessary to ascertain).
Vitamin B_{12} (cyanocobalamin)	Lower than normal levels of serum B_{12} have been reported in about half of users of oral contraceptives.	Absorption may be impaired.
Vitamin C (ascorbic acid)	Lower levels of ascorbic acid in leukocytes, platelets, and plasma.	May either increase the catabolism of ascorbic acid or change tissue distribution; raises levels of ceruloplasmin, a catalyst of ascorbic acid oxidation.
Riboflavin	Decreased excretion of urinary riboflavin and decreased activity of erythrocyte glutathione reductase, an enzyme used to determine riboflavin nutriture.	Related in some way to increased plasma cortisol level in users and to increased vitamin B_6 requirements.
Vitamin A	Increased plasma vitamin A levels except in users of parenterally administered, long-acting progestin.	Currently unclear, probably related to increase in lipoprotein bound to vitamin A and induced by estrogen.
Vitamin K	Increased serum levels of vitamin K-dependent clotting factors.	Unclear, but appears to be related to the risk of thromboembolic phenomena associated with oral contraceptives containing estrogen.

Table 5-16 The Effects of Oral Contraceptives on Nutritional Status (Continued)

Nutrient	Effect	Mechanism
Zinc	Controversial—increased zinc requirements have been suggested since lower plasma levels have been reported, but other reports have shown increased plasma zinc levels in users of combination-type pills.	There may be a redistribution of zinc between red cells and plasma rather than a depletion.
Copper	Marked elevation of serum copper and ceruloplasmin follows use of estrogen-type pills.	Copper absorption may be increased, since no change occurs in urinary excretion.
Calcium	No blood responses.	Radiocalcium studies indicate that intestinal absorption of calcium is improved in users of oral contraceptives.
Iron	Iron binding and serum iron levels increase; serum iron elevation appears to be related to diet since it occurs only in some women.	Decreased menstrual blood loss.

lead to the development of pernicious anemia. Vitamin supplements should be given when these drugs are prescribed.[108]

Anticonvulsants   Anticonvulsant drugs have an antagonistic effect on vitamin D, and epileptic patients have been reported to develop rickets after receiving these drugs.[109] Anticonvulsants can increase susceptibility to early development of osteomalacia.[110] Deficiencies of vitamins K and B_6 and folic acid have been reported in conjunction with use of anticonvulsant drugs, as has an elevated incidence of birth-defective offspring.[111]

Drugs of Abuse   Alcohol used in large quantities can lead to tissue depletion of such nutrients as folate, thiamine, magnesium, and zinc, either because of the increased need for these nutrients to metabolize the alcohol or because the diets of alcohol abusers are frequently deficient in these nutrients. Alcohol, particularly when used excessively, has profound effects on the gastrointestinal system and liver and creates consequent disturbances in nutrient utilization. The increasing incidence of alcohol use and abuse among children and adolescents and the apparent spread of alcoholism across age and socioeconomic categories underline the need for educating young people about the nutritional consequences as well as the other hazards of alcohol ingestion.

Cigarette smoking, as is widely known, depresses appetite and consequently can interfere with adequacy of dietary intake. Vitamin C requirements are increased by smoking.

Narcotics, stimulants, and depressants may markedly disturb nutritional status, both by their direct pharmacologic effects on body utilization of nutrients and because the life-style, including eating behavior, of abusers is often incompatible with obtaining an adequate diet. Diet therapy is an essential component of treatment and rehabilitation of substance abusers. Drug use is discussed in Chapter 6 and treatment of abusers in Chapter 17.

Drugs in Combination   Drug-drug interactions and their consequences have come under increasing scrutiny in recent years. When several drugs are used in combination, they may interact with one another to produce complex effects on nutrient needs and nutritional status. Dietary assessments should be carried out on adolescents who use combinations of medicines or other drugs. A monograph on nutrition and drug interrelations,[112] now in preparation, will provide up-to-date information and recommendations for prevention and treatment of nutritional problems.

NUTRITION EDUCATION FOR ADOLESCENTS

The objective of nutrition education is to provide information and promote attitudes that will enable persons to make informed and healthful decisions about their dietary practices. The strategy for attaining this goal with educational programs for adolescents is to appeal to their developmentally characteristic interests and motives and to find ways around the age-typical qualities that act as deterrents to learning and to behavior change. Adolescents have great potential as learners and in some ways are more amenable to nutrition education than people at other stages of life. For one thing, adolescents are in a state of change and as a consequence are often especially receptive to "new" ideas. Teenagers themselves are quite well aware that they are changing, and their awareness produces both curiosity and anxious eagerness for a satisfactory outcome; both these attributes contribute to readiness to learn. In addition, teenagers' drive for self-determination, their newly developing cognitive capacity for gathering and processing information, and their self-interest are among the developmental avenues that can be used for teaching about nutrition.

Educational Offerings Must Be Relevant to the Students

When nutrition education programs are relevant to the interests and activities of the learner, they are quite enthusiastically received. Young adolescents, who are anticipating or experiencing the physical changes of puberty, usually are highly interested in physical function and physical appearance. Their concern about growth rate, body size and configuration, skin changes, and all kinds of physiological activities is often intense. Interest in body image runs high. These young people are quite responsive to information about the role of nutrients in body-building, weight control, new physiologic experiences such as menstruation, and old but previously relatively unnoticed body functions such as gastrointestinal activity. Dental health is also of interest to many young or middle adolescents, both because they wish to project a winning smile and because they may have experienced the dental caries peak of adolescence and the attendant discomforts of treatment. (An excellent teaching aid about diet as it pertains to dental health is available from the Nutrition Today Society.[113])

The preeminent interests of high-school-age young people usually revolve around issues of independence, sex role behavior, and peer acceptability. They are still quite receptive to information about the relationship between diet and appearance and between diet and performance (i.e., intellectual or physical performance). In addition, they are often on their own with regard to food selection for one or more meals daily, many are spending their own money for those meals, and they usually have a

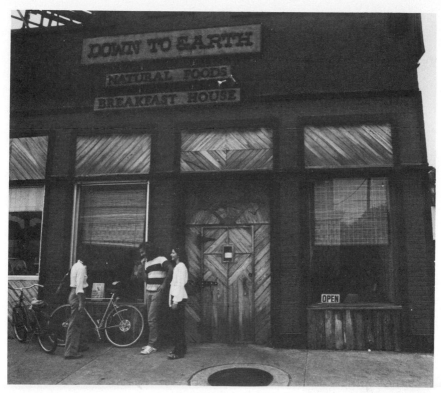

Adolescents gradually assume responsibility for their own food selection. Knowledge with which to make informed choices is a major tool for health promotion. Nutrition education must accommodate to the fact that diet is heavily influenced by the ethical, esthetic, and political values that develop during adolescence. (*Copyright © 1980 by Anne Campbell.*)

choice about where and what they eat. High-school-age youth also are conscious of and critical of the ethics of social policy, and they can become interested in social issues such as consumer influence on the prepared food industry, food additives, ecology as it pertains to food supply, and so forth.

College-age young men and women, whether or not they are in school, are involved in defining a life-style for themselves as persons who for the most part independently select their objectives and autonomously work toward them. Major interests of late adolescents include career choice (and preparation for functioning in the selected work role) and love relationships, perhaps by now narrowed to one particular person. Many of the earlier-mentioned concerns, of course, continue into adulthood.

Finally, adolescents are, like people of other ages, greatly influenced in their attitudes and interests by their cultural and experiential back-

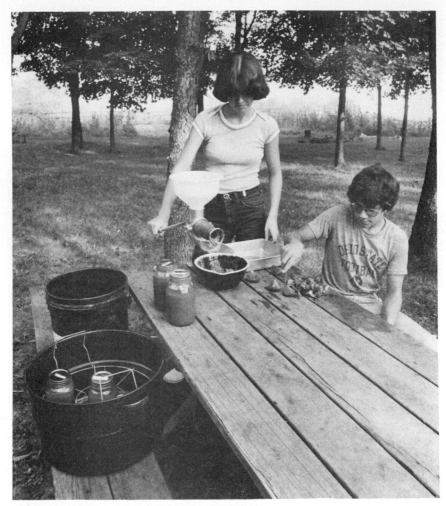

Educational programs are most effective when they deal with material that is directly related to the learners' personal interests and objectives. For example, young people who seek economic self-sufficiency or avoidance of chemical additives in commercially prepared foods may welcome learning projects related to gardening and food preservation. (*Copyright* © *1980 by Anne Campbell*.)

grounds. As Hofmann, Becker, and Gabriel[114] point out, rural and small-town young people tend to mature in their interests more slowly than inner-city youth, who are likely to become independent in their financial affairs, social roles, and living arrangements at an earlier age. Ethnic membership and socioeconomic status are obvious modifiers of interest, attitude, objectives, and rate and direction of psychosocial development. The political and economic tone of the current social scene (unemployment, the energy crisis, political scandal, the "back to the land" movement, women's rights, and so forth) also color young people's thinking and behavior. Some if not all of these diverse factors impinge upon attitudes and practices related to food use. Nutrition education, like other educational areas, must take into account the personal interests and outlooks of learners if it is to be effective.

At all ages, adolescents (again like others) are interested in information that they feel particularly pertains to their own current situation, especially if the information offers hope of personal betterment: solution to a problem, improvement in appearance or performance, and so forth. Those who smoke, drink, use oral contraceptives, train for sports or engage in other forms of physical culture, have specific health disorders, or are pregnant, for example, may be especially responsive to the aspects of nutrition education that pertain to their personal circumstances. Because they tend to be quite present-oriented, most adolescents are far more interested in the relatively short-range effects of nutrition practices than in long-range matters such as longevity.

Approaches to Teaching

Several useful articles have recently appeared in the literature to describe effective approaches to nutrition education for young people. Rice[115] discusses ways to make consumer education relevant through discovery techniques and by involving students in the identification of key problems by using situation solutions. This method can be adapted to teaching facts about vegetarian diets, diets to maximize athletic performance, or diets for other content areas of concern. Nutrition games have been successfully used to familiarize students with the nutrient content of foods. Class gardening projects have integrated the study of several sciences with nutrition to produce and analyze favorite dishes, which are then eaten by all in a festive setting.[116] Additional innovative teaching approaches have been designed around real life situations, simulations of reality, and abstractions from reality.[117] Some adolescents have identified films as a preferred method of receiving new information.[118]

Table 5-17 is a summary of the nutrition education services provided to nurses and others by four major resource organizations. A virtually unlimited range of information and teaching materials, along with consultation about their selection and use, is available through these organizations either free or at nominal cost.

Content Areas for Nutrition Education

The topics previously discussed—nutrient needs, weight control, drug-nutrient interrelationships, diet during pregnancy, diet for athletes—are obviously suitable topics for nutrition education programs for teenagers. In addition, since snacking is a way of life during the adolescent years,

Table 5-17   Nutrition Education Materials: A Guide to Libraries and Clearing Houses That Offer Information on Nutrition Education Materials*

I. The Nutrition Information and Resource Center
   Beecher-Dock House
   The Pennsylvania State University
   University Park, Pa. 16802   Telephone: (814) 865-1751 or 865-6323

   This center was recently established under the Nutrition Education Grant to the Nutrition Program, College of Human Development at Pennsylvania State University, provided by the Heinz Endowment and given through the Nutrition Foundation. It is a working collection of nutrition education materials, staffed by nutritionists.

   Special Service Features:
   1. Makes its services available to teachers, university faculty and students, professionals in other agencies, and the public at large.
   2. Receives requests by letter, phone, or personal visit for help in identifying and selecting reliable nutrition information and educational materials.
   3. Assists client in making arrangements, if needed, to secure nutrition education materials by loan or purchase.
   4. Provides consultation to those planning a nutrition education exhibit, learning center, etc.
   5. Provides referral to other professionals and agencies when appropriate.

II. The Food and Nutrition Information and Educational Materials Center (FNIC)
    The National Agricultural Library, Room 304
    Beltsville, Md. 20705   Telephone: (301) 344-3719

    This center was established to select, collect, maintain, and lend resource materials for use in training school food service personnel and by the nutrition education community. The FNIC collection includes both print and nonprint materials related to food service and nutrition. Print materials include books, journal articles, pamphlets, government documents, special reports, proceedings, bibliographies, etc. Types of nonprint materials maintained are films, filmstrips, slides, games, charts, audiotapes, and video cassettes.

    Special Service Features:
    1. Maintains this collection and lends primarily to the following groups:
       a. Employees of the Food and Nutrition Service, USDA.
       b. State school food service directors and staff.
       c. County, city, or district school food service personnel.
       d. Colleges and universities offering courses applicable to school food service training.
       e. Professional societies and research institutions involved in school food service and related subject areas.
       f. Selected libraries with which FNIC shares reciprocal arrangements.
    2. Accepts requests by mail, telephone, or personal visits.
    3. Lends materials gratis.
       a. Print materials for one month
       b. Nonprint materials for two weeks (no more than three nonprint media lent at any one time to one person; films cannot be scheduled more than one month in advance)
    4. Makes available a catalog of the FNIC collection.
       a. Materials are indexed according to specialized vocabulary as well as by author and title.
       b. Materials are abstracted, extracted, or annotated to provide descriptive information including intended audience.

Table 5-17   Nutrition Education Materials (*Continued*)

5. Makes available a separate catalog, "Audiovisual Guide to the Catalog of the FNIC."
6. Issues from time to time *Cumulative Indexes* to update and supplement the *Catalog*.
7. Maintains a 24-hour telephone monitor; regular office hours are 8 A.M. to 5 P.M., Monday through Friday.

III. The National Nutrition Education Clearing House (NNECH)
2140 Shattuck Avenue, Suite 1110
Berkeley, Calif. 94704   Telephone: (415) 548-1363

This is a service of the Society for Nutrition Education which provides reference to nutrition education materials (print and nonprint) judged by qualified nutritionists to contain accurate information. Special services such as preparation of bibliographies, selection and abstraction of materials, administration of nutrition education questionnaires, etc., can be contracted through the NNECH staff. NNECH is not a lending library. Reference lists and bibliographies prepared by the staff are offered at modest cost.

Special Service Features:
1. Provides extensive annotated bibliographies on such topics as food habits, methods and kinds of nutrition education, and nutrition education for Spanish-speaking Americans.
2. Provides selected teaching/counseling materials and background reference lists for nutrition educators. Print and nonprint materials as well as selected journal articles are included.
   a. Subject matter is described by key words.
   b. Publication date, cost, and ordering information are given for each item.
3. Provides two leaflets (one for professionals and one for laypersons) listing reliable nutrition resources.

IV. The Office of Education and Public Affairs
The Nutrition Foundation, Inc.
888 Seventeenth Street, N.W.
Washington, D.C. 20006   Telephone: (202) 872-0778

This foundation, created and supported by leading companies in the food and allied industries, is a public, nonprofit institution. The Foundation is dedicated to the advancement of nutrition knowledge and to its effective application in improving the health and welfare of all persons.

Special Service Features:
1. Produces *The Nutrition Foundation Index to Nutrition Education Materials*, which lists entries according to source, subject matter, readership level, audiovisual materials, and alphabetical order by title (including pertinent information about the publications); also lists addresses of additional sources of nutrition education materials, information, and personal contacts. (*Note*: materials have not been evaluated for content and are not necessarily recommended by the Nutrition Foundation.) Cost of $5.00/copy is below cost of production.
2. Produces other nutrition education materials on various topics and makes available a catalog and order sheet for these items. Cost is modest.
3. Produces *Nutrition Reviews*, a recognized publication used widely by nutritionists.

*Provided through the courtesy of the Nutrition Information and Resource Center, Pennsylvania State University.

"snacker's education" about the relationship of snacks to total food intake is an important part of nutrition education. This subject matter can often be tied to the topic of consumer competence or consumer power, since adolescents' interest in influencing "the establishment" and/or in getting the most for their money is easily aroused. The fast-food industry's expansion is apparent throughout the United States, and market projections for prepared snack foods predict a growth rate of 6 percent per year. Adolescents compose a major segment of the buyers of these products.

Vending machine foods typically are high in salt, sugar, and calories, and low in vitamins, minerals, and proteins. Vending machine snackers need to be cautioned against overuse of high-salt and high-sugar products and should be informed of their need to obtain fruits and vegetables from other sources during the day. If consumers choose the more nutritious of the available foods, vendors will replace the products that have poorer nutritional value. The consumer's voice is heard by business and industry today, as is evidenced, for example, by the growth and current wide distribution of "natural foods." In many universities and public places, machines carrying vegetable and fruit juices, yogurt, soups, sandwiches, and fresh fruit have become popular with all age groups. Consumer groups, which can certainly include adolescent groups such as student organizations and others, can request that vending companies provide nutritious items in the machines provided for their use. Fast-food chains, popular with adolescents, are increasing the number and variety of foods offered. Whether the nutrient quality of fast foods and snack products will be improved depends on the demands the public places on industry and the activism of both consumer and professional groups to have high-quality food made available. Fleck's[119] helpful suggestions for improving the nutrient quality of snacks can be used by both groups.

Adolescents need to become able to select an adequate diet for themselves. As a means to this end, they need to learn how to make substitutions to utilize a variety of foods in their diet and how to interpret nutrition labels on processed foods. Most elementary school nutrition education programs emphasize the basic four food groups; nutrient content of foods follows well as a focus of junior high school and high school programs.

Ethical Considerations

Nutrition education, like other areas of education, aims at making adolescents aware of the relationships between phenomena so that they may be well informed about the choices they make and the outcomes that are predictable from those choices. Nutrition education can expand young people's understanding about food use as an influence on such major aspects of their lives as health, economics, and personal satisfaction. However, most adolescents know more about nutrition than they apply.

The gap between understanding and practice exists for many reasons: habits, social influences, differences in availability of foods, and myriad others. One of those factors that should not be overlooked, particularly with adolescents, is the satisfaction obtained from eating. The educator must help the learner examine the pros and cons of making (or not making) changes in this highly personal and symbolic area of behavior. Will a modified diet be equally satisfying? What benefits can be expected to accrue? What will they cost? These questions cannot always be answered, but their exploration is highly desirable from an ethical standpoint and lends a dimension of depth to the adolescent's learning and decision-making.

REFERENCES

1 J. J. Sternlieb and L. Munan, "A Survey of Health Problems, Practices, and Needs of Youth," *Pediatrics*, **49**:177–186, February 1972.
2 "Teens Want to Be Thin, Health Survey Finds," *Family News and Features*, August 1976.
3 H. E. C. Millar, *Approaches to Adolescent Health Care in the 1970s*. Rockville, Md.: USDHEW, PHS, HSA Pub. No. (HSA) 75-5014, 1975.
4 G. Christakis, "Nutritional Assessment in Health Programs," *Journal of the American Public Health Association*, **63**:1–82, November 1973, Supplement.
5 S. J. Fomon, *Nutritional Disorders of Children—Prevention, Screening and Follow-up*. Rockville, Md.: USDHEW, PHS, HSA Pub. No. (HSA) 76-5612, 1976.
6 "Guidelines for Diet Counseling," *Journal of the American Dietetic Association*, **66**:571–575, June 1975.
7 "The Nurse's Role in Health Assessment and Promotion," *The Canadian Nurse*, **73**:40–41, March 1977.
8 Committee on Nutrition Advisory to CDC Food and Nutrition Board, *Comparison of Body Weights and Lengths or Heights of Groups of Children*. Atlanta, Ga.: USDHEW, PHS, Center for Disease Control, March 1974.
9 Center for Disease Control, *Sources of Error in Weighing and Measuring Children*. Atlanta, Ga.: USDHEW, PHS, Nutrition Surveillance, September 1975.
10 Fomon, op. cit.
11 P. V. V. Hamill, T. A. Drizd, C. L. Johnson, R. B. Reed, and A. F. Roche, "NCHS Growth Charts, 1976," *Monthly Vital Statistics Report*, **25**(3), Supplement, June 22, 1976.
12 Center for Disease Control, *Nutrition Indices*. Atlanta, Ga.: USDHEW, PHS, Nutrition Surveillance, June 1977.
13 Fomon, op. cit.
14 Christakis, op. cit.
15 National Academy of Sciences, *Recommended Dietary Allowances*, 8th rev. Washington, D.C.: National Research Council, Food and Nutrition Board, 1974.

16 Health and Welfare Canada, Committee for Revision of the Canadian Dietary Standard, *Dietary Standard for Canada*, rev. ed. Ottawa, Canada: Bureau of Nutritional Sciences, 1974.

17 National Institutes of Health, *How Children Grow*. Bethesda, Md.: USDHEW Pub. No. (NIH) 73-166, 1972.

18 H. N. Munro, "Formulation of Research Priorities," in J. I. McKigney and H. N. Munro (eds.), *Nutrient Requirements in Adolescence*. Cambridge, Mass.: M.I.T. Press, 1973.

19 National Institutes of Health, *How Children Grow*, op. cit.

20 Ibid.

21 Munro, op. cit.

22 V. A. Beal, "Nutritional Intake," in R. W. McCamnon (ed.), *Human Growth and Development*. Springfield, Ill.: Charles C Thomas, 1970.

23 B. Wait and L. J. Roberts, "Studies in the Food Requirement of Adolescent Girls. I. The Energy Intake of Well-Nourished Girls 10 to 16 Years of Age," *Journal of the American Dietetic Association*, 8:209, 1932.

24 National Center for Health Statistics, *Preliminary Findings of the First Health and Nutrition Examination Survey, United States, 1971–72: Dietary Intake and Biochemical Findings*. Rockville, Md.: USDHEW Pub. No. (HRA) 76-1219-1, 1976.

25 Beal, op. cit.

26 National Center for Health Statistics, *Preliminary Findings of the First Health and Nutrition Examination Survey*, op. cit.

27 B. Wait, R. Blair, and L. J. Roberts, "Energy Intake of Well-Nourished Children and Adolescents," *American Journal of Clinical Nutrition*, 22:1383–1396, October 1969.

28 M. C. Hampton, R. L. Huenemann, L. R. Shapiro, and B. W. Mitchell, "Calorie and Nutrient Intakes of Teenagers," *Journal of the American Dietetics Association*, 50:385–396, May 1967.

29 O. C. Johnson, "The Food and Drug Administration and Labeling," *Journal of the American Dietetic Association*, 64:471–475, May 1974.

30 Food and Drug Administration, *Nutrition Labels and U.S. RDA*, rev. ed. Rockville, Md.: PHS, HEW Pub. No. (FDA) 76-2042, January 1976.

31 J. I. McKigney and H. N. Munro, *Nutrient Requirements in Adolescence*. Bethesda, Md.: DHEW Pub. No. (NIH) 76-771, 1976.

32 Ibid.

33 R. Howard and N. Herbold, *Nutrition in Clinical Care*. New York: McGraw-Hill Book Co., 1978.

34 R. L. Pike and M. L. Brown, *Nutrition: An Integrated Approach*, 2d ed. New York: John Wiley and Sons, 1975.

35 E. N. Todhunter, *A Guide to Nutrition Terminology for Indexing and Retrieval*. Washington, D.C.: DHEW, PHS Contract No. Ph 43-67-1449, 1970.

36 Center for Disease Control, *Ten-State Nutrition Survey, 1968–1970; V— Dietary*. Atlanta, Ga.: DHEW Pub. No. (HSM) 72-8133, 1972.

37 National Center for Health Statistics, *Preliminary Findings of the First Health and Nutrition Survey*, op. cit.

38 McKigney and Munro, op. cit.

39   Ibid.

40   H. Guthrie, *Introductory Nutrition*, 3d ed. St. Louis: The C. V. Mosby Co., 1975.

41   E. R. McAnarney, "Adolescent Pregnancy: A Pediatric Concern?" *Clinical Pediatrics*, **14**(1):19–22, January 1975.

42   National Center for Health Statistics, *Natality, Volume I*. Washington, D.C.: DHEW, PHS, 1976.

43   A. D. Hofmann, "Identifying and Counseling the Sexually Active Adolescent Is Every Pediatrician's Responsibility," *Clinical Pediatrics*, **11**:625–629, November 1972.

44   T. F. McDonald, "Teenage Pregnancy," *Journal of the American Medical Association*, **236**(6):598–599, August 9, 1976.

45   S. J. Ventura, "Teenage Childbearing: United States, 1966–1975," *Monthly Vital Statistics Report, Natality Statistics*, Vol. 26, No. 3 (supplement), September 8, 1977.

46   J. F. Jekel, N. C. Tyler, and L. V. Klerman, "Induced Abortion and Sterilization among Women Who Became Mothers as Adolescents," *American Journal of Public Health*, **67**(7):621–625, July 1977.

47   D. Rush, A. C. Higgins, M. D. Sadow, and S. Margolis, "Dietary Services during Pregnancy, and Birth Weight: A Retrospective Matched Pair Analysis," *Pediatric Research*, **10**(4), 1976 (abstract).

48   G. A. Webb, C. Briggs, and R. C. Brown, "A Comprehensive Adolescent Maternity Program in a Community Hospital," *American Journal of Obstetrics and Gynecology*, **113**:511–523, June 15, 1972.

49   A. B. Dott and A. T. Fort, "Medical and Social Factors Affecting Early Teenage Pregnancy: A Literature Review and Summary of the Findings of the Louisiana Infant Mortality Study," *American Journal of Obstetrics and Gynecology*, **125**(4):532–536, June 15, 1976.

50   A. M. Thompson, "Pregnancy in Adolescence," in J. I. McKigney and H. N. Munro (eds.), *Nutrient Requirements in Adolescence*. Cambridge, Mass.: M.I.T. Press, 1973.

51   T. Brewer, "Metabolic Toxemia, the Mysterious Affliction," *Journal of Applied Nutrition*, **24**:56, 1972.

52   H. Jacobson, "Nutrition and Human Reproduction Workshop" (workshop summary), Buffalo, N.Y.: Lakes Area Regional Medical Program, Inc., 1974.

53   Thompson, op. cit.

54   Ibid.

55   National Academy of Sciences, *Recommended Dietary Allowances*, op. cit.

56   Thompson, op. cit.

57   M. Winick and J. A. Brasel, "Nutrition and Cell Growth," in R. S. Goodhart and M. E. Shils (eds.), *Modern Nutrition in Health and Disease*, 5th ed. Philadelphia: Lea and Febiger, 1973.

58   E. S. Holey, "Promoting Adequate Weight Gain in Pregnant Women," *American Journal of Maternal Child Nursing*, **2**(2):86–89, March-April 1977.

59   R. E. Hytten and I. Leitch, *Physiology of Human Pregnancy*, 2d ed. Philadelphia: Lippincott, 1971.

60   Christakis, op. cit.

61 National Academy of Sciences, *Maternal Nutrition and the Course of Pregnancy*, Washington, D.C.: National Research Council, Pub. No. 1761, 1970.

62 Ibid.

63 Ibid.

64 R. R. Streiff and A. B. Little, "Folic Acid Deficiency in Pregnancy," *New England Journal of Medicine*, **276**:776–779, April 6, 1967.

65 S. B. Kahn, S. Fein, S. Rigberg, and L. Brodsky, "Correlation of Folate Metabolism and Socioeconomic Status in Pregnancy and in Patients Taking Oral Contraceptives," *American Journal of Obstetrics and Gynecology*, **108**:931–935, November 15, 1970.

66 R. E. Hodges, "Vitamin and Mineral Requirements in Adolescence," in J. I. McKigney and H. N. Munro (eds.), *Nutrient Requirements in Adolescence*, Cambridge, Mass.: M.I.T. Press, 1973.

67 A. Giroud, *Nutrition of the Embryo*. Springfield, Ill.: Charles C Thomas, 1970.

68 M. D. Lindheimer and A. I. Katz, "Sodium and Diuretics during Pregnancy," *New England Journal of Medicine*, **288**:891–894, April 26, 1973.

69 Guthrie, op. cit.

70 C. T. Torre, "Nutritional Needs of Adolescents," *American Journal of Maternal Child Nursing*, **2**(2):118–127, March-April 1977.

71 B. Luke, "Lactose Intolerance during Pregnancy: Significance and Solutions," *American Journal of Maternal Child Nursing*, **2**(2):92–96, March-April 1977.

72 B. Luke, "Understanding Pica in Pregnant Women," *American Journal of Maternal Child Nursing*, **2**(2):97–100, March-April 1977.

73 National Institutes of Health, *How Children Grow*, op. cit.

74 Pike and Brown, op. cit.

75 National Academy of Sciences, *Recommended Dietary Allowances*, op. cit.

76 Ibid.

77 Guthrie, op. cit.

78 Pike and Brown, op. cit.

79 U.S. Department of Agriculture, *Essentials of an Adequate Diet*, rev. ed. Washington, D.C.: USDA, 1971.

80 N. Smith, *Food for Sport*, Palo Alto, Calif.: Bull Publishing Co., 1977.

81 Ibid.

82 R. Mullis and F. W. Thye, *The Nutritionist's Game Plan*. Blacksburg, Va.: Virginia Polytechnic Institute and State University, Extension Service, 1977.

83 Ibid.

84 E. Darden, *Nutrition and Athletic Performance*. Pasadena, Calif.: The Athletic Press, 1976.

85 American Association for Health, Physical Education and Recreation, *Nutrition for Athletes: A Handbook for Coaches*. Washington, D.C.: AAHPER, 1971.

86 National Institutes of Health, *How Children Grow*, op. cit.

87 G. McBride, "Human Appetite, Eating Behavior Complexities Tantalize Scientists," *Journal of the American Medical Association*, **236**:1433–1445, September 27, 1976.

88   M. Winick (ed.), *Childhood Obesity*. New York: John Wiley and Sons, 1975.
89   E. M. Poskitt and T. J. Cole, "Do Fat Babies Stay Fat?" *British Medical Journal*, 1(6052):7–9, January 1, 1977.
90   F. P. Heald, "Juvenile Obesity," in M. Winick (ed.), *Childhood Obesity*. New York: John Wiley and Sons, 1975.
91   G. Ravelli, Z. A. Stein, and M. W. Susser, "Obesity in Young Men after Famine Exposure in Utero and Early Infancy," *New England Journal of Medicine*, 295(7):349–353, August 12, 1976.
92   J. C. Knittle, "Basic Concepts in the Control of Childhood Obesity," in M. Winick (ed.), *Childhood Obesity*. New York: John Wiley and Sons, 1975.
93   Heald, op. cit.
94   C. C. Seltzer and J. Mayer, "A Simple Criterion of Obesity," *Postgraduate Medicine*, 38:A-105, 1965.
95   Heald, op. cit.
96   H. Bruch, *Eating Disorders*. New York: Basic Books, 1973.
97   R. B. Stuart and B. Davis, *Slim Chance in a Fat World*. Champaign, Ill.: Research Press Co., 1972.
98   A. J. Stunkard, "New Therapies for the Eating Disorders: Behavior Modification of Obesity and Anorexia Nervosa," *Archives of General Psychiatry*, 26:391–398, May 1972.
99   Ibid.
100 Stuart and Davis, op. cit.
101 L. S. Levitz, "Application of Behavioral Therapy to Obesity," *Journal of the American Dietetic Association*, 62:22–26, January 1973.
102 H. A. Jordan, "In Defense of Body Weight," *Journal of the American Dietetic Association*, 62:17–21, January 1973.
103 I. Gross, M. Wheeling, and K. Hess, "The Treatment of Obesity in Adolescents Using Behavioral Self-Control," *Clinical Pediatrics*, 15:920–924, October 1976.
104 National Academy of Sciences, *Maternal Nutrition and the Course of Pregnancy*, op. cit.
105 D. A. Roe, *Drug-Induced Nutritional Deficiencies*. Westport, Conn.: Avi Publishing Co., 1976.
106 Guthrie, op. cit.
107 Roe, op. cit.
108 Ibid.
109 Ibid.
110 C. Christiansen, P. Rodbro, and M. Lund, "Incidence of Anti-Convulsant Osteomalacia and Effect of Vitamin D: Controlled Therapeutic Trial," *British Medical Journal*, 4:695–701, December 22, 1973.
111 R. C. Theuer and J. J. Vitale, "Drug and Nutrient Interactions," in H. A. Schneider, C. A. Anderson, and D. B. Coursin (eds.), *Nutritional Support of Medical Practice*. New York: Harper and Row, 1977.
112 J. N. Hathcock, *Nutrition and Drug Interrelations*, Nutrition Foundation Monograph. New York: Academic Press, in preparation.
113 D. P. DePaola and M. C. Alfano, "Diet and Oral Health," *Nutrition Today*, 12:6, 1977.

114 A. D. Hofmann, R. D. Becker, and H. P. Gabriel, *The Hospitalized Adolescent: A Guide to Managing the Ill and Injured Youth*. New York: The Free Press, 1976.

115 A. S. Rice, "How Do You Know It's Relevant?" *Forecast for Home Economics*, **19**:F103, 1973.

116 S. Held, "How I Teach Nutrition: Nutrition Facts Can Bloom in Your Garden," *Forecast for Home Economics*, **20**:F26, 1975.

117 H. T. Spitze, "Innovation Techniques for Teaching Nutrition," *Journal of Nutrition Education*, **2**:156, 1971.

118 S. E. Weiss, "Generating Nutrition Awareness in Tenth Graders through a Discussion-Initiating Film," unpublished master's thesis, Virginia Polytechnic Institute and State University, Blacksburg, Virginia, 1977.

119 H. Fleck, *Introduction to Nutrition*. New York: Macmillan Publishing Co., 1976.

BIBLIOGRAPHY

Caghan, S. B.: "The Adolescent Process and the Problem of Nutrition," *American Journal of Nursing*, **75**(10):1728–1731, 1975.

Dickens, G. and W. H. Trethowan: "Cravings and Aversions during Pregnancy," *Journal of Psychosomatic Research*, **15**:259, 1971.

Food and Agricultural Organization: *Handbook on Human Nutritional Requirements*. Rome, Italy: FAO-WHO Nutritional Studies, No. 28, 1974.

Fregly, M. J. and M. S. Fregly: *Oral Contraceptives and High Blood Pressure*. Gainesville, Fla.: The Dolphin Press, 1974.

Garrow, J. S.: *Energy Balance and Obesity in Man*. New York: American Elsevier Publishing Co., 1974.

Getchell, E. and R. Howard: "Nutrition in Development," in G. Scipien et al., *Comprehensive Pediatric Nursing*, 2d ed. New York: McGraw-Hill Book Co., 1979.

Gifft, H. H., M. B. Washbon, and G. G. Harrison: *Nutrition, Behavior and Change*. Englewood Cliffs, N.J.: Prentice-Hall, Inc., 1972.

Huenemann, R. L., M. C. Hampton, A. R. Behuke, L. R. Schapiro, and B. W. Mitchell: *Teenage Nutrition and Physique*. Springfield, Ill.: Charles C Thomas, 1974.

Jelliffe, D. B.: *The Assessment of the Nutritional Status of the Community*. Geneva, Switzerland: World Health Organization, 1966.

Kretchmer, N.: "Lactose and Lactase," *Scientific American*, **227**:70, 1972.

National Center for Health Statistics: "Dietary Intake of Persons 1–74 Years of Age in the United States," *Advance Data*, No. 6, March 1977.

Nutrition Staff, Bureau of Community Health Services: *Preliminary Guide for Developing Nutrition Services in Health Care Programs*. Rockville, Md.: USDHEW, PHS, HSA, 1976.

"Will a Fat Baby Become a Fat Child?" *Nutrition Reviews*, **35**:138, 1977.

World Health Organization: *Energy and Protein Requirements*. Geneva, Switzerland: FAO-WHO Technical Report Series No. 522, 1973.

Chapter 6

Substance Use and Abuse

Dee Williams

The use and abuse of chemical substances is being recognized as a topic of concern by nurses in all areas of practice. The nurse who deals with adolescents, regardless of clinical setting, needs to be knowledgeable about drugs, their uses and abuses, and ways to assist young people in developing informed and responsible behavior in regard to them. This chapter describes drug use patterns and undertakes to present a comprehensive compilation of the information nurses and adolescents need to know about psychoactive drugs and the outcomes of using them. Prevention and treatment of abuse are introduced here, and treatment is dealt with in greater depth in Chapter 17.

DEFINITIONS

A lack of uniform definitions creates difficulty in discussing substance use and abuse. For the purposes of this chapter, a *drug* will be defined as any chemical substance other than food that significantly alters the bodily functions or structures of an organism. *Psychoactive drugs* are those that result in changes in perception, feelings, mood, or behavior. The central nervous system is their principal site of action. The psychoactive drugs are the ones most commonly abused. *Drug use* refers to the voluntary taking of a drug and is not evaluative with regard to legality, social acceptance, or medicinal value. *Drug misuse* describes the "periodic or occasional improper or inappropriate use" of a chemical substance.[1]

The word *addiction* is perhaps one of the most emotionally charged terms associated with drug use. Its connotations include illegal and criminal activities as well as morally objectionable behavior. In 1950 and 1957, the World Health Organization Expert Committee on Addiction-Producing Drugs defined and redefined the terms *addiction* and *habituation*. Neither term proved adequate to describe the varied types and patterns of drug use and abuse observable even in 1957. In 1964, the WHO Expert Committee thus coined a new term, *drug dependence*, to be used instead of addiction and habituation. The new label was introduced not because it seemed to fit the observed patterns of abuse, but as an attempt to escape the connotations and confusion associated with the two previous terms. Drug dependence was defined generally as "a state arising from repeated administration of a drug on a periodic or continuous basis. . . . Its characteristics will vary with the agent involved and this must be made clear by designating the particular type of drug dependence in each specific case—for example, drug dependence of the morphine type, of cocaine type, of cannabis type, of barbiturate type, etc."[2]

Though the new term, dependence, did avoid some of the pitfalls of its predecessors, it did not seem to indicate what was felt to be the seriousness of the drug problem at the time. The term *drug abuse* began appearing spontaneously in the 1960s. It often went undefined, yet seemed more popular than previous terms. Depending on the "authority" quoted, the criteria necessary for establishing drug abuse may include legal, social, moral, or medical issues. For the purposes of this chapter, *drug abuse* will refer to the use of any drug to the extent that it interferes with an individual's social, economic, or physical functioning.

Two other terms, *psychological dependence* and *physical dependence*, are frequently used in discussing psychoactive drugs. Psychological dependence refers to a strong psychological drive to continue the use of a chemical. Though anxiety may result if the drug is discontinued, there is no associated physical symptomatology. Physical dependence is confirmed when the user experiences a set of symptoms, a withdrawal syndrome, if the drug is abruptly discontinued.

Substance use and *substance abuse* have recently achieved popularity. Although all substances of abuse are by definition drugs, the term *drug abuse* as often used has come to be restricted to references to the illegal and socially unacceptable psychoactive drugs. *Substance use* and *substance abuse* have been adopted as broader terms which do not exclude

legal and accepted chemicals such as alcohol and drugs obtained by prescription. However, in this chapter *substance use* and *abuse* are inter-
changeable with *drug use* and *abuse*.

INCIDENCE OF DRUG USE AND ABUSE

There is no doubt that ours is a drug-taking society. In 1970, a total of
$32,589,000,000 was spent by American consumers on alcohol, tobacco,
and prescription and over-the-counter drugs.[3] Caffeine, nicotine, and alcohol are definitely the most commonly used psychoactive drugs in the
United States. The physical harm incurred as a result of their use vastly
exceeds that which results from the use of all other psychoactive drugs
combined.[4]

   In 1970, the National Institute of Mental Health began its "Psychotropic Drug Study." The part of the study aimed at determining the extent
of drug use in the adult population was conducted by Drs. Hugh J. Parry
and Ira H. Cisin. Results of the study indicated that some 82 percent of
the 2,552 respondents drank coffee and 52 percent drank tea during the
previous year. Twenty-five percent drank six or more cups of either or
both daily. With regard to nicotine, 43 percent of the male and 34 percent
of the female respondents were current smokers. Though the percentage
of smokers is less than that of coffee and tea drinkers, the total doses of
nicotine consumed each year far exceed the doses of caffeine. The Parry-
Cisin study further documented that only 22 percent of the male and 37
percent of the female respondents had consumed no alcoholic beverages
in the previous year, with some 34 percent of the males and 14 percent
of the females falling into the heavy or very heavy drinker categories.
Psychoactive prescription drugs were used by 13 percent of the males and
29 percent of the females in the previous year. A substantial proportion
of those persons reported only occasional use. The most frequently used
psychoactive prescription drugs were the sedatives and antianxiety
agents.[5]

   A large market also exists for illegally obtained drugs. There are
generally two ways in which these substances become available. One is
the so-called gray market. A person for whom a drug is prescribed passes
it on to a friend or acquaintance either free or at a cost. The second way
to obtain drugs illegally is "on the street," through the black market.
Drugs for sale on the black market come from two sources. Prescription
items illegally diverted for sale on the street (e.g., barbiturates, diet pills,
synthetic narcotics) constitute one source. The second source is the group
of substances whose possession and sale are illegal under any circumstances (e.g., heroin, LSD, cocaine). The latter group also includes "bootleg" drugs manufactured by illicit chemists and sold as a variety of

substances, including imitations of prescription compounds. Bootleg drugs may or may not contain the active ingredients they promise.

Figures regarding the frequency of illegally obtained drugs are estimates at best. In the early 1970s, the New York State Narcotic Addiction Commission conducted a survey regarding the use of psychoactive drugs. Regular users (at least six times a month) ranged from 0.1 percent for controlled narcotics to 4.0 percent for antianxiety agents. Needless to say, drugs such as marijuana, LSD, heroin, and cocaine were obtained illegally. More surprising, however, is the fact that from 50 to 95 percent of the persons using drugs available on prescription (barbiturates, tranquilizers, amphetamines, sedative-hypnotics) also obtained them illegally.[6]

The incidence of substance use and abuse among adolescents varies. An extensive survey of adolescent drug usage was conducted in San Mateo County, California, grades 7 through 12, over the 4-year span between 1968 and 1971. The results, when combined with similar information from Massachusetts, Maryland, Utah, Idaho, and New York, led to several useful generalizations. Compulsive drug use, or abuse, by adolescents occurs in a small percentage of cases. Periodic use is somewhat higher, but experimental use accounts, by far, for most adolescent drug use. Approximately 60 to 80 percent have tried alcohol, 40 to 60 percent tobacco, 5 to 30 percent marijuana, 1 to 25 percent LSD, 5 to 20 percent amphetamines, 3 to 15 percent barbiturates, and 0.5 to 3 percent heroin. Only 20 percent of the San Mateo County high school students reported no drug use whatsoever. Three percent used only tobacco and 13 percent only alcohol and tobacco. The percentages of total abstainers were greatest in the lower grades, gradually decreasing by the twelfth grade to 16 percent. Moderate alcohol use seems to be a norm, particularly among adolescent males. Use in excess of ten times the previous year was reported by approximately 13 percent of the seventh graders and by approximately 40 percent of the twelfth graders. Experimental use increased from 46 percent in the seventh grade to 78 percent in the twelfth grade. Adolescent males tended to use drugs more frequently than females, and usage patterns tended to vary with social, racial, economic, religious, and ethnic factors.[7]

Most persons reporting the use of psychoactive drugs have tried more than one substance. Many experimental users take whatever is available in their setting. More experienced users may have a drug of choice, that is, one they would prefer if several were available. Substance abusers may substitute a second drug for the preferred one if supplies are low. Others have abuse patterns that involve alternating drugs.

If the use of psychoactive drugs is common to both adolescents and adults, and if few young people engage in substance abuse, then why is there a preoccupation with the youth drug scene? Some adults are now concerned with adolescent drug use because the availability of substances with abuse potential appears to be greater than ever before. Almost any adolescent can obtain practically any drug he or she wants. Adolescents also tend to use different drugs than adults do, and that creates concern because adults lack personal experience with those substances and are inclined to be uneasy about the unknown. Many adults have accepted misinformation and developed misconceptions regarding those drugs and have reacted to hearsay about their side effects and dependency potential.

A third factor that creates anxiety is that a larger proportion of young people than adults obtain their drugs illegally. The strictly illegal substances such as marijuana, LSD, heroin, and cocaine are of course available only through the black market, and a greater percentage of young people than adults have at least tried those drugs. In addition, adolescents are likely to obtain even the legalized psychoactive prescription drugs illegally. One study conducted in 1967–1968 in San Francisco revealed that of those people under 30 years old who reported use of psychoactive prescription drugs, 51 percent had acquired them illegally.[8] Thus, young people tend to operate outside the law while their parents get prescriptions from physicians. Certain ironies of the law, furthermore, have created resentment and rebellion among youth: (1) some drugs (e.g., liquor and tobacco) are legal for adults but illegal for adolescents, and (2) those substances that are illegal have not always been so, but have been illegalized by adult legislators.

Etiology of Adolescent Drug Use

Why, then, in the face of adult disapproval as well as legal risks, do adolescents use drugs? For most young people, substance use is part of the attempt to facilitate completion of adolescent developmental tasks. The establishment of oneself as an individual separate from one's parents, the clarification of a value system, and the establishment of intimate interpersonal relationships outside the family are tasks that, for successful resolution, bring current-day adolescents into encounter with drugs in some form.

Some young people use drugs as a temporary relief from the internal or external pressures they feel. Some use drugs as a way of establishing themselves in a certain group. Some are merely curious and experiment with various drugs as a way of satisfying that curiosity. Drugs may be used to relieve boredom or for pure physical pleasure. The use of illegal chemicals may represent a rejection of adult values.

At what point, then, does substance use become substance abuse? Simply put, when the use of chemicals begins to interfere with the adolescent's forward movement and development, there is cause for concern. Though most young people use drugs as but one part of the maturational

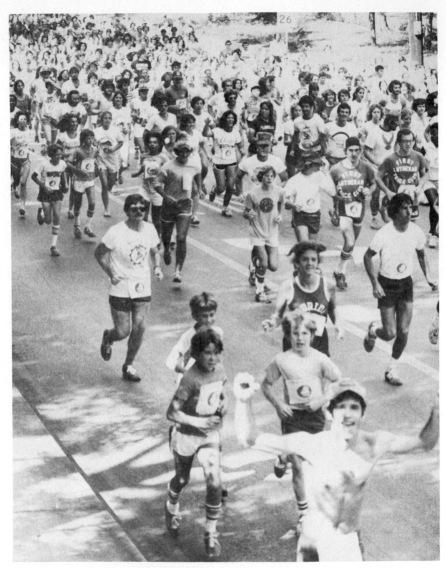

Almost all adolescents (indeed, almost all people) have used psychoactive drugs at some time. The commonly used ones, and those responsible for more physical harm than results from use of *all* other psychoactive drugs, are alcohol, nicotine, and caffeine. Actual abuse of these or other drugs involves a very small percentage of adolescents. (*Copyright © 1980 by Anne Campbell*.)

process, a small number come to depend on chemicals. Abuse exists when (1) a young person`s overriding concern involves the acquisition and use of drugs, or (2) drug use causes family and other interpersonal relationships to become unimportant and decisions regarding occupation or school to be postponed. Certainly if the adolescent becomes involved with the law or shows any signs of physical dependence or deterioration due to drug use, then the situation has gotten out of hand and warrants immediate attention.

No one set of psychological or sociocultural circumstances exists as a predictor of substance abuse, but there may be some identifiable factors which make one adolescent more susceptible than another to drug dependence. These same factors, however, can exist in adolescents who do not become drug abusers.[9] Family systems that block communication or in which much tension exists may contribute to substance abuse. Parents who themselves are drug abusers may foster the same in their children. This is most readily seen in the case of alcohol.[10] Young people who are unable to form close interpersonal relationships or who are particularly intolerant of frustration may abuse chemicals as a way of avoiding tension. Psychologically disturbed adolescents may use drugs as an attempt to exert some control over reality, or as self-medication for the relief of anxiety.[11] Social factors such as extreme poverty may also contribute to drug abuse. Feelings of hopelessness and entrapment associated with inner-city ghetto life are temporarily forgotten, especially when drugs are readily available and subculturally accepted.[12]

THE DRUGS

The Drug Experience

The experience an individual has when using a particular drug is dependent on a number of factors. These include the drug itself, the dosage, route of administration, the user's expectations, previous drug experience, and the environment in which the drug is used.

The intensity of a specific drug experience is determined largely by the dose administered. Usually, an increase in the dose results in an increase in the effects. The relationship between the dosage used and the reactions produced is represented in a dose-response curve, the lower end being the threshold dose, or smallest amount needed to measure a response. *Effective dose* refers to the amount of drug necessary to produce a desired effect. *Lethal dose* refers to the amount of drug which results in death. Average effective doses are compared with the lowest known lethal dose to determine the safety margin of a particular drug. *Potency* refers to the amount of drug needed to produce a specific effect. The smaller the dose required, the more potent the drug. Potency is not directly related to effective dose or to the lethal dose.

The rate of onset of the effects of psychoactive drugs, and to some extent the intensity of those effects, is partially determined by the route of administration. The most commonly used methods of administering drugs are inhalation, ingestion, and injection (subcutaneous, intramuscular, and intravenous).

Inhalation and ingestion are the oldest routes of administration. Inhalation is second only to intravenous injection for rapidity of onset of effects. Inhalation is used for drugs which exist as true gases or for those which vaporize or produce smoke or fumes when heated. Within seconds the drug is exposed to the alveolar surface of the lungs where it has immediate access to the bloodstream.

When swallowed, a drug is usually absorbed in the upper portion of the small intestine. The rate at which this occurs depends on how rapidly the drug moves through the stomach. In general, a drug is made available to the small intestine more rapidly if ingested on an empty stomach. Liquids are more readily absorbed than drugs in solid form. Oral ingestion provides the slowest rate of onset of effects.

Another route of administration involves placement of a solution or crystalline drug compound in direct contact with the nasal mucosa. The drug is not inhaled but is absorbed directly into the blood vessels in the nostrils. Comparably, the sublingual route of administration involves placement of a solid drug under the tongue, allowing it to dissolve and be absorbed by the blood vessels in the mouth. Both of these methods provide more rapid access to the bloodstream than does ingestion.

Of the three forms of injection, the intravenous route produces the fastest results. Intramuscular injections are next and the subcutaneous route is third. Within seconds of an intravenous injection maximal effects are felt. It takes approximately 20 to 30 minutes for the effects of an intramuscular or subcutaneous injection to reach a peak.[13]

Serious side effects may develop as a result of certain drugs and their route of administration. For instance, excessive nasal inhalation of cocaine may result in perforations of the nasal septum. Alcohol, a gastric irritant, can cause ulcerations of the stomach wall. Physical damage associated with injection is related to the drugs used and also to the life-style of the user. Many preparations sold on the street contain substances that are irritants to the skin or blood vessel walls. When injected, these can result in scarring and abscesses. In addition, needles and syringes passed from person to person with little regard for sanitation leave all involved susceptible to serum hepatitis, endocarditis, tetanus, cellulitis, thrombophlebitis, and embolic pneumonia.[14]

The metabolism of a drug begins as soon as it enters the body. Metabolism occurs at a slower rate than absorption until maximum effects are reached. Different drugs have different metabolic rates and there is little that can be done to accelerate or retard that process.

Certain drugs, such as aspirin, reach their maximum effectiveness at a specific dosage level. If more of the drug is taken the only likely outcome is an increase in side effects. Other drugs, such as alcohol, do show an increase in the effects as the dose is increased. Some drugs when taken together, for example alcohol and barbiturates, have additive effects. They produce changes which are greater than those expected from either drug.

Tolerance is another concept related to time and metabolism. For some drugs, repeated use of the same dose produces a decrease in the desired effect, so that an increase in dose is necessary to produce the same effect. With some drugs, e.g., LSD, tolerance can develop quickly. Other drugs require regular use over longer periods of time before tolerance develops, and for some substances there appears to be no decrease in effects regardless of frequency of use or dose.[15]

The individual drug user's expectations and previous drug experience definitely play a role in the way a drug experience is perceived. The first time some drugs are used the experience may not be a particularly pleasant one. Part of the subjective reaction depends on the user's knowledge of the drug and how realistic his or her expectations are. Often this knowledge is supplied by more experienced users. Individuals therefore learn what effects to look for and which ones to tolerate or ignore.[16]

One phenomenon that warrants mention here is the placebo effect. A placebo is an inert substance thought to be a drug. One may experience certain effects based on what one thinks one is taking rather than on what the substance actually is. This occurs more frequently with inexperienced users, particularly adolescents, who are tricked into buying and taking inert substances. Also, some individuals report a response disproportionate to the amount of drug taken. This is most easily seen in the use of alcohol. A person who desires to be intoxicated may feel so after only one or two drinks.[17]

Environment is also influential in some drug experiences. In stressful situations certain drugs may produce unpleasant effects. There are other substances, however, whose use seems totally independent of the environment. Once under the influence of the drug, the user either discounts or ignores the environment. It is almost impossible to predict an individual's response to the environment, changes in perceptions, or subjective evaluation of a particular drug experience.[18]

Classification of Substances

Psychoactive drugs may be classified in several different ways. The system used in this chapter is based on the pharmacological properties, with one exception. The first drugs discussed, the "nondrugs," are placed together because they are viewed similarly by society, not because they are pharmacologically similar. The rest of the psychoactive drugs are grouped according to pharmacological criteria, which include the type of effect produced, therapeutic uses, and mechanism of action. Tolerance to one drug in a particular category usually implies some degree of tolerance to others in the same group. Likewise, physical dependence on the effects of one drug usually means the same for others in that category. Cross-tolerance and cross-dependence have important implications for substance abuse and treatment.

The Nondrugs   Caffeine, nicotine, and over-the-counter preparations are not generally thought of as drugs by our society. Their use is socially acceptable, at least for adults.

Caffeine   Caffeine is one of the xanthines, the oldest known stimulants. It is commonly associated with coffee, but is available as the main ingredient in certain over-the-counter preparations and is found in cola drinks. The xanthines also include theobromine and theophylline, which are found, along with caffeine, in chocolate and tea, respectively. Caffeine is the most potent and theobromine the least potent with regard to central nervous system effects. Theophylline has the most potent effect on the cardiovascular system.[19]

The xanthines have as their main action, via stimulation of the cerebral cortex, the alleviation of fatigue and drowsiness and an increase in rapidity and clarity of thought processes. Motor activity correspondingly increases but coordination and timing may be impaired. The xanthines affect heart rate, blood vessel diameter, blood pressure, heart rhythm, urination, circulation, and gastric secretion. These effects are observed after the ingestion of one or two cups of coffee or tea.[20] Absorption of caffeine occurs rapidly after oral ingestion, with peak blood levels reached in 30 to 60 minutes. Maximal central nervous system effects occur about 2 hours after intake.[21]

Psychological dependence, evidenced in statements such as "I can't do a thing before I've had my two cups of morning coffee," is possible. Physical dependence can occur in persons who drink five or more cups of coffee a day. The most clearly documented symptom, headache, develops after about 18 hours of abstinence.[22] Some persons also report nausea and lethargy. Tolerance develops to certain effects of caffeine, most notably to increases in urinary output and salivation, but is less noticeable regarding central nervous system stimulation. The xanthines are cross-tolerant as a group.

Certain toxic effects manifest themselves after the ingestion of one gram of caffeine (7 to 10 cups of coffee). Insomnia, excitement, and restlessness are the initial symptoms. Chronic overindulgence results in sleep disturbances, restlessness, anxiety, and cardiac irregularities. The estimated fatal dose taken orally is ten grams (70 to 100 cups of coffee). One known human death followed the intravenous injection of 3.2 g of caffeine.[23,24]

Nicotine   Nicotine is commonly associated with tobacco. It is consumed by inhalation (e.g., cigarette smoke), exposure to the oral mucosa (e.g., snuff, chewing tobacco), or some combination of the two (e.g., cigar smoking). Tolerance does develop to its effects, as do physical and psychological dependence. A variety of symptoms are reported by those who abruptly discontinue the use of nicotine. These include nervousness, drowsiness, anxiety, lightheadedness, headache, fatigue, gastrointestinal disturbances, insomnia, dizziness, sweating, cramps, tremors, and palpitations. Nicotine is extremely toxic. A cigar contains two lethal ingestion doses, about 120 mg. Luckily, when tobacco is smoked, not enough of the drug is absorbed quickly enough to cause death. At low doses, nicotine causes an increase in respiratory rate and coronary blood flow, vasoconstriction in the skin, and increased heart rate and blood pressure.[25]

Though some have begun to view smoking as a physical and psychological dependence on nicotine, most continue to discount the role of nicotine itself, admitting only that the process of smoking is hazardous to health. Since the publication of the 1964 *Report of the Surgeon General's Advisory Committee on Smoking and Health*, smoking has been directly linked to heart disease, emphysema, bronchitis, and various forms of cancer, most notably lung cancer. Adolescents, though convinced that cigarette smoking is dangerous, are not generally aware of the dependency-producing properties of nicotine. Most adolescent smokers believe that they will smoke for several years and then quit. They do not acknowledge the fact that they may be unable to stop. In the 1970 Lieberman Report, conducted for the National Clearinghouse for Smoking and Health, young people said they began smoking because their elders and peers did. A definite increase in the proportion of adolescent smokers was noted despite active antismoking educational campaigns.

Over-the-Counter Drugs   Over-the-counter drugs include a host of preparations, some of which contain psychoactive substances. They are approved by the Food and Drug Administration for use by the general public when taken as directed. Their proper use depends upon competent self-diagnosis and treatment of common, minor ailments. For this reason, the FDA is concerned with adequate labeling and information delivery on over-the-counter drugs. One result of governmental controls is that false claims and comparisons have decreased. There is growing concern, however, that advertisements now imply instant solutions to life's problems rather than alleviation of particular symptoms and encourage people to expect that chemicals will provide easy answers to everyday frustrations. Nevertheless, over-the-counter drugs are more likely to be misused than abused.[26]

Depressants   Generalized central nervous system depressants can be subdivided into (1) sedative-hypnotics, and (2) volatile solvents and aero-

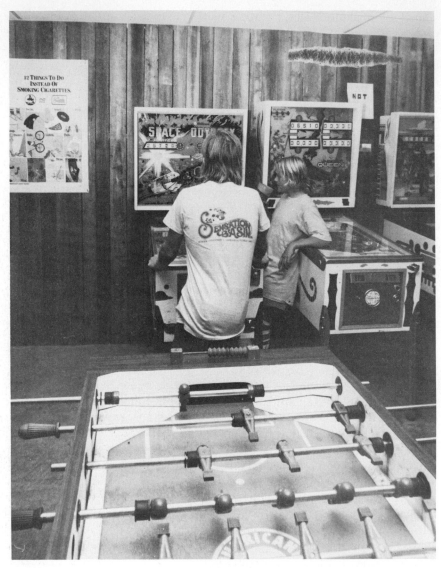

Businesses, schools, and recreational establishments that cater to young people can do far more than they traditionally do to try to discourage drug use and promote health in other ways. This recreation hall forbids smoking and displays the American Cancer Society poster, "12 Things To Do Instead Of Smoking Cigarettes." (*Copyright © 1980 by Anne Campbell*.)

sols. Depressants, which at small therapeutic doses produce a calming effect, or sedation, and at higher doses induce sleep, or hypnotic effects, include alcohol, barbiturates, and similar drugs. These drugs are more widely abused and are implicated in more drug-related deaths than any others in Western society. The volatile solvents and aerosols will be discussed separately.

Alcohol The process of fermentation, which forms the basis for all alcoholic beverages, has long been recognized. There are, chemically speaking, several different kinds of alcohol. Ethyl alcohol, or ethanol, is the form found in alcoholic beverages. Alcohol is taken almost exclusively by ingestion. It is unique in that it can be absorbed through the stomach lining as well as in the small intestine. Once in the bloodstream, alcohol goes almost immediately to the liver, where it is acted upon by the enzyme alcohol dehydrogenase. This enzyme is the primary factor which determines the rate of alcohol metabolism. Most moderate drinkers can metabolize a maximum of 0.25 to 0.33 oz of pure alcohol an hour. Heavy drinkers may metabolize alcohol more rapidly if no liver damage or metabolic disorders exist. If intake occurs more quickly than metabolism, the blood alcohol concentration rises.[27]

Alcohol dehydrogenase oxidizes the alcohol to form acetaldehyde, which is metabolized to form acetic acid and, ultimately, carbon dioxide, oxygen, and energy. An ounce of pure alcohol provides about 200 cal. It has no nutritional value. Very little alcohol is excreted unchanged by the body, perhaps only 2 percent in most situations.[28]

Alcohol is a central nervous system depressant. Though it may appear behaviorally to stimulate, alcohol actually depresses the inhibitions. For some persons this results in an increase in activity. If ingestion continues, more basic behaviors are depressed, ultimately resulting in decreased motor function, loss of consciousness, or even death. The behavior which emerges when inhibitions are depressed varies with the psychological makeup of the individual. Also, the more rapidly the blood alcohol concentration rises, the more drastic the behavioral changes.[29, 30]

An excessive intake of alcohol usually results in a hangover. These symptoms may constitute a mild withdrawal syndrome. The thirst probably results from the movement of intracellular fluid to extracellular spaces. Alcohol decreases the output of an antidiuretic hormone and causes the body to excrete more fluid than is ingested. The nausea and stomach upset are the results of the gastric irritant properties of alcohol. Headaches may be a reaction to the *congeners* in the beverage. (Congeners are natural products of fermentation and processing; some are quite toxic.) A hangover may also be the result of fatigue for those who exert themselves physically when drinking.[31]

Adolescent alcohol abusers do not demonstrate the long-term sequelae of chronic alcoholism, for the obvious reason that those effects take a number of years to appear. Youths *are* subject to the nausea and anorexia that result from alcohol's gastric irritant qualities, and to hepatic changes. When alcohol ingestion interferes with dietary intake, nutrition suffers.

When alcohol intake is abruptly discontinued in physically dependent drinkers, the withdrawal syndrome begins. The initial symptoms of anxiety and tremors develop within 3 to 36 hours of abstinence. Hallucinations may occur over the next day or two. Insomnia, nausea, vomiting, and feelings of unreality are common. Unless treatment is instituted, delirium tremens (''DT's'') or convulsions may develop. Some persons with delirium tremens die as a result of hyperthermia, peripheral vascular collapse, or self-inflicted injuries. The central nervous system symptoms seen in withdrawal are probably the result of the body's ability to compensate for the depressant effects of high levels of alcohol: Though the drug is discontinued the nervous system continues its increased activity until it has a chance to readjust. The severity of the withdrawal syndrome depends on the degree of physical dependence but is more severe and life-threatening than withdrawal from the narcotics.[32, 33] Chapter 17 discusses detoxification care and rehabilitation.

Barbiturates   Barbiturates are medically prescribed for anxiety, insomnia, and epilepsy and are used in anesthesia. They are classified according to their duration of action. The longer-acting barbiturates, e.g., phenobarbital, are infrequently abused. The shorter-acting ones, such as pentobarbital, secobarbital, and amobarbital, are those preferred by drug users.

Most barbiturates, including those used illegally, are taken by mouth. Some abusers inject their doses subcutaneously and a smaller number use them intravenously. When the drugs are taken orally, absorption is in part dependent on stomach contents. The longer-acting barbiturates are absorbed more slowly than the shorter-acting ones. The barbiturates are distributed to various parts of the body, including the brain, and are ultimately circulated to the liver, where they are deactivated. Barbiturates are metabolized almost completely, very little being excreted unchanged in the urine. The short-acting barbiturates are deactivated at the rate of about 2.5 percent per hour and the longer-acting types at about 0.7 percent per hour.[34]

For use as sleeping aids, barbiturates are not without drawbacks. One side effect is the ''barbiturate hangover,'' the residual sedation that exists the next morning. Some people begin to use an amphetamine or other stimulant to counteract this, the result being a cycle of drug use. With barbiturate-induced sleep, dreaming time is reduced.[35] Research indicates that dreamless sleep is not as restful. When barbiturates are used over an extended period of time, symptoms of sleep deprivation may result.

Barbiturate abuse may develop gradually, with the individual increasing the dose over time. Misused barbiturates are often taken in the same way as alcohol and many of the same effects are noted. The individual appears intoxicated, the effects lasting about 4 to 5 hours. Barbiturates may be abused in combination with alcohol or heroin. They are the single most frequently used drug for suicide, accounting for one-fifth of all completed suicides in the United States.[36] Death results from respiratory depression in cases of overdose.

The barbiturates generally depress the central nervous system, resulting in a decrease of inhibitions. Physical dependence and tolerance develop with repeated, continuous use of high doses. Repeated use of barbiturates seems to result in an increase in the production of the hepatic enzymes necessary for their deactivation. Certain tissues also apparently develop a resistance to the effects of the drug. Tolerance to the lethal dose, however, does not seem to increase significantly with physical dependence.[37]

The withdrawal syndrome is similar to that associated with alcohol dependency. The severity of withdrawal symptoms is proportional to the amount of drug regularly taken and the length of time since the last dose. Anxiety, insomnia, weakness, anorexia, nausea, vomiting, tremors, and muscle twitching appear after about 8 to 24 hours of abstinence. Unless the adolescent is treated, convulsions may occur on the second or third day. An acute psychosis similar to delirium tremens then develops; death can result. The peak intensity of withdrawal symptoms occurs about 30 to 40 hours after onset. Chapter 17 includes information about management of barbiturate withdrawal.

Barbiturate abusers face many of the same difficulties as do alcohol-dependent persons. Employment becomes impossible, the incidence of traumatic injuries increases and personal care declines. Unlike most alcohol abusers, however, barbiturate abusers may maintain an adequate diet. Psychoses seen in barbiturate abusers are probably the result of preexisting psychological impairments.[38]

Other Sedatives and Hypnotics Included in this category are the nonbarbiturate drugs used for sedation and sleep. Three of these, chloral hydrate, paraldehyde, and the bromides, were in use prior to the barbiturates. Paraldehyde and chloral hydrate behave much like alcohol. They have both been used as anesthetics, but the former has a very disagreeable taste and odor and the latter produces considerable gastric upset. The bromides, when used in hypnotic doses over several days, tend to accumulate and produce a toxic state, bromism. The symptoms of bromism include dermatitis and constipation initially, but can progress to motor disturbance, delirium, and psychosis if use continues. These three drugs are rarely used today.[39]

In 1941, the barbiturates came under attack, yet the demand for sedatives and hypnotics continued. Glutethimide (Doriden), ethinamate

(Valmid), ethchlorvynol (Placidyl), methaqualone (Quaalude), and methyprylon (Noludar) were developed and advertised as safe substitutes for the barbiturates. Though not chemically similar, these drugs are pharmacologically equivalent to the barbiturates and alcohol, producing the same sort of intoxication, physical dependence, and resultant withdrawal syndrome.[40]

Inhalants, Volatile Solvents, and Aerosols   This section includes those substances that are inhaled, glue being the most publicized example. The first inhalant widely used for intoxication without the unpleasant side effects of alcohol was nitrous oxide ("laughing gas"). Effects begin within 30 seconds of inhalation and reach a peak within 2 or 3 minutes. There appears to be no tendency to increase the dose. Nitrous oxide was discovered in 1776 and was first used as a general anesthetic in 1844. It is still used at times during dental work and childbirth. In combination with other, longer-lasting anesthetics it may be used in surgery. Ether is another inhalant with a long history. Introduced in liquid form in the early 1700s, ether was used as an analgesic and later as a recreational drug. Ether vaporizes easily and was used as an inhalant beginning in the nineteenth century. Chloroform is the third of the older inhalants. Discovered in 1831 and used immediately for its intoxicating effects, chloroform was also used as a general anesthetic. It soon fell into disfavor because of the hazard of overdose. Nitrous oxide, ether, and chloroform are still used recreationally on occasion. Use occurs most frequently among persons with ready access to them, notably anesthetists, anesthesiologists, and others in the health professions.[41]

The more commonly used inhalants today are products with no known medical uses. These include gasoline, cleaning solvents, lighter fluid, paint and lacquer thinners, aerosol sprays, and, of course, glues. Twenty-three solvents are known to have been used as inhalants, but substances containing toluene seem to be preferred. Toluene has few irritant effects, vaporizes rapidly, and produces pleasurable psychoactive sensations.[42]

There were no reports of the use of solvents or aerosols until a nationwide scare campaign in 1960; then the use of glue in particular soared. Corporations that produced glues began to work on safeguards against their abuse. Several states enacted laws to control solvent inhalation. Meanwhile, young people discovered that aerosol inhalation also produced intoxication. Most reports of solvent and aerosol inhalation involve boys between the ages of 10 and 15 years in what seems to be an activity usually abandoned by midadolescence.[43,44]

Semiliquid solvents, such as glues and cements, are usually squeezed into a paper or plastic bag, which is then held tightly over the mouth and/or nose. The vapors are inhaled until the desired effects are attained. Liquid solutions are inhaled directly from their containers or are placed on cloth or gauze. The cloth is placed in a bag or held directly over the mouth or nose. Most aerosol users attempt to separate the propellant from the solid contents of the can. Volatile solvents may be warmed before inhalation as this increases concentration of the substance.[45]

The inhalants are general central nervous system depressants though each produces other effects as well. These range from feelings of dizziness to delusions of strength to hallucinations. Users experience impaired judgment, feelings of drunkenness, euphoria, giddiness, ataxia, and slurred speech. Some youths inhale the solvent until they lose consciousness. The effects last about 15 to 45 minutes, followed by 1 or 2 hours of drowsiness. Total or partial amnesia may exist for the period of intoxication. Unpleasant side effects such as irritation of the eyes, tinnitus, sneezing, photophobia, diplopia, nausea, coughing, diarrhea, vomiting, and chest, muscle, and joint pain may be experienced during the period of intoxication and for some time afterwards.[46]

There is little evidence of physical dependence with solvent or aerosol inhalation. Tolerance does develop to the central nervous system effects after prolonged and frequent use. Persons who are psychologically dependent may spend most of their waking time intoxicated. Except for trichloroethylene, trichloroethane, and fluorinated hydrocarbons used in some aerosols, the inhalants and solvents seem to carry little risk of producing permanent organ damage. Death, however, has occurred during or after use of the inhalants. The user may lose consciousness with the bag still tightly sealed around the mouth and nose and become asphyxiated. Cardiac arrest is associated with the use of the halogenated hydrocarbons found in some aerosol propellants and cleaning solvents. The third cause of death associated with the inhalants remains something of a mystery. Persons who use trichloroethane or fluorohydrocarbons immediately following physical activity or stress have been known to appear suddenly startled or frightened, look panicky, and run away a short distance before collapsing and dying.[47]

Antianxiety Agents   The antianxiety agents, also known as minor tranquilizers, were synthesized and marketed in the 1950s to compete with barbiturate sales. The first one introduced was meprobamate (Miltown, Equanil). Others include chlordiazepoxide (Librium) and diazepam (Valium). A dose of the antianxiety agents sufficient to reduce anxiety does not seem to produce the degree of drowsiness that barbiturates do. The antianxiety agents are also less likely to result in death following an overdose. Other differences between the two are insignificant. The antianxiety agents are just as likely to cause physical dependence resulting in a severe withdrawal syndrome; tolerance develops with frequent use.[48]

The drugs are usually taken by mouth. Most users, typically female adults, are introduced to them by doctors. More prescriptions are written each year for these drugs than for all other psychoactive drugs combined. Not generally associated with the youth drug scene, they are more likely to be misused than abused. The use of antianxiety agents is considered socially acceptable and receives little attention.[49]

Stimulants   Drugs used to improve mental and physical performance when one is fatigued are usually central nervous system stimulants. The most widely used group, the xanthines, was discussed earlier. Cocaine, a naturally occurring stimulant, is in a category of its own. The amphetamines constitute the third group and are the second most frequently used stimulants.

Cocaine   Cocaine, used in Peru since about 500 A.D., is naturally formed in the coca plant. The active ingredient in coca leaves was isolated in 1844. In 1883, a German doctor gave cocaine to Bavarian soldiers on maneuvers and reported increases in their ability to perform when fatigued. Sigmund Freud was one of many to read of this account. He proceeded to treat himself, his family, and many of his friends with cocaine for fatigue and depression. He strongly believed that cocaine was not addictive and that it could, in fact, be used to aid in the withdrawal from narcotics. Freud encouraged his medical colleagues to prescribe cocaine for morphine withdrawal and for neurasthenia. He is probably the one man most responsible for the popularization of cocaine in Europe.[50]

In the 1870s an American surgeon demonstrated that cocaine, when injected near a nerve, produced local anesthesia. It was used for that purpose until more reliable drugs became available. In 1885, however, accusations concerning the addictive properties of cocaine began.

Freud discontinued both personal and professional use of the drug in 1887 when a close friend experienced a cocaine psychosis. Nevertheless, the use of cocaine in nerve tonics, patent medicines, other home remedies, and Coca-Cola continued until 1914. Though it does not fit the pharmacological definition of a narcotic, cocaine is legally described and controlled as such.[51]

If it were not so expensive and inconsistently available, cocaine would probably be used more frequently. Many have described it as the "king of drugs." It is generally inhaled through the nose but may be injected. Cocaine is not taken orally because it is inactivated by gastric secretions.[52]

Cocaine increases motor activity and heart rate at moderate doses. At high doses, convulsions can occur and the heart may stop. Respiratory rate is increased only at high doses. Cocaine is inactivated quickly, so inhalations or injections every 15 to 20 minutes are required to maintain its euphoric effect.[53]

Cocaine is sometimes used with other drugs, such as heroin. Those who abuse the drug may develop a psychotic state consisting of hallucinations, paranoid delusions, and impulsive, violent behavior which usually clears within a few days of abstinence. Some abusers risk the dangers associated with injection; others, who inhale instead, may develop perforations of the nasal septum.[54]

The question of physical dependence on cocaine is unsettled. There is no dramatic withdrawal syndrome, but a user may experience fatigue and an increase in appetite following abstinence. A period of depression may also occur, encouraging repeated drug use. Some maintain that tolerance develops to the euphoric effects; others deny that this is so.[55]

Amphetamines   Synthesized in the 1920s, the amphetamines are recent additions to the drug world. By the 1930s, the major effects were documented. Several products containing amphetamines appeared as over-the-counter drugs, e.g., inhalers for bronchial congestion and pills for fatigue. Amphetamines were used extensively in World War II to increase soldiers' performance and factory workers' production. After the war, tons of surplus pills were marketed as over-the-counter antidotes for drowsiness and depression. In 1948, certain restrictions were imposed, yet the use of amphetamines continued to rise.[56] Currently approved medical uses are restricted to the treatment of narcolepsy and, paradoxically, hyperkinetic behavior in children.

Prior to the 1960s almost all amphetamines, though perhaps illegally obtained, were legally manufactured and taken orally. In the 1960s, injections and the manufacture of bootleg amphetamines gained popularity. First administered in combination with heroin by narcotics abusers, and as a "cure" for heroin addiction by some physicians, the intravenous use of amphetamines ultimately produced the "speed freak" phenomenon.[57]

Those people who inject amphetamines every 2 to 4 hours for several days may take hundreds of milligrams at a time. Tension, tremulousness, and the chances of developing an amphetamine psychosis increase. Hallucinations and paranoid delusions are sometimes accompanied by violent, impulsive behavior. These symptoms usually subside within several days of abstinence though some 5 to 15 percent of persons with this symptomatology do not recover completely.[58]

Amphetamines are rapidly absorbed when taken orally. Maximum effects—a state of alertness, arousal, and euphoria—occur about two to three hours after ingestion. Improvements in performance otherwise affected by fatigue or boredom occur. Amphetamines also decrease hunger, elevate blood pressure, and increase heart rate. They are inactivated largely by the liver, with one-half the dose being excreted unchanged in the urine.[59]

Tolerance develops to the appetite-depressant qualities of amphetamines within 4 to 6 weeks when the drug is taken as prescribed for obesity. Tolerance to the cardiovascular effects develops more rapidly than tolerance to the arousal and euphoria. Abrupt abstinence is accompanied by depression, fatigue, and an increase in appetite, though it is debatable whether this constitutes a withdrawal syndrome.[60]

Those who inject the drug are susceptible to the health hazards associated with injections. Chronic speed users are frequently 20 to 30 pounds underweight and suffer from poor nutrition. Though some persons have died following high doses of amphetamines, the overdose phenomenon is generally manifest in severe chest pain and several hours of unconsciousness.[61]

Narcotics   Narcotic drugs are those used to relieve pain and induce sleep. There are three groups of narcotics: (1) the naturally occurring ones such as opium and its derivatives, morphine and codeine; (2) the semisynthetic ones, which include heroin, oxycodone (Percodan), and hydromorphone (Dilaudid); and (3) the synthetic ones, such as meperidine (Demerol), methadone, and pentazocine (Talwin).[62]

Opium, Morphine, and Codeine   Opium is extracted from the poppy, *Papaver somniferum*, grown most extensively in Asia Minor and the Far East, with Turkey being the largest producer of opium in the world.[63] Opium itself is usually smoked in the Far East but is not very popular in the United States. It can be taken orally but, like all the narcotics, is greatly inactivated by digestion. Morphine and codeine are two naturally occurring alkaloids found in the poppy plant. Morphine is used medically to relieve pain; codeine is used as an analgesic and as a cough suppressant. Illegal morphine use to any degree is found only among those with ready access to the drug, i.e., health professionals. Most street users in the United States claim a preference for heroin. Adolescents are perhaps the only group likely to abuse codeine, doing so by drinking one or two bottles of a codeine-containing cough syrup, e.g., elixir of terpin hydrate with codeine.[64]

Heroin   Heroin was first synthesized from morphine in 1874. There are three known, measurable differences between the two: (1) heroin is two to four times more potent as an analgesic, (2) the effects of a heroin injection are more quickly noticed, and (3) the effects of heroin last about 3 to 4 hours and those of morphine last about 4 to 5 hours. The other important features of the two drugs are very similar. Heroin is usually "snorted" (inhaled) at first, but it can be smoked. Some users inject the drug, usually subcutaneously or intravenously.[65]

The distribution and metabolism of heroin in humans are poorly understood. In the body heroin is quickly converted to 6-mono-acetylmorphine (6-MM) which seems equipotent with heroin. Then 6-MM is converted to morphine, which is further metabolized and excreted. Heroin is almost completely metabolized in the body. Morphine and trace amounts of 6-MM appear unchanged in the urine.[66]

When heroin is injected intravenously, its effects are felt almost immediately and are very intense. The initial effect is described as similar to a sexual orgasm felt in the entire abdomen. The body quickly releases histamine, which results in itching, a reddening of the eyes and a fall in blood pressure. Until tolerance to the central nervous system depressant effects develop, the user becomes heavily sedated. After tolerance develops, heroin produces euphoria in which anxiety, appetite, and sexual desire are greatly diminished.[67]

Heroin is a general central nervous system depressant causing decreases in respirations, miosis (constriction of the pupils), and decreases in gastric motility and peristalsis. Heroin frequently produces nausea and vomiting. Regular use of heroin results in tolerance to many of its effects, most significantly to the depressant responses of sedation, analgesia, euphoria, and respiratory depression. Consequently, the user may increase the dose.[68]

Physical dependence occurs with repeated, regular use. The severity of the withdrawal syndrome is directly proportional to the amount of drug used. Though not usually life-threatening, heroin withdrawal is decidedly unpleasant, and many abusers continue their drug use in order to avoid the withdrawal process. Most heroin is of such poor quality that some persons have likened the withdrawal syndrome to a bad case of flu. About 4 to 10 hours after the last dose, the abuser experiences rhinorrhea, lacrimation, restlessness, insomnia, yawning, perspiration, and drug craving. Sleep may follow for 10 to 15 hours. Anorexia, nausea, vomiting, and diarrhea occur. Pupillary dilation, increased heart rate, hot and cold flashes, increased blood pressure, and involuntary twitching or kicking result as a rebound effect of central nervous system depression. Spontaneous orgasm may occur. Excessive fluid loss resulting in acid-base imbalance can, but rarely does, end in cardiovascular collapse and death. The withdrawal symptoms reach peak intensity within 36 to 72 hours, then gradually subside. Most symptoms disappear within 5 to 10 days of abstinence.[69] Care during withdrawal is discussed in Chapter 17.

There is no evidence whatsoever that heroin itself is responsible for any long-term organ damage in the user. Physical problems associated with heroin abuse are the results of the intravenous route of administration and the life-style of the user. The mortality rate among abusers is, however, high. Eighty-seven percent of those deaths have been attributed to heroin overdose. This diagnosis seems inconsistent with the observation that many heroin abusers are able to take extremely high doses with no untoward effects. The poor quality of heroin available on the street makes it unlikely that a user could secure enough of the drug to overdose. Alternative explanations suggest that such deaths may be the result of allergic reactions to other substances mixed with the heroin, or that heroin when used along with alcohol may result in death.[70]

Synthetic Narcotics   The synthetic narcotics include meperidine (Demerol), methadone (Dolophine), and pentazocine (Talwin). Though they may be used when heroin is in short supply, these drugs do not constitute any significant proportion of the youth drug scene.[71]

Meperidine was originally introduced as an analgesic comparable to morphine but without its shortcomings. Many of the original claims soon proved false. Physical dependence is possible and tolerance develops with repeated, regular use. There are two factors, however, which decrease the abuse potential of meperidine; it is a tissue irritant, producing skin ulcers and tissue damage where injected, and it has a short duration of action, 3 hours or less. Supplies of meperidine are usually limited, so most users are persons in the health care professions.

Pentazocine is one of the newest synthetic narcotics. It does not seem to produce the euphoria sought by narcotics users. Physical dependence can result with high doses on a daily basis.[72]

Methadone is a synthetic narcotic developed by the Germans in World War II. It was introduced in the United States in the 1950s for use in withdrawal from heroin. Methadone at low oral doses prevents the occurrence of narcotic withdrawal symptoms. At high oral doses it blocks the euphoric effects of other narcotics if they are also taken. If injected, methadone produces the same effects as heroin. The potential for physical dependence exists regardless of the route of administration. Side effects reported by those in methadone withdrawal and maintenance programs include weight gain, constipation, increased fluid intake, delayed ejaculation, increased frequency of urination, numbness of hands and feet, and hallucinations. It is difficult to determine whether such symptons existed prior to methadone use.[73]

The availability and subsequent abuse of methadone began as a result of poorly and naively run withdrawal and maintenance programs. Heroin abusers in treatment began injecting their methadone, using it in addition to heroin, or swapping it for other narcotics. As a result, methadone programs came under considerable attack and many were closed, thereby decreasing methadone abuse on the streets.[74]

Hallucinogens   The hallucinogens are those drugs with the potential to cause varying distortions in perception. They have also been called *phantasticants, psychotomimetics*, and *psychedelics*. Hallucinogens are found naturally in a variety of plants and can be manufactured synthetically.

Natural Hallucinogens   The peyote cactus, whose primary active ingredient is mescaline, is one of the most widely known natural hallucinogens. The crown is harvested, sliced into discs, and dried to produce mescal buttons. The peyote cactus is used legally in certain religious ceremonies of the Native American Church of the United States. There are no accepted medical uses for the plant.[75]

When the mescal buttons are eaten, mescaline is readily absorbed. Maximum concentrations appear in the brain within 30 minutes to 2 hours. About half of the drug is excreted within 6 hours, with small amounts still present up to 10 hours after ingestion.[76]

At low doses, mescaline produces euphoria. At doses of 5 mg per kilogram of body weight, hallucinations begin. Pupils dilate, pulse rate and blood pressure increase, and there is an elevation of body temperature. Death can result from convulsions and respiratory arrest. Nausea and sometimes vomiting are unpleasant side effects which accompany mescaline use. Tolerance develops with regular, repeated use, but there is no evidence of a withdrawal syndrome. Mescaline is cross-tolerant with LSD.[77]

Certain members of the potato family contain hallucinogenic substances. *Atropa belladonna*, or the deadly nightshade, *Hyoscyamus niger*, or henbane, *Mandragona officinarum*, or the mandrake plant, and many of the *Datura* species produce distortions in perception when ingested. They each contain atropine, scopolamine, and hyoscyamine as active ingredients. These plants are not used with any degree of regularity today. Most were used as poisons in the past.[78]

The seeds of the morning glory species *Rivea corymbosa* are hallucinogenic. The plant was most widely used in Mexico for religious ceremonies. The morning glory seeds sold in the United States are of the *Ipomoea violacea* species and do not produce perceptual distortions if eaten.[79]

There are a few varieties of mushrooms that possess hallucinogenic properties. The *Amanita muscaria* has been used mostly in Russia and Scandinavia. More well known in the United States is the *Psilocybe mexicana* mushroom. The active ingredient, psilocybin, was isolated in 1958 by Albert Hofmann, the discoverer of LSD. Ingested orally, psilocybin mushrooms produce effects very similar to LSD and mescaline; the three are cross-tolerant. Once absorbed, psilocybin is converted to psilocin. Effects begin within 10 to 15 minutes and are dose-related. They range from mild, pleasant, relaxing experiences to hallucinations and changes in body image. Physical dependence has not been demonstrated.[80]

LSD   LSD, or d-lysergic acid diethylamide, is perhaps the best known and most widely used hallucinogen. Albert Hofmann, a Sandoz chemist working in Switzerland in 1938, is credited with the discovery of LSD. Five years later, Dr. Hofmann experienced the hallucinogenic properties of the drug. In 1953, Sandoz laboratories applied to the Food and Drug Administration for rights to study LSD. Large quantities were distributed to scientists throughout the world. By 1966, LSD was available on the black market.[81]

The popularization of LSD was closely tied to the work of Timothy Leary and Richard Alpert. Though criticized by the scientific and legal communities, Leary and Alpert conducted experiments comparing many hallucinogens. They espoused a philosophy of life based on what they claimed to be the religious and mystical qualities of these drugs. The life-style called in part for a rejection of traditional values and behavior. The "tune in, turn on, drop out" philosophers began to lose their appeal in the late 1960s.[82]

LSD was used experimentally by the medical profession for the treatment of schizophrenic patients. It has also been used to treat the terminally ill, but neither use is currently sanctioned. LSD has always been a legally controlled substance.[83]

When taken orally, LSD is absorbed from the gastrointestinal tract rather rapidly. Little is known regarding its metabolism and excretion. Certain effects are perceptible within 30 to 40 minutes. Rises in blood pressure and heart rate, pupillary dilation, flushing, increased salivation, trembling in the extremities, and occasionally vomiting are evident 1 to 3 hours after ingestion and disappear within 6 hours. The psychic effects—feelings of unreality, depersonalization, and other perceptual distortions—may persist for 8 to 12 hours.[84]

If LSD is taken daily, tolerance develops within 5 days. It likewise disappears within a few days of abstinence. There is no evidence of physical dependence. Two deaths have been attributed to LSD, but these claims are suspect. The lethal dose of LSD is considered far in excess of that needed to produce psychological effects.[85,86]

One of the most frequent untoward effects of LSD use is the "bad trip," which consists of anxiety, paranoia, feelings of loss of control, or fears of insanity while under the influence of the drug. Though psychically painful, the feelings usually disappear within 8 to 12 hours. Susceptibility to a bad trip may depend on emotional well-being and sense of security at the time the drug is taken. Whether or not LSD use can result in longer-lasting psychotic symptoms is unsettled. Those who experience such symptoms may have had a tenuous hold on reality prior to use of the drug. Flashbacks, or the uncontrolled, spontaneous recurrence of LSD experiences, may occur, most frequently in times of fatigue or stress. Such experiences represent a loss of control and are extremely upsetting for some users.[87,88]

The so-called amotivational syndrome is sometimes associated with LSD use. The individual appears apathetic and ineffectual with a low frustration threshold and little desire to move in any direction regarding important decisions. Whether this is a direct result of LSD use is questionable.[89]

In the late 1960s, the mass media charged LSD with producing chromosomal damage in users and with causing birth defects in babies born to LSD-using mothers. Both claims represent distortions of scientific data.

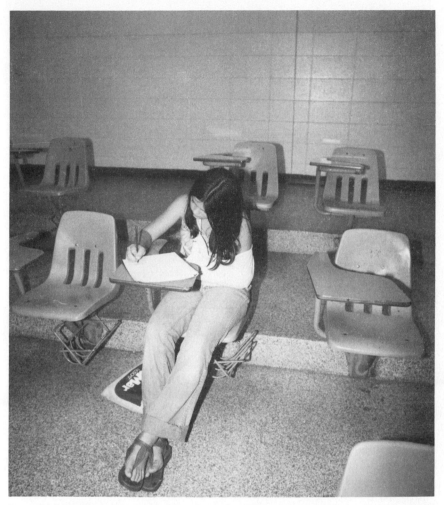

Drug use by teenagers is not usually of psychopathological origin but is rather one of the experiences undertaken in the process of growing up. Drug *abuse* is probably best understood if viewed as an unhealthy reaction to stress. A particular adolescent chooses drug abuse rather than some other form of behavioral maladaptation because of a myriad of social, physical, familial, and personal factors that are thus far poorly understood. (*Copyright ©* *1980 by Anne Campbell.*)

Experiments with animals seem to demonstrate these possibilities, but no data exist to corroborate these findings in human beings.[90]

Other Synthetic Hallucinogens   DMT, or N, N-dimethyltryptamine, is not a widely used drug in the United States. Though found in many plants and extracted for use by some South American and Caribbean Indians, DMT is also synthesized. Ineffective if taken orally, it must be smoked, inhaled nasally, or injected. DMT has been nicknamed "the businessman's trip" because its effects last such a brief time (about 1 or 2 hours) that it can be used at lunchtime.[91]

DOM, or 2, 5-dimethyloxy-4-methylamphetamine, commonly known as STP, is a synthetic hallucinogen that produces effects similar to those of LSD. The effects of DOM begin within 1 hour of ingestion, reach maximum intensity in 3 to 5 hours, and subside in 7 to 8 hours. Physical dependence probably does not develop, and it is unknown whether tolerance results from repeated use. Most of the substances sold on the street as mescaline are probably DOM.[92]

Marijuana and Hashish   Marijuana is the common name for the hemp plant, *Cannabis sativa*, and also refers specifically to its dried leaves and tops. Hashish is the extracted resin of the plant. Grown easily in temperate and tropical climates, hemp is used commercially in making rope, twine, and cord. Marijuana has been used medicinally to treat a vast number of illnesses, including gout, hysteria, convulsions, depression, tetanus, and rheumatism.[93]

In 1935, the commissioner of the Federal Bureau of Narcotics began a media campaign against marijuana. By 1937, 46 states had laws against the use of the plant. Though lacking support from the medical community, the commissioner began pushing for federal antimarijuana laws. Between 1937 and 1970, most state and federal laws equated the possession and sale of marijuana with that of heroin. In 1970, the Comprehensive Drug Abuse Prevention and Control Act reduced federal penalties for the possession of marijuana.[94] State laws vary.

Regardless of the laws and the campaigns against marijuana, its use has continued to increase. It is the fourth most frequently used psychoactive drug (after caffeine, nicotine, and alcohol). In 1969, the director of NIMH reported that between 8 million and 12 million Americans had tried marijuana at least once. Of those, 65 percent were classified as experimenters, 25 percent as social users, and 10 percent as chronic users. Polls taken in various colleges in 1969 reported that 15 to 25 percent of the respondents had tried marijuana. One year later, those estimates increased to 16 to 70 percent.[95]

Once dried, the leaves and tops of the *Cannabis* plant are smoked or eaten. There are about 20 chemical compounds, cannabinoids, in the plant, of which tetrahydrocannabinol (THC) is believed to be primarily responsible for its psychoactive effects. The potency of any given batch of marijuana or hashish is dependent on the percentage of THC present. By weight, hashish may contain 5 to 12 percent THC. Marijuana plants grown in the United States usually have less than 0.2 percent, Mexican plants less than 1 percent, but some Jamaican plants contain as much as

4 to 8 percent. Climate, soil, harvesting, and drying techniques affect THC concentrations.[96]

The effects of marijuana, felt almost immediately after the smoke is inhaled, reach a peak in about 70 minutes and disappear in 3 to 4 hours. When the substance is eaten, the effects begin within 30 minutes to 2 hours and last no more than 6 hours. Hashish is generally smoked. Although some claim to have purchased THC in liquid or tablet form, this is doubtful. The procedure for synthesizing the chemical is so complicated that the price would be prohibitive.[97]

Physiologically, THC produces increases in heart rate and peripheral blood flow, and injection of the conjunctiva. Minor changes occur in blood pressure, respiration, and body temperature. Dryness of mouth and increased appetite are reported by some but not all users. Psychologically, marijuana produces a sense of well-being, relaxation, and tranquility for most. Vision seems sharper and sound more distinct. Time seems to pass very slowly. Sleepiness may occur.

Persons who are depressed, apprehensive, or angry may experience an intensification of those feelings during marijuana use. When taken in extremely large amounts, marijuana can cause hallucinations and result in a bad trip similar to one resulting from LSD use. Flashbacks and the amotivational syndrome have been associated with chronic use; however, few adverse effects persist if use is discontinued. There have been no reported deaths due to overdose.[98]

There is no evidence that physical dependence develops with marijuana use. The question of tolerance is unclear. In animals, daily doses of THC seem to produce progressively weaker effects. Human subjects, however, report an increase in effect as they become more experienced users. This phenomenon is referred to as reverse tolerance.[99]

Major Tranquilizers, Mood Elevators, and Lithium   There are two categories of psychoactive drugs that are not commonly abused. One is the major tranquilizers, used primarily in the treatment of psychotic symptoms. These drugs include the phenothiazines, e.g., chlorpromazine (Thorazine), fluphenazine (Prolixin), thioridazine (Mellaril); the butyrophenones, e.g., haloperidol (Haldol); the thioxanthenes, e.g., thiothixene (Navane); the oxoindoles, e.g., molindone (Moban); and the rauwolfia alkaloids, e.g., Reserpine. Such drugs when taken by nonpsychotic persons act as sedatives but do not seem to produce the euphoria associated with drugs of abuse.[100] The second category of psychoactive drugs not commonly abused is comprised of the medications used to treat mood disorders. Antidepressants, which include the tricyclics, e.g., imipramine (Tofranil), amitriptyline (Elavil), and doxepin (Sinequan), and the monoamine oxidase inhibitors, e.g., phenelzine (Nardil) and tranylcypromine (Parnate), are used therapeutically in the treatment of depression. Lithium carbonate, though not chemically similar to the antidepressants, is used to treat manic-depressive disorders and is also not popular among drug abusers.[101]

PREVENTION AND TREATMENT

Drugs, in and of themselves, are neither good nor bad, and it appears, after their centuries-long history, that they are here to stay. For all drugs, legal and illegal, there will be abstainers, users, and abusers. The prevention of adolescent drug use entirely is an unrealistic goal, but efforts to decrease use and to prevent abuse are likely to yield positive results.

Prevention occurs on three levels. Primary prevention involves efforts, mostly educational, to help all young people make responsible decisions regarding the use of psychoactive substances *before* using them. Secondary prevention efforts are aimed at those adolescents already identified as drug users, the goal being to prevent abuse. Tertiary prevention involves treatment of drug-abusing adolescents in order to prevent deterioration in personal, social, economic, and/or physical functioning.[102]

For nurses to be effective in drug abuse prevention and treatment they must be comfortable both with themselves and with adolescents in general. They must examine their value systems, prejudices, motives, goals, and limitations. Nurses must seek to correct misconceptions and to fill in gaps in knowledge regarding adolescents and drugs. In addition to utilizing traditional forms of education, such as college courses, public lectures, and professional reading, nurses can increase their knowledge and experience by working with adolescents in free clinics, runaway shelters, and rap houses. These settings provide excellent opportunities to assess one's own strengths and weaknesses in dealing with the problems of young people, one of which is drug use.

Primary Prevention

Nurses can involve themselves in the prevention and treatment of drug abuse on all three levels. Viewed as experts in health care, they may be sought as consultants on the topic of drug use. School and community health nurses are in excellent positions to initiate or offer assistance in developing educational programs for students, faculty, and parent-teacher organizations. On a less formal basis, nurses can make use of opportunities to correct misconceptions and foster open discussions about the issues of drug use with individuals or groups. Nurses who have regular contact with adolescents can set aside preannounced times in which any topic of concern can be discussed, one of which is bound to be drugs. Above all, educational efforts must seek to impart knowledge, not to moralize or present only the dire consequences of drug abuse. The opinions of young people must be heard and respected. Too often adolescents have discovered that information presented by adults was biased, only partially correct, and delivered in a way that negated their own judgment. They have therefore tended to disregard the facts with the fiction, and have consequently been left less than well prepared to make responsible decisions regarding drug use.

Secondary Prevention

Nurses may also identify those adolescents already using drugs. An experimental or periodic drug user may present in a state of intoxication, one example being the adolescent who is referred to the school nurse because of apparent intoxication in class. Far more frequently, however, adolescents will reveal their drug taking only to trusted adults. If a nurse is available and has managed to establish a relationship with the adolescent, then the nurse may be that adult. The building of such relationships can occur in a variety of settings—school, practitioner's office, inpatient unit, clinic. The most important ingredients are a genuine interest in the adolescent and an ability to convey that interest in a straightforward manner.[103,104]

Any young person who seeks nursing or medical attention should be routinely asked about the use of drugs, legal and illegal. The more comfortable a nurse is in asking such questions, the more likely that nurse is to get honest answers. At the outset of the interview, the nurse should briefly explain the limits of confidentiality laws regarding treatment of minors. This enables the adolescent to decide what he or she is willing to reveal. Questions specifically regarding drug use need not be prefaced with further assurances of confidence unless the adolescent asks for reassurance or clarification. Though nurses must develop their own interview techniques, the following questions are suggested as guidelines for obtaining useful information about drug use.

1   Do you take any prescribed medication now? In the recent past? What? How much? For what?
2   Are you allergic to any medication?
3   What other drugs have you used? Do you use them now? How much? How often?
4   How much alcohol do you use? What kind? How often?
5   Have you ever had a bad reaction to any drugs?
6   Have you ever had trouble stopping the use of any drugs?

Most adolescents who use drugs are not completely honest about it, particularly with a strange adult. They may minimize answers for fear of discovery or exaggerate in order to impress. In certain situations, it may be appropriate to ask friends or family members to comment on various parts of the assessment findings. Direct questions such as the ones above are applicable in those situations. Questions about the behavior of a particular adolescent may also help identify drug use as a possibility.

Once adolescent drug users are identified, nurses may work with them individually or in groups, formally or informally, in an effort to prevent the development of drug abuse. Educational efforts and discussions for individuals, peer groups, and families are appropriate interventive approaches.

Treatment

Tertiary prevention, or treatment, for adolescent drug abusers may occur in a variety of settings, as described in Chapter 17. Abuse must first be documented by history, physical assessment, or laboratory assessment.

Assessment   As mentioned previously, the reliability of information elicited from the adolescent may be questionable, though it acquires more validity when substantiated by family or friends.

The practitioner is perhaps more likely to see physical evidence of drug use in the abuser than in the experimental user. Evidence of intoxication at the time of the assessment manifests itself in various ways, depending on the drug. Slurring of speech, inappropriate affect, and decreased attention span may indicate use of a central nervous system depressant. In the absence of the smell of alcohol, the possibility of use of barbiturates, of other sedatives and hypnotics, or, in younger adolescents, of inhalants, solvents, or aerosols should be entertained. In cases of severe central nervous system depression, the adolescent may present with decreases in blood pressure, pulse, and respirations. Pupillary constriction is specific to the use of the narcotics. Mydriasis (dilated pupils) and photophobia may accompany use of the hallucinogens. Though not intoxicated at the time of assessment, users of hallucinogens may evidence flashback experiences by seeming momentarily disoriented and unable to think clearly. Persons on central nervous system stimulants may appear extremely energetic or nervous. Amphetamine use also produces tachypnea.[105]

In the absence of intoxication during the assessment, certain other physical findings should raise the practitioner's awareness to the possibility of drug abuse. Any evidence of trauma, e.g., bruises, sores, or burns, should be explored, as these could have occurred during intoxication. Perforations or ulcerations of the nasal septum may indicate excessive cocaine use. Scars, abscesses, and new needle marks may indicate the injection of drugs by the adolescent. Pulmonary infection, thromboses, or granulomas with resulting decreases in pulmonary function may occur as a result of drug injection. Scleral icterus, decreases in liver function, or hepatomegaly may indicate hepatitis secondary to unsterile injection techniques.[106]

Several laboratory techniques are available to analyze blood and urine for the presence of drugs or their major metabolites. Thin-layer chromatography (TLC) and gas-liquid chromatography (GLC) are the best known procedures. TLC is fast, less expensive, and relatively simple. False negatives may occur if drugs are present in amounts below the sensitivity of the equipment used. False positives are possible when two or more drugs can occupy the same position on the filter paper, e.g., cocaine and diazepam (Valium) can occupy the same spot as methadone, and glutethimide (Doriden) may be mistaken for barbiturates. GLC is more sensitive and identifies a wider variety of drugs but is very expensive. Another procedure used solely in the detection of heroin use involves fluorescence of the urine at a specific wavelength. A measurement is taken with a fluorospectrophotometer. The process is less complicated than TLC and provides the same degree of accuracy, but the machinery is very expensive. Hemoglobin values, red blood cell indices, white blood cell counts, and conventional urinalyses are not specific indicators of drug use. Seven to 10 days of abstinence usually render the body drug-free.[107]

Intervention   The treatment of drug abusers occurs on two levels, emergency intervention and long-term rehabilitation. Emergency care may be necessary during acute intoxication or during the withdrawal process, or both, depending upon the drug used.

Toxicity following the use of large amounts of any chemical can require treatment and may actually constitute a medical emergency. The emergency situations most commonly associated with drug abuse in adolescence include overdoses of barbiturates or narcotics, the temporary psychotic episodes resulting from excessive amphetamine use, and the bad trips associated with LSD. Other emergencies may arise from overdose of the major tranquilizers, mood elevators, lithium, or the antianxiety agents. Any adolescents who are seen in any of these situations should be questioned about drug use in general once the emergency is over. Follow-up contact and possibly referral for drug abuse treatment should occur. Both short- and long-term interventions are discussed in Chapter 17.

CONCLUSION

Certain generalizations emerge when the youth drug scene is considered in its entirety. The most basic of these is that drugs are here to stay. Prohibition efforts have never worked. Brecher's discussion of the consequences of the United States' alcohol prohibition period from 1920 to

1933 (continued availability and use of beverage alcohol, crippling and death resulting from use of unsafe bootleg liquor, inroads made by crime syndicates, adoption and popularization of other legal and illegal drugs) is illustrative.[108]

Societal attitudes about adolescent drug use have been detrimentally influenced by the fact that adults and adolescents use different drugs. Adults harbor many myths about the drugs with which they are unfamiliar. Laws are then based on misinformation and a fear of the unknown. Consequently, most of the physical, financial, and social risks of illegal drug use are a direct result of their illegality. Another fact that seems evident is that as long as there are drugs there will be drug users and abusers. Adolescents seek to meet certain personal needs through their drug-taking behavior. Until those needs are met in other ways, the use will continue. Lastly, it appears that the drugs that cause the most physical and psychological damage are those which are available legally, yet most of our law enforcement and educational efforts are aimed at curbing the use of illegal drugs.

It seems that some broad recommendations are in order. For one, adults must stop perpetuating myths and misinformation regarding adolescents and the drugs they use. Laws must not continue to be based on erroneous data. Adults and adolescents need to learn the facts about psychoactive drugs, not the horror stories. Efforts to help young people make decisions regarding drug use need to be local and educational rather than federal and legal. Of utmost importance is a process which allows the adolescent to examine and solidify a value system based on responsible decision making.

REFERENCES

1 H. J. Cornacchia, D. J. Bentel, and D. E. Smith, *Drugs in the Classroom*. St. Louis: C. V. Mosby Co., 1973, p. 32.
2 F. G. Hofmann, *A Handbook on Drug and Alcohol Abuse*. New York: Oxford University Press, 1975, p. 25.
3 Cornacchia et al., op. cit., p. 9.
4 E. M. Brecher, *Licit and Illicit Drugs*. Boston: Little, Brown and Co. 1972, p. 475.
5 Brecher, op. cit., pp. 476–479.
6 Cornacchia et al., op. cit., p. 10.
7 Cornacchia et al., op. cit., pp. 13–16.
8 Brecher, op. cit., p. 487.
9 Hofmann, op. cit., p. 50.
10 O. S. Ray, *Drugs, Society and Human Behavior*. St. Louis: C. V. Mosby Co., 1972, p. 92.
11 Hofmann, op. cit., pp. 50–51.

12 Hofmann, op. cit., p. 52.
13 Hofmann, op. cit.
14 Hofmann, op. cit.
15 Ray, op. cit., pp. 63–64.
16 Hofmann, op. cit., pp. 46–48.
17 Hofmann, op. cit., p. 45.
18 Hofmann, op. cit., pp. 48–49.
19 Ray, op. cit., pp. 109–115.
20 Brecher, op. cit., p. 199.
21 Ray, op. cit.
22 Ray, op. cit.
23 Brecher, op. cit.
24 Ray, op. cit.
25 Ray, op. cit., pp. 103–105.
26 Ray, op. cit.
27 Ray, op. cit., pp. 85–86.
28 Ray, op. cit., p. 86.
29 Hofmann, op. cit.
30 Ray, op. cit.
31 Ray, op. cit., pp. 86–87.
32 Hofmann, op. cit., p. 111.
33 Ray, op. cit., p. 93.
34 Ray, op. cit., p. 173.
35 Ray, op. cit., p. 175.
36 Ray, op. cit., p. 176.
37 Hofmann, op. cit., pp. 121–125.
38 Hofmann, op. cit., pp. 125–126.
39 Ray, op. cit., pp. 172–173.
40 Brecher, op. cit., p. 256.
41 Brecher, op. cit., pp. 312–318.
42 Hofmann, op. cit., p. 131.
43 Brecher, op. cit., pp. 321–324.
44 Hofmann, op. cit., p. 132.
45 Hofmann, op. cit., pp. 133–135.
46 Hofmann, op. cit., pp. 135–137.
47 Hofmann, op. cit., pp. 137, 145–146.
48 Brecher, op. cit., pp. 256–259.
49 Brecher, op. cit., pp. 256–259.
50 Brecher, op. cit., pp. 272–274.
51 Brecher, op. cit., pp. 275–276.
52 Hofmann, op. cit., pp. 240–242.
53 Ray, op. cit., p. 161.
54 Hofmann, op. cit., p. 242.
55 Hofmann, op. cit., p. 242.
56 Brecher, op. cit., pp. 278–279.
57 Brecher, op. cit., pp. 281–282.
58 Brecher, op. cit., pp. 281–285.

59   Ray, op. cit., pp. 166–170.
60   Hofmann, op. cit., pp. 235–236.
61   Hofmann, op. cit., pp. 237–239.
62   Hofmann, op. cit., p. 69.
63   Ray, op. cit., p. 181.
64   Hofmann, op. cit., pp. 88–89.
65   Hofmann, op. cit., p. 72.
66   Hofmann, op. cit., pp. 78–79.
67   Hofmann, op. cit., pp. 74–78.
68   Hofmann, op. cit., pp. 74–80.
69   Hofmann, op. cit., pp. 80–84.
70   Brecher, op. cit., pp. 21–32, 101–114.
71   Hofmann, op. cit., p. 90.
72   Hofmann, op. cit., pp. 90–93.
73   Brecher, op. cit., pp. 135–139, 153.
74   Hofmann, op. cit., pp. 163–175.
75   Ray, op. cit., pp. 215–217.
76   Ray, op. cit., p. 219.
77   Ray, op. cit. pp. 219–220.
78   Ray, op. cit., pp. 220–224.
79   Ray, op. cit., pp. 228–229.
80   Ray, op. cit., p. 227.
81   Ray, op. cit., pp. 233–234.
82   Ray, op. cit., pp. 234–237.
83   Brecher, op. cit., pp. 349–356.
84   Ray, op. cit., pp. 241–242.
85   Hofmann, op. cit., p. 169.
86   Ray, op. cit., p. 238.
87   Hofmann, op. cit., pp. 159–161.
88   Ray, op. cit., pp. 245–246.
89   Hofmann, op. cit., pp. 164–165.
90   Hofmann, op. cit., pp. 166–169.
91   Ray, op. cit., pp. 229–230.
92   Ray, op. cit., p. 220.
93   Brecher, op. cit., pp. 397–412.
94   Brecher, op. cit., pp. 413–421.
95   Brecher, op. cit., p. 422.
96   Hofmann, op. cit., pp. 185–196.
97   Hofmann, op. cit.
98   Hofmann, op. cit., pp. 209–217.
99   Hofmann, op. cit., pp. 208–209.
100 Ray, op. cit., pp. 143–149.
101 Ray, op. cit, pp. 149–152.
102 Cornacchia et al., op. cit., pp. 10–11.
103 P.K. Burkhalter, *Nursing Care of the Alcoholic and Drug Abuser*. New
     York: McGraw-Hill Book Co., 1975, pp. 41–47.
104 Hofmann, op. cit., p. 259.

105   Hofmann, op. cit., pp. 247–259.
106   Hofmann, op. cit., pp. 247–259.
107   Hofmann, op. cit., pp. 259–263.
108   Brecher, op. cit., pp. 265–266.

BIBLIOGRAPHY

Brecher, Edward M.: *Licit and Illicit Drugs*. Boston: Little, Brown and Co., 1972.
Burkhalter, Pamela K.: *Nursing Care of the Alcoholic and Drug Abuser*. New York: McGraw-Hill Book Co., 1975.
Cornacchia, Harold J., David J. Bentel, and David E. Smith: *Drugs in the Classroom*. St. Louis: C. V. Mosby Co., 1973.
Hofmann, Frederick G.: *A Handbook on Drug and Alcohol Abuse*. New York: Oxford University Press, 1975.
Irwin, Samuel: *Drugs of Abuse: An Introduction to Their Actions and Potential Hazards*. Beloit, Wis.: Student Association for the Study of Hallucinogens, Inc., 1973.
Ray, Oakley S.: *Drugs, Society and Human Behavior*. St. Louis: C. V. Mosby Co., 1972.

Chapter 7

The Adolescent with Mental Retardation

Susan Ann Clemen
Ann Wizinsky Pattullo

In the past, the adolescent with mental retardation was segregated from the mainstream of experience and provided with minimal, if any, opportunity to cope with the developmental tasks of adolescence. Today adolescents with retardation can identify with peers in ways that were not previously possible. Revolutionary changes occurring in the field of mental retardation are emphasizing similarities rather than differences. Integration of persons with retardation into the community is a major thrust. Environmental factors are under closer scrutiny so that those facilitating average ("normal") development can be provided. The protective and restrictive milieu of the segregated institution has been recognized as a significant barrier to the attainment of optimally average life experiences. A major vehicle for promoting integration or access to average life experiences is the movement out of the institution and into the community. The community provides the least restrictive, most facilitative environment for maturation. This can be true even when the community setting is a nursing home, if the major goal of the setting is programming for the highest attainable level of independent functioning.

As with average adolescents, the degree to which any retarded adolescent successfully adjusts as a social being varies according to the
nature and quality of previous and current life experiences and physical,
emotional, and cognitive status. This chapter describes areas in which
these factors often differ from those of the average adolescent and discusses ways the nurse can effectively intervene to minimize these differences. Current issues in the field of mental retardation will be explored
to help the reader identify why some of the differences in life experiences
have occurred for adolescents with mental retardation.

Typically, the differences are weighted in a negative direction. In
general, the magnitude of the differences is influenced by the timing of
diagnosis; the earlier the condition is diagnosed, the greater the possibility
that the severity of retardation is pronounced. Physical stigmata and/or
muscular dysfunction evident at birth influence how the environment perceives and treats the individual, and, in turn, the way the environment
treats the individual influences how the child experiences his or her world.
Later recognition reduces the frequency of nonaverage life experiences
and increases the possibility that adjustment to the requirements and
expectations of society will come closer to that of the average adolescent.
Less severe mental retardation is most often not accompanied by physical
stigmata or noticeable developmental delay, so it may not be recognized
until the child enters school. The more evident the retardation is at birth,
the less likely it is that the individual will proceed through the average
socialization process. Early case finding and *intervention* can, of course,
maximize child and family functioning.

Clinical experience reveals that often the mentally retarded adolescent's socializing experiences during childhood have been deficient in
both quantity and quality. As a result, it can be expected that during the
chronological pubescent period this individual may still be working on
earlier life tasks. Not only may the psychological and social problem-
solving processes be delayed in their inception, but the processes may be
prolonged and may never be totally accomplished. The latter is true of
any adolescent, but it is more likely to be the case with the mentally
retarded adolescent whose condition and life experience differ significantly
from the average.

Even though the process of psychosocial development may be delayed, the majority of adolescents who are mentally retarded must deal
with the same developmental tasks as other adolescents. Success in their
struggle to achieve social adequacy is measured by the same parameters
used with any adolescent: ability to gratify sexual needs within socially
acceptable norms, productive use of personal capacities, realistic perceptions of self and environment, regard for self and others, and some
degree of self-sufficiency in current and future functioning. The present-

day difficulties for retarded adolescents and their families can be expected to lessen in the future as the new emphasis on similarities rather than differences is experienced throughout childhood.

Because the new focus on the need for average rather than deviant life experiences is in its early phase of implementation, the environmental risk of conditioning "retarded" behavior must constantly be kept in mind. Interactions with mentally retarded adolescents must occur in the context of the "hall of mirrors" question posed by Fishman and associates, who ask how much the social context, which reflects many persons' diminished expectations of retarded people, produces "retarded" behavior.

> In other words, to what extent is retardation a function of being treated as a retarded person? Conversely, how much does the learning deficit [when apparent] serve to organize people in the social context to treat him as retarded?[1]

The concept that individual differences are a function of being human must take precedence over stereotypic ideas about mental retardation. The "hall of mirrors" must reflect the retarded person's human strengths and needs.

Too often, the world of the adolescent who has mental retardation has been, and is still at risk of being, organized in accordance with the narrow perspective of the retardation label. Self-fulfilling prophecies deter these adolescents from fulfilling their potential.

The phenomenon of the "hall of mirrors" experience is not unique to persons who have labels that carry negative connotations. Individuals who are dependent on the approval of others often respond to even the most subtle messages. Messages can be communicated by averted eyes, crossed arms, frowns, smiles, and other body language. Receiving these messages is a common experience for all adolescents in their search for peer group approval. It occurs as a major influence of this stage of their socialization even when there is no other label attached to their person-hood. Many readers can attest to this from personal experience.

Other experiences of the reader may further clarify the significance of the process of social signaling. We have all, at some time and to some degree, been "mentally retarded" in some social contexts. We may have been too anxious during a test to solve a problem that had been so easy to do just the day before. We may have been too overwhelmed, too frightened, or too confused to do what we knew we were capable of doing under different circumstances. Others in our environment did not expect us to continue to behave in certain ways just because we were temporarily distraught and disorganized; we were not expected to be consistently deficient in our functioning. Our label was "student," "newcomer," "nurse," or any word that carried the expectation of potential for more competence, under different circumstances, in another place or at another time. Thus, we knew that our "retarded" behavior was not expected to continue; our social contexts did not treat us as "retarded." We did not remain captive in a suppressive "hall of mirrors." We were allowed to demonstrate our real selves and our real potential. We became appropriately adaptive.

Adolescents with mental retardation need the same opportunities to demonstrate what they are capable of achieving. Some will need more support and specific guidance than others. The degree of guidance needed, however, must be determined on the basis of *demonstrated performance* rather than by assumptions made from the label "retarded."

During this period of nationwide transition from segregation to integration in the field of mental retardation, concepts regarding change have considerable relevance. Exposure to the average human experience represents a significant change in life-style for many of these adolescents. This change in life-style presents potential problems as well as solutions. Problems arise when the change occurs with such rapidity that the gap between learned adaptive capacities and environmental expectations is too great. This is true of any adolescent. Other chapters in this book describe the "crisis" nature of this stage of human development for any adolescent; the concept of change is a pervasive theme. This concept has more critical relevance and influence for the adolescent who is mentally retarded than for any other, because almost every sphere of influence in the lives of these individuals is being reexamined and modified.

The holistic perspective of nursing equips the reader to be instrumental in assisting both adolescents and their families to benefit from the new philosophies and approaches that have had such a critical impact on their lives. Many of the nursing skills and approaches described in other chapters of this book can be applied here. The major differentiating characteristic of this group of adolescents lies in their intellectual capacity and their ability to adapt to the social demands of the average environment. Neither intelligence nor adaptive capacity is static. Therein lies the impact that nursing can have in the lives of these adolescents.

DEFINING MENTAL RETARDATION: SOME PERSPECTIVES AND ISSUES

Defining mental retardation has posed a major problem to society, professionals, and the individuals who are assigned to this minority group. Ambiguity, disagreement, and confusion abound. In over 2,500 years of attempts, no single, universally recognized definition has been developed.[2] In 1976, Jordan identified 13 types of definitions, "each reflecting the views of a particular theoretician and each generally incompatible with those of any other."[3] Despite the disagreement and ambiguity that prevail, each definition of mental retardation that has been made public has influenced societal attitudes and professional functioning. Several motivations for definitions, and several outcomes, have been noted in the literature. The writer of the definition may originally have had altruistic intentions, such as identification of retarded people for the purpose of helping them, both as individuals and as a group. The original intent may have been technical and humanistic—for purposes of understanding, intervention, and social and economic decision making. However, once a label is known, it is no longer private; it is in the public domain, and both positive and negative results can ensue. Appropriate administrative decisions may be made, but discrimination and loss of freedom may occur. The individuals who are labeled have attention drawn to their particular needs for socialization and health maintenance but risk emphasis on their deficits rather than a balanced look at their needs, strengths, and potential.

A critically pervasive influence on educational decisions is the reliance on intelligence tests.[4] Early influential definitions of mental retardation differentiated average individuals from individuals who are mentally retarded solely by scores on intelligence tests. "The use of standardized tests scores for determining special class placement has been and continues to be an integral part of the public education system."[5] Labels such as mildly, moderately, severely, and profoundly retarded were applied to individuals whose intelligence quotient (IQ) score fell into highly specific ranges that varied in their cutoff points. One such series was 52–67, 36–51, 21–35, and 0–20. On the basis of these labels, individuals were assigned specific classroom placements by the educational system. Mildly retarded individuals, for example, were considered to be educable and thus were placed in a special classroom in the regular school setting.

Too often, it is still not recognized that the IQ classification system used to describe mental retardation contains very little useful information. The boundaries between "average" and "mentally retarded" are not clear or precise. In addition, particularly in relationship to categories or degrees of function or deficit, the parameters are very imprecise. Different disciplines use different numerical cutoff points. In some schools, only persons who achieve a score of 70 or less on an IQ test would be put into a special education classroom. If another test, or the same test, were given by someone from another discipline under different internal or environmental conditions, one of these same students might make a score of 75. The student would then remain in an average classroom, even if he or she was not functioning well in this classroom. This practice of placing children in classroom settings solely on the basis of IQ scores has resulted in some individuals' being provided special educational placements when they do not need them and other individuals' being denied special educational opportunities when they do need them.

The most advanced thinking about IQ is summarized in a new and comprehensive reference for judges, attorneys, law students, parents, professionals, advocates, and others concerned with the legal rights of citizens who are mentally retarded. In the introductory chapter, IQ is not mentioned until it becomes necessary to make a point about its relevance to the reader:

> An I.Q. is one of the least helpful facts available to the professional. It gives little information or guidance although it provides a basis for stereotyping. . . . These characteristics of I.Q. . . . work to the disadvantage of the person to be served. . . . An I.Q. represents the score that an individual obtains on a specific test under certain standardized conditions. . . .[6]

It must be emphasized here that the validity of IQ testing is not only a function of the test questions but also of the internal and external environments of the individual being tested.

> The score may predict performance in some areas, but it is of very limited value in most areas of human functioning. A parallel would be to time a person's running speed over a measured distance under specific conditions of temperature, humidity, and wind velocity and then to use the resultant time (score) to determine what the person would be permitted to do. Those with slow times would not be permitted to make contracts, marry, handle their assets, have children or attend regular classes in public school.[7]

This advanced thinking is not always reflected in current practice. Many school systems and professionals involved in helping individuals who are mentally retarded still use IQ scores and derived categorization as a basis for planning their professional interventions.

There are, however, numerous leaders in the field of mental retardation striving to move away from the traditional IQ classification system. The American Association on Mental Deficiency (AAMD), the interdisciplinary professional organization in the field, has been active in the process of definition and classification of mental retardation. In 1959, AAMD required, for the first time, measurement of both intellectual functioning and *adaptive behavior functioning* at the time of diagnosis. This recommendation was based on the belief that individual abilities are greatly influenced by experiences in different environments. Currently, the most widely used definition of mental retardation is the one developed by AAMD in 1973. This definition is as follows:

> Mental retardation refers to significantly subaverage general intellectual functioning existing concurrently with deficits in adaptive behavior, and manifested during the developmental period.[8]

The "significantly" was added to modify "subaverage general intellectual functioning" found in the AAMD's 1959 definition. Significantly subaverage refers to test performance that is two or more standard deviations from the population mean, whereas subaverage referred to only one standard deviation. Thus, the behavioral category of borderline retardation was eliminated. This reflected the changing philosophy and knowledge of the seventies. A more optimistic perspective of the social capabilities of the person with low intelligence began to prevail.

This major change, however, had a detrimental effect on American society's provision of services to this group.[9] Individuals who formerly qualified for vocational rehabilitation services, and who still needed these services, were declared ineligible when "borderline retardation" was eliminated from the definition. It is eminently clear that elimination of this group "does not mean that such individuals are free from problems of learning and social adaptation, or that they do not require appropriate supporting services."[10]

However, because we have no standardized way of assessing learning and social adaptation problems, the "significantly subaverage general intellectual functioning" is currently used as a major criterion for determining society's standards for provision of health and educational services.

In recognition of this major problem for all individuals whose intellectual and adaptive learning needs still exist, AAMD has reappointed Grossman's task force to issue a supplement to the 1973 *Manual on Terminology and Classification*.[11] Until such time as adaptive functional assessments become standardized, it is essential for professional nurses to use their clinical judgment and expertise to determine service needs of clients. Provision of services should be based on an accurate, individualized nursing assessment rather than on guidelines contained in a definition. Limitations in both intelligence and adaptation should be identified.

Adaptive behavior is defined by AAMD as "the effectiveness or degree with which the individual meets the standards of personal independence and social responsibility expected of his age and cultural group."[12] Other definitions or descriptions of adaptive behavior tests convey essentially the same message: "primarily refers to the effectiveness of an individual in coping with the natural and social demands of his or her environment,"[13] and, somewhat more explicitly, "typical behavior observed during mealtimes," "under *optimal* conditions," and "representative toileting behaviors during day and night shifts using a standardized interview" with familiar ward personnel.[14] Also, from Balthazar's tests of adaptive behavior:

> . . . objective measures of coping behaviors . . . specifically . . .
> > (1)   Unadaptive Self-Directed Behaviors;
> > (2)   Unadaptive Interpersonal Behaviors;

(3)   Adaptive Self-Directed Behaviors;
(4)   Adaptive Interpersonal Behaviors;
(5)   Verbal Communication;
(6)   Play Activities; and
(7)   Responses to Instructions[15]

It should be made clear here that the last three descriptive quotations were not stated as "definitions" in original texts. Balthazar was describing *what* his scales were measuring. He clearly states, in his description of purpose, that they measure the person's "*representative* behavior" only and make no claim to "evaluate aptitude or 'intelligence' in terms of any external standards or norms."[16]

It is important for the nurse in the community to know that community standards or norms are different from those under which Balthazar's scales were developed. He points out that his scales were developed on a population of severely or profoundly retarded individuals who were residents in institutions.[17]

Balthazar's model of identifying specific behaviors to observe when assessing adaptive functioning provides useful *guidelines* for nurses who are developing an assessment framework. However, it is crucial for the nurse to remember that the *norms* discussed in Balthazar's work can be applied to only a very limited population, that is, residents in institutions who demonstrate severe to profound levels of deficiency. This point is being emphasized here to stress the fact that environment critically influences behavior.

It should be clear to the reader at this point that defining mental retardation and differentiating adolescents who are mentally retarded is a complex process greatly compounded by a lack of operational clarity. Without question, a highly individualized and relevant assessment must be made before specific modes of professional intervention are selected. Before discussing assessments and interventions for retarded adolescents, we must examine another perspective of the problem of defining mental retardation: Mental retardation must be differentiated from mental illness and developmental disability.

DIFFERENTIATION FROM MENTAL ILLNESS AND DEVELOPMENTAL DISABILITY

Mental illness, developmental disability, and mental retardation are frequently confused or erroneously used as synonyms. Mental illness covers a wide range of personal and social problems that can result in distorted perceptions of self, others, and objects. Major categories of mental illness are neurosis and psychosis. Mental retardation is not a mental illness. Indeed, mental retardation is not an illness, but individuals who have mental retardation can also have mental illness.

Differentiating mental retardation and developmental disabilities is more difficult. More issues are involved when other handicaps are introduced. Among these issues are "questions of economy in the spread of resources among competing needs, and of effectiveness of general versus specialized approaches to prevention and management."[18] Additional factors influencing preference for the term "developmental disability" are primarily legal or attitudinal. It is a term that is sufficiently malleable to encompass a large number of widely different disorders and combinations of these disorders. One reason it is used as a synonym for mental retardation is that the term "developmental disability" carries less stigma. The stigmatic nature of mental retardation is reflected in changes in both terminology and treatment over time. The trend is definitely in the direction of positive humanism. Often, attitudes of parents, professionals, and governmental agencies are being reflected when "developmental disability" and "mental retardation" are used synonymously. They are not synonymous. Concern with stigma and thoughtful, disciplined use of language is appropriate. However, using "mental retardation" and "developmental disability" synonymously does a disservice to both. Operational clarity and the human value of the individuals with both conditions suffer when the reality of the specific handicap is thus denied. The developmental disability label has been used to designate individuals with the following problems: blindness, autism, mental retardation, cerebral palsy, learning disabilities, and epilepsy. In 1978 a new definition of developmental disability was written into federal legislation as an amendment to the Rehabilitation Act of 1973, section 503:

The term "developmental disability" means a severe, chronic disability of a person which—

    a.   is attributable to a mental or physical impairment or combination of mental and physical impairments;

    b.   is manifested before the person attains age 22;

    c.   is likely to continue indefinitely;

    d.   results in substantial functional limitations in three or more of the following areas of major life activity:

        i.   self-care

        ii.   receptive and expressive language

        iii.   learning

        iv.   mobility

        v.   self-direction

        vi.   capacity for independent living, and

        vii.   economic sufficiency; and

    e.   reflects the person's need for a combination and sequence of special, interdisciplinary, or generic care, treatment, or other services which are of lifelong or extended duration and are individually planned and coordinated.[19]

Frequently, cerebral palsy and mental retardation are used synonymously. Some individuals who have cerebral palsy also have mental retardation. There are, however, many individuals with cerebral palsy who have no intellectual deficiencies. In fact, we know of individuals with cerebral palsy who have attained a Ph.D. If individuals with mental retardation and cerebral palsy are placed in the same category, the developmental disability category, will the myth that all cerebral palsy individuals are mentally retarded be perpetuated?

MAJOR TRENDS IN THE FIELD
OF MENTAL RETARDATION

The goal of full appreciation of the individuality of people who are retarded has not yet been achieved. The use of the term *retardates* does not convey the concept of unique personhood. The use of this term in the literature to refer to people who have retardation as one of their characteristics implies that there are some professionals in the field who, at some emotional level, have retained a dehumanizing perspective of the people who are supposed to benefit from their interventions. However, changes are occurring.

Sweden has strongly influenced the life-styles of people who are retarded and of the people who influence their development. It is in large part due to the leadership demonstrated in that country that "normalization" and "humanization" have become increasingly evident in the language and behavior of those in the field in the United States. The normalization principle for intervention in mental retardation has had a major impact on the improvement of services and community attitudes. As a liberalizing humanistic movement, normalization was first conceptualized by Bank-Mikkelson in Denmark and was made law in that country in 1949.[20] It was elaborated upon in the literature by Nirje in 1969, following its implementation and legalization in Sweden in 1967.[21] Normalization is "utilization of means which are as culturally normative as possible in order to establish and/or maintain personal behaviors which are as culturally normative as possible."[22] Or, put more simply, "Let a retarded person live as normal a life as he possibly can in as normal a setting as possible. That person is more prone to live up to this normal environment and those normal expectations."[23]

The establishment of specialized facilities specifically to serve the needs of persons who are retarded is in direct contradiction to the principle of normalization, because segregating them from average peers restricts their opportunities for the common, everyday experiences that help them become normalized. Normalization requires instead that, insofar as their ability permits, persons with retardation receive their educational and other services from the same agencies that serve ordinary people and in the same settings. Agencies and services that are designed and operated for the public as a whole rather than for any special subgroup, such as retarded people, are referred to in common usage and throughout this chapter as *generic*.

Two terms have come into use to describe the process of normalization, particularly as it applies in legal and educational matters: *least restrictive alternative* and *mainstreaming*.

1 Least restrictive alternative: At this time new laws affecting the living experience of individuals with retardation are being formulated in this country, largely in terms of securing normalizing experiences for them. This process uses the principle of the least restrictive alternative: "When government does have a legitimate communal interest to serve by regulating human conduct, it should use methods that curtail individual freedom to no greater extent than is essential for securing that interest."[24] Or, again more simply, "When you swat a mosquito on a friend's back, you should not use a baseball bat."[25]

2 Mainstreaming: Mainstreaming means that people who are retarded should be permitted to use generic services insofar as possible.[26] Although the concept refers to *all* generic services, it is currently most widely used by educators. It was within the perspective of the school system that the word *mainstreaming* was coined.[27] The federal government reinforced this concept through the passage of the Education for All Handicapped Children Act (Public Law 94-142) on November 29, 1975. This act mandates that all handicapped children from 3 to 21 years of age be provided a free education. School systems that do not have appropriate diagnostic and therapeutic facilities and personnel are legally bound to purchase whatever is required. In addition to full educational opportunities, other rights are covered by law: due process safeguards, which assist parents in challenging decisions regarding their children; education in the mainstream to the fullest extent possible; assurance that tests and other evaluation materials do not reflect cultural or racial bias; and a "child-find" plan to identify all children within the state who have special needs.

Increased numbers of mentally retarded people who were formerly segregated from mainstream contact are now living in neighborhood communities among nonretarded people. Some have come into the community after years of institutional living, and others have not been accepted by institutions that have recently restricted their population. These changes have affected communities in many ways. Professionals, parents, citizens, and those who provide service in the community, with no former real experience with people who are retarded, are not only being required to expand and improve services but are also being required to reexamine their attitudes toward these people and what they are capable of achieving.

Attitude reassessment is still occurring in most communities, but there is a beginning movement toward acceptance of mentally retarded individuals.

CHARACTERISTICS OF
MENTALLY RETARDED ADOLESCENTS

In order to establish a satisfying role in the community, the mentally retarded adolescent must, to the highest degree possible, accomplish the same developmental tasks that face others. The commonalities between retarded teenagers and their average peers are far more numerous than are the characteristics and needs that distinguish retarded young people from others. The great majority of adolescents who are retarded are only mildly so. For most of these adolescents, there may be only mild delay in the development of socially adaptive behaviors. These adolescents' greatest need is access to the world of average adolescent experiences.

Distinguishing characteristics are more likely to be exhibited by those individuals whose variation from the average in past and current functioning is greatest, a minimal percentage of all afflicted. This section will describe areas in which the experience of the mentally retarded adolescent may differ from the average. The paucity of data regarding the psychosocial development of the retarded adolescent and the magnitude of the differences among these individuals require that the perspective of individual variability be maintained, in terms of both the individual and the socializing milieu.

Individual Factors

The developmental tasks of adolescence will be examined with the goal of identifying the special problems that might be encountered by the retarded adolescent, the parents, and the nurse. Problems in handling adolescent tasks are often related to the level of cognitive functioning and to a diffused or negative sense of identity.

Cognitive Functioning　The transfer from simple, concrete thinking to the more complex intellectual functioning required for abstract thinking typically occurs during adolescence. Mental retardation interferes with this process, reducing the retarded adolescent's ability to plan activities, make judgments, transfer acquired skills from one function to another function independently, and understand the physical and emotional changes that are taking place.

In terms of cognitive functioning, the gap between the average person and the mentally retarded person becomes more evident during adolescence. Because the mentally retarded adolescent has adultlike physical features, there is a corresponding expectation by significant others that there will also be adultlike social behavior. During adolescence, it is no longer socially accepted for the mentally retarded adolescent to interact with children much younger than his or her chronological age. If previous life experiences did not provide this adolescent with the skills needed to interact with average adolescent peers, social isolation is likely to occur.

Richardson has focused on the problem of adolescents of borderline intelligence who are not labeled or who have never been labeled mentally retarded and who remain ineligible for remedial programs.[28] These "borderline" adolescents, as many educators will attest, experience severe difficulty in achieving success and legitimate status in school. Their poor performance is frequently attributed to inattention, poor study habits, or laziness. They too readily become the scapegoats of peers and teachers and develop a resentment toward authority figures. Some seek to achieve status among their peers through deviant and delinquent behavior. Because they are not identified as a population with special needs, they are not subjected to the stigmatization of a label, but they do not receive the benefits of specialized services. Their situation in some ways resembles the one in which those individuals found themselves when the definition of mental retardation was changed to exclude the borderline category. The reader will recall that needed rehabilitation services were thereby denied to less severely retarded adolescents and young adults. A major difference between the groups, which has implications for nurses, is that the never-labeled do not have special education classrooms. The adolescent tasks of establishing a personal identity, a role in the community, independence, authority coping, peer acceptance, and a positive sexual identity are all hindered with this group.

Developing a Positive Personal Identity   It is during adolescence that young people who are retarded are most forcefully confronted with the many ways they differ from others. Concrete evidence of these differences is manifest in the many adultlike activities that peers and siblings are often permitted the opportunity to participate in but are denied to these adolescents. Driving a car, dating, traveling alone, using the telephone, remaining alone at home, and having a group of friends the same age are some of these activities. Adolescents may not understand why they are not permitted to take the same risks and enjoy the same activities as their chronological peers. Vulnerability to suggestion and modeling may predispose their parents to unverified fears, as in the following example:

> Mrs. Cardan always personally took Keith, her 13-year-old mentally retarded adolescent, to social functions, believing that the only time Keith had socially acceptable behavior was when she was physically present in the situation. It was not until she was ill one night and her husband insisted that Keith be

allowed to go to a party with a friend and the friend's mother that Mrs. Cardan learned that Keith could handle social activities without her constant supervision.

A common stereotype that inhibits the promotion of a positive self-concept is that of the weak ego status that is often viewed as inherent in mental retardation. The ego of this adolescent is not a static entity, immune to change. The changes that do occur are the result of social conditioning processes. Unfortunately, many of the people who influence development throughout childhood and who still are involved in this adolescent's social conditioning processes do not believe that change can occur.

Anxiety is frequently experienced by anyone who approaches a new task. Retarded adolescents often do not have a repertoire of skills developed to the level of habit patterns that average adolescents apply to new skills automatically. Simpler tasks assume a complexity that increases retarded adolescents' feeling of certainty that they will fail. This may result in failure to try to do something new. Anxiety may cause them to be easily distracted, frustrating others so that they give up working with these adolescents rather than trying to increase their comfort by trying alternative strategies.

Tasks may be presented in language they may not understand and with a rapidity that leaves them confused so that they resort to defense mechanisms that reduce the stress encountered. Withdrawal is often the defense used. This is manifest in several ways: nodding eye contact that simulates understanding but may actually be a pretense, silence, avoidance of eye contact, a quick lift of the shoulder accompanied by "I dunno," or a physical exit from the situation. Scratching the hair or skin, frowning, and saying "What?" usually indicate the adolescent is trying to handle the confusion. This response is often met with impatience, if it is recognized at all as an attempt to handle the problem.

Inability to verbalize needs may be the result of expressive speech problems or may be caused by lack of opportunities to articulate needs. The adolescent's opinion about what is happening to him or her may not be sought, thus compounding feelings of anxiety. Even when these adolescents can speak, adults, including professionals, may seek information from their parents in their presence, ignoring the possibility that the adolescents have valid knowledge about themselves to contribute. This considerably reduces feelings of self-worth.

Opportunities to be instrumental in determining what happens to them are often lacking for mentally retarded individuals. Average childhood experience in making simple choices is reduced or denied. Under these circumstances, it is difficult to achieve a sense of mastery in relation to self and the environment.

Concrete experiences in making choices may still be absent or diminished in adolescence. Decisions about what to do or what to wear may be made by parents and other adults, without identifying cause-and-effect relationships in ways that can be comprehended by these adolescents.

The need for time to process new information and to respond is often met with impatience. Basic strategies for making choices and decisions with awareness of real or possible contingencies are often not developed. Lack of opportunity to experience themselves as capable contributes to a lack of confidence and to a diminished ability to be realistic about their capabilities.

Self-perceptions are often poor, enhancing difficulties in dealing with the reality of the true self. Defining self can be very threatening, especially when variations from average are great. A frequent experience of these adolescents is to hear others use terms that communicate to them that they are objects rather than persons. In referring to them, often in their presence, even professionals use terminology such as "a trainable," "a retardate," "an educable," "a Down's," or "a Mongoloid."

These adolescents often have had little experience that would contribute to their understanding of what mental retardation is. They have had concrete experiences that communicate that it is negative: ridicule from average peers, and avoidance of discussions about it with adults who themselves find it painful to deal with. As a result, they may deny this component of their personhood.

Others in the adolescent's immediate environment may attend to only negative aspects of his or her appearance, personality, and behavior, contributing to the perception of self as "bad." Sincere compliments in recognition of major accomplishments may not be forthcoming because, in comparison with what others of that age can do, this adolescent's achievements are so minimal that they do not seem significant.

Personal space is used to reflect self. With these adolescents, particularly those who have grown up in institutions, experience in the ownership of space may be limited to a bed that is no different from a multitude of others in the same room. When bedrooms are partially or totally owned in homes, decor often reflects the childlike percept of others or of self. Retarded adolescents' rooms often have stuffed animals or dolls in them. Rejection may be communicated through the quality of space. Walls may be drab and furniture old and used. The opportunity to choose paint colors, furnishings, and other decorative objects that reflect personal taste and feelings about self may be absent.

Respect for self is also reflected through experiencing privacy. This is particularly important when one is involved in a personal and intimate activity. It is not unusual to observe these adolescents toileting themselves without closing the bathroom door when others, even strangers, are around. When this happens, it is often ascertained, upon questioning, that this member of the family is the only one for whom closing the door is not required.

Personal space, when owned, is often invaded without permission. Parents often report that they have seen their sons or daughters masturbate because they opened bedroom doors without knocking or without waiting for a response after knocking. Apologies for this behavior, which is considered rude when done to the average person, are not made to this adolescent. This kind of modeling reduces opportunities for these adolescents to learn age-appropriate respect for the privacy of others.

Very often this adolescent is conditioned to be agreeable and conforming. Saying "yes" throughout childhood may have been a major source of acceptance, both in institutions and in family homes. Fear of nonacceptance of a negative response interferes with reality experiences in developing assertiveness. "Passive" is an adjective often used to describe retarded adolescents.

Experience in negotiating and compromising is often foreign to these adolescents. Their solution for conflict is often physical and concrete: fight or flight. These actions are not always understood by other people as natural outcomes of inexperience. If fight is used as a way to deal with conflict, the adolescent is labeled an angry, hostile individual.

Absence of encouragement to verbalize feelings allows no alternative but to act them out in ways that are viewed as childish and bizarre. Frustration, a common experience, may be dealt with through crying or withdrawal. The difference between having feelings and expressing these feelings responsibly is not made clear to retarded teenagers. Opportunities are lost to help the adolescent understand that having negative feelings is human and acceptable; the ways the feelings are expressed are immediately censured. Parents often report that they do not model ways to handle feelings appropriately.

Physical appearance plays a prominent part in the development of the self-concept during adolescence. Changes in physique bring about changes in what significant others expect in terms of behavior and what they permit in terms of social activities. Societal norms for sex-appropriate behavior become more evident. Adolescents who have retardation are pressured to conform to masculine and feminine roles, just as average adolescents are.

To a greater degree than average peers, the mentally retarded adolescent has limited understanding of the physical changes that are occurring in his or her body. Reassurance that these are a normal part of growing up is less available. Preparation for the changes is often absent, and assurance from parents and others that these changes are normal is often lacking. In contrast to other adolescents, retarded adolescents cannot find reassurance in reading magazines that address the commonality of changes, nor do they have the benefit of having a group of peers who describe the changes they are experiencing and the confusions and uncertainties that these changes arouse in them.

Understanding the changes is often made more confusing by lack of reinforcement of the idea that childish behavior is no longer acceptable. A school social worker reported that during the Christmas season a conflict often occurs among teachers and between teachers and parents as to whether or not an adolescent's fantasy about Santa Claus should be encouraged. Fear of being "cruel" by denying these adolescents the opportunity to sit on Santa's knee outweighs the adolescents' need to be confronted with the reality of responsibility to fulfill their own desires. They have little idea of how to get what they want.

Clothing and adornment may perpetuate the concept of self as child. Mentally retarded adolescents can be observed wearing Mickey Mouse barrettes in their hair and ankle socks instead of hose when they are 16 years old.

The adolescent girl may wish to use makeup. The parents of average adolescents are often horrified by the mannequinlike look of their daughters as they leave home, but they know that others will not consider them bad parents because of the way their daughters look. If this does happen, secure parents will know the problem lies with the critic. The parent of the adolescent who is retarded may not feel so secure. The adolescent may never have been allowed to choose between two lipsticks, with information given about the factors to be taken into consideration, such as skin tone, hair color, and color of clothing. If the adolescent chooses the inappropriate color, the parent may withdraw the choice and buy the more appropriate lipstick, thus contributing to the inadequate perception of self of the adolescent. Some adolescents are denied the opportunity to use makeup because its use reaffirms the fact that the risks of maturity, particularly sexuality, must be confronted.

Developing Independence   The mentally retarded adolescent's ability to experience self as independent is impeded, both by the common experience of being treated like a child and by the adolescent's perceptions of adults. These adolescents often see adults as omnipotent and not subject to rules. They may be unaware of the fact that adults are sometimes punished. This misunderstanding, coupled with their observations that children and they themselves are punished for infractions, reinforces their perception of themselves as dependent children.

It is difficult to conceptualize separation from parents when one does not perceive oneself as capable of being critical of all-powerful adults. Similarly, when this adolescent's daily experience includes parent participation in self-care tasks, confidence that one can function without parents is absent.

Lack of practice in attempting or completing tasks is the most frequent reason for the adolescent's failure to assume completely independent functioning. Parents often assume responsibility for part or all of a task for several reasons. The adolescent's readiness to assume greater responsibility for self may not be evident, because signs of readiness are often very subtle and the parent may not be alert to them. Parents need to help their retarded adolescents practice frequently and be constantly alert to the subtlest approximation to a task. This requires patience and persistence and can be accompanied by frustration and a conflicting desire to perform other necessary activities. It is often easier and more expedient for the parent to do the task.

Fear that the adolescent will be ridiculed and that others will think the parent is neglecting the child may motivate the parent to intervene to try to assure social acceptance. For example, a mother may continue to lay out clothing that matches when the adolescent has demonstrated capability in accomplishing all other aspects of dressing. If a parent has not done this and the adolescent chooses his or her own clothing, the prophesied fears may materialize: The adolescent may be ridiculed by peers. This may result in the adolescent's asking the parents' advice in choosing matching clothes, thus perpetuating dependency. If the adolescent comes home angry or crying, the parents' tendency may be to view the event as a painful failure, reinforcing the need to revert to the "necessary" protective pattern of putting out the clothes.

Mentally retarded adolescents often do not have some of the self-help skills usually learned during childhood. They may be unable to conceptualize in the abstract, and skills learned in one task are not likely to be transferred automatically. Parents may not know how to help the adolescent and may be frustrated by repeated failure experiences. They may perceive inability as stubbornness or unwillingness to learn.

Parents can easily lose patience, particularly when they feel they must carry out a task they had assigned to the adolescent. They tire of repeating simple instructions and give in to frustration. These occasions are particularly confusing to this adolescent, whose child-adult inner vacillations are worsened by lack of follow-through. A feeling of childish hopelessness can result.

The perception of childish inability may carry over into lack of confidence in retarded adolescents' ability to assume responsibility for some of the tasks that are shared by all family members, or even responsibility for caring for their own rooms. These adolescents see their siblings being required to do what they are not allowed to do. This experience, repeated many times, reaffirms the feeling of being different and not belonging.

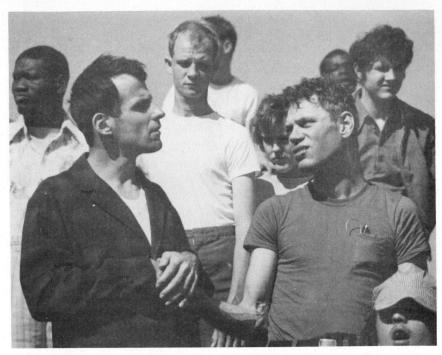

Peer companionship and the expression of feelings are necessary for adjustment and at-tainment of developmental tasks among retarded as well as unretarded young people. (*Copyright* © *1980 by Anne Campbell.*)

Dependence on others to move around the community severely limits the adolescent's independence. This adolescent is frequently transported by the family or accompanied by someone the family trusts when public transportation is used. Arrangements for transportation may become habitual and stereotyped, reflecting a pattern of treating the adolescent like a child. Cues of adolescent readiness to assume responsibility are often missed. An adolescent may have been participating in a work activity center for months, and the staff may continue to remind the adolescent when it is time to clean up the work area so that he or she will be ready for the bus. This habit serves the staff more than it does the adolescent.

Mobility around a building or a neighborhood requires that the adolescent become able to interpret traffic signals and other signs that enable people to reach their intended destinations. Because of the risks involved in moving around independently, this adolescent is often accompanied by an adult who acts on signs and other cues without identifying these to the adolescent. This minimizes the risk that the adolescent will be hit by a car, get lost, or go into the wrong building or room, but it deprives him or her of the opportunity to learn about relevant cues for mobility. When going to a new place, average adults often draw maps clearly identifying major reference points. Some adults even take out the map prior to returning home. Opportunities to prevent anxiety and acquire a feeling of independence by using this same strategy often are not made available to the adolescent. Adults are aware of the value of approaching strangers to ask directions. Fear of the adolescent's vulnerability to strangers and a lack of confidence in the ability to discriminate a safe adult to approach may prevent the parent from teaching the adolescent how to do this. Some adolescents may have been taught how to identify police officers, but opportunities to practice application of this knowledge may not be made available. The benefits of rehearsal and role-play may not be appreciated by parents.

This adolescent often has a severely restricted set of alternatives for use of leisure time. After-school activities are often limited to playing with younger children outdoors, playing with toys in his or her room, or watching television. This restrictive pattern is useful in that it is safe and involves minimal time and energy expenditure on the part of the parents. Parents may be aware of the social, emotional, and cognitive benefits to be gained by enlarging the number of activities available, but they may be more influenced by fears of the adolescent's inability to make appropriate choices and to plan for activities. Usually these fears are the result of inadequate demonstration by the adolescent of the ability to do so when appropriate support is provided, and the parents fear that the adolescent may experience painful disappointment in a new social experience. It is easy to forget that most, if not all, adults have experienced indecision and anxiety before entering a new experience and that their fears of rejection have sometimes been realized and pain experienced. Eventually awkwardness is overcome and pleasant feelings replace anxiety. However, the parent of the mentally retarded adolescent, when focusing on the vulnerability and the inadequacy of social skills, concentrates on the negative aspects of a new social experience and often does not make the choice available.

Preparation for Vocation   Sustained dependency, particularly in self-help skills (such as grooming) and peer interaction skills, is a major hindrance to successful vocational preparation. Self-care skills and awareness of rights and responsibilities of self and others greatly influence job retention. The adolescent who never learns to set an alarm is less likely to be on time for work. The same applies to one who has never risked use of public transportation. How does this adolescent get to work when the family car isn't working?

Childish behavior often reinforced earlier may be repeated in the job situation. If an adolescent has been allowed to interrupt conversations between two adults in the home setting, he or she may not realize that this is considered inappropriate in another setting.

Parents may have conflicting feelings about having the adolescent prepare for work because of their lack of confidence in the possibility of success when the adolescent competes in the job market and the threat of loss of Social Security income if money is earned.

Retarded adolescents often need to learn how to contribute services to others. They may not have experienced opportunities to assist in cooking and housework and to learn how much their work helped the parents and other family members. Opportunities are lost to teach these adolescents to be aware of others' needs and of the give-and-take of shared work situations.

Expression of Sexuality Much of what has already been said in terms of developing a positive identity and independence is relevant to how this adolescent handles developing sexuality. Special needs, parental concerns, and suggested strategies for nursing intervention have been extensively described by Pattullo.[29-33]

When private and intimate activities related to self-help are assumed by parents or siblings of the opposite sex, explicit messages are given that this adolescent is not a sexual being. Fathers may be fastening brassieres and brothers bringing a forgotten towel into the bathroom.

Participation of opposite-sex family members in intimate self-care activities may also be a clue to the possibility of incest. Sexual abuse of the mentally retarded adolescent girl by family members may occur for the same reasons it does with average adolescents. However, the vulnerability of adolescents who are retarded is increased. They are often even more in need of the demonstration and verbalization of affection that accompanies this practice. They often are more vulnerable to threats of recrimination and may not understand the significance of the conflicting messages they receive with this activity. Karen, a 13-year-old adolescent girl known to us, was sexually molested for a year by her stepfather before she told her mother. She feared her stepfather's threat to put her into an institution if she told anyone about their sexual activities.

The sexuality of persons who are retarded has been the subject of myths that are often not only untrue but contradictory. Retarded people have been described as undersexed, oversexed, asexual, infertile when retardation is severe, and late in maturing.[34] In spite of evidence to the contrary, the myths are pervasive and are even described in the professional literature.[35] Mattinson's study of formerly institutionalized adults impressed her with the quality of the affectional relationships she saw during her interviews with retarded couples.[36]

Parents' feelings about their adolescents' sexuality are influenced by many factors. Parents may not be comfortable with the reawakening of their own adolescent conflicts or with having to deal with an area that is causing them personal distress in their own lives at the time of their sons' and daughters' pubescence. They may be experiencing emotional trauma related to their own life changes, which may be viewed as loss of sexual attractiveness, at the same time that physical evidence indicates their sons and daughters are developing what they are losing.

Parents may not have had the opportunity to learn that their fears of the risks involved for their adolescents when they become involved in caring relationships are quite usual. Perske has recognized the difficulties parents experience in permitting their adolescents to take the risks involved in interdependent, caring relationships.[37] Professionals rarely open up this area as one that is legitimate for direct discussion. This only serves to reinforce the parents' feelings that the sexual nature of their sons and daughters should be denied or repressed. Professional insecurities do not help parents learn how to help themselves and their adolescents. Parents commonly worry about vulnerability to sexual exploitation, public masturbation or exposure of the genitals, difficulties with self-care during menstruation, socially disapproved ways of dealing with sexual curiosity, and pregnancy.

Parents who attend workshops on sexuality may feel threatened by what they perceive to be an irresponsibly liberal perspective that is in conflict with their own values. Exclusion of their input into sex education programs conducted in schools or sheltered workshops compounds their fears and increases their anger with those who are presumptuous enough to assume this prerogative without their sanction. The excluded parent who is denying the sexuality of sons or daughters may fear that learning about sex may stimulate ideas and activities that would otherwise not occur.

Assumptions regarding parents' knowledge about sex may be unfounded. When such an assumption is communicated, it is more difficult for the parents to ask for the help they need to assist their sons and daughters.

The adolescents themselves may feel confused about their erotic impulses, particularly when they receive mixed messages regarding how to deal with them. The opportunity to learn that all of these feelings are manifestations of attributes they have in common with other people is lost when sexuality is not discussed with them.

Visualizing internal organs is difficult for the average adolescent. The use of diagrams that show the pelvic area may be conceptually integrated by the average adolescent, but to the mentally retarded adolescent they may have no meaning in relation to self. Diagrams that show the pelvic region in relation to the total human body are more meaningful to the retarded adolescent.

Peer Relationships   Mentally retarded adolescents have little or no peer contact outside the school setting, both in direct interactions and by telephone. Average adolescents use the telephone to extend contact with others who are going through this very confusing stage and are thus reinforced that they are not alone in what they are experiencing. The mentally retarded adolescent may not even know how to use a telephone independently. Speech difficulties may have resulted in the abrupt termination of conversation by someone who misunderstood the hesitancy or poorly articulated speech. Feelings of rejection related to phone experiences may inhibit attempts to learn how to use it independently.

Developing friendships is a complex process involving subtle behaviors, which average adolescents learn over time with and from peers their own age. Mentally retarded adolescents' friends are usually younger children with whom they feel more comfortable but from whom they do not learn the increasingly complex stages of developing reciprocally responsible friendships. A parent proudly related that her son had an average friend his age. When asked what they did together, the parent replied, "Oh, they wrestle."

Average chronological peers may ridicule the appearance and awkward behavior of retarded adolescents. Clothing selected for them may not be like that worn by chronological age peers, further setting them apart. Opportunities to demonstrate success in peer-related activities are often lacking because parents fear ridicule and competition.

Retarded adolescents may describe, to parents and others, peer activities that lead the adults to assume the adolescent is involved in activities that are age appropriate. One parent reported that her daughter went to teen dances. Discussion with the daughter revealed that she was a passive observer.

Health Promotion   Adolescents' past experiences with health professionals greatly influence how motivated they are to become involved in health maintenance activities. Past experiences often have been negative and are remembered as anxiety producing. Often these adolescents have been excluded from any participation in the management planning process, even to the point of not being told why they are going to a particular health care facility. Even for adults, going for care is a major adjustment accompanied by anxiety, and adults at least know why they are going and what to expect when they get there. Letters regarding appointments are often addressed to parents without even adding the name of the adolescent in the salutation.

Health promotion needs are greatest in the areas of nutrition and dentistry. Obesity is a frequent problem, a result of lack of exercise and a high carbohydrate intake. Candy is often given to adolescents by parents to help make up for the positive experiences they are missing in their lives.

These adolescents may not have developed the habit of brushing their teeth as the last part of the total process of eating. Developing such a pattern as a habit is not so necessary for average adolescents, because they can more readily conceptualize the cause-and-effect relationship between plaque formation and painful decay. The retarded adolescent may avoid going to the dentist, and the parent may not require it. This may be avoidance of exposure to a painful experience, but the possibility that the parent or dentist questions whether the adolescent is worthy of costly attention should also be considered.

In general, it is known that there is an increased possibility of the presence of physical deviation among individuals with mental retardation. Some of these physical deviations are growth failure, cerebral palsy, fine and gross motor deficits, congenital heart problems, and dental abnormalities.[38]

It is generally observed that neurological problems are increased in this population. Functions that may be affected include physical growth, fine and gross motor activity, vision, hearing, speech, and the ability to attend to relevant stimuli. Hammar and Barnard found that 70 percent of the adolescents who were receiving services in a specialized clinic had signs of central nervous system dysfunction and/or physical defects.[39] Nurses working with mentally retarded adolescents to promote health maintenance should be alert to their need for a complete physical evaluation.

Socializing Milieu

Deficiencies and delays in the retarded child's functioning influence parents to alter their childrearing approaches to accommodate the child's deficiencies. By adolescence, parenting patterns aimed at reducing risk to the child and anxiety in the parent have been reinforced so frequently that they become automatic means of preventing and ameliorating problems. At adolescence, the child's response to internal and external changes, coupled with the parent's focus on vulnerability and deficiency, heightens the potential for protective patterns to become exaggerated to the extent that they may assume a defensive rigidity that interferes with the adolescent's opportunities to take the risks necessary to adapt to the more complex demands of the larger social milieu. Parents are often unaware of the degree to which protective management patterns increase the frequency of problems encountered by their adolescents.[40]

Many parents were advised, at the birth of the child, that their children would never mature. It is less likely that these parents, by the time the child reaches adolescence, have resolved the dynamic conflict that surrounds having a retarded child. Indeed, the conflict may be exacerbated: "Pubescent changes tend to catalyze problems and perceptions of him in others which were dormant or non-existent previously."[41] The "others" in the statement include nurses and other professionals, parents, siblings, peers, other nonfamilial but professionally concerned persons, and the general community.

In spite of recent legislative advances such as Public Law 94–142, the parents' search for appropriate training programs for their retarded sons and daughters still occurs. Acute shortages of recreational, vocational, and social services exist, particularly for those with additional handicaps.[42]

Even families that initially receive comprehensive medical diagnostic evaluations often fail to obtain follow-up medical guidance and counseling later. Hence, families often are without help from a physician or other health professional and are ill-prepared for the difficulties that may arise with pubescent growth and sexual maturation.[43] Professionals, as well as parents, may be responsible for the failure to maintain health services and developmental guidance.

Rarely throughout their child's lifetime are parents involved as significant participants in the process of determining the services they and their child receive, yet the ultimate responsibility for care rests with them. Lack of opportunity for participation with professionals in planning care deprives parents of needed experiences that would help them to be more informed and qualified in carrying out parental responsibilities. More than frustrating exclusion by self-protecting professional experts is involved. Parents *do* have feelings and observations to contribute, and involving parents in planning gives an explicit message of their worth and dignity.[44]

Often professionals do not involve the parents in planning because of their own unresolved feelings about mental retardation. Professionals, like parents, do have positive or negative feelings, which either facilitate or inhibit therapeutic intervention. It is essential for nurses to analyze their feelings and develop appropriate ways to deal with negative feelings so that they do not interfere with the therapeutic process.

NURSES' FEELINGS

There are a number of factors that cause nurses to experience a variety of feelings in the early stages of working with mentally retarded adolescents. Integration into the mainstream of average experience for children who are mentally retarded is a relatively recent phenomenon. It is unlikely that nurses have had, during their own childhood period of attitude development, opportunities for balanced experiences with mentally retarded children—experiences that would have allowed for an appreciation of

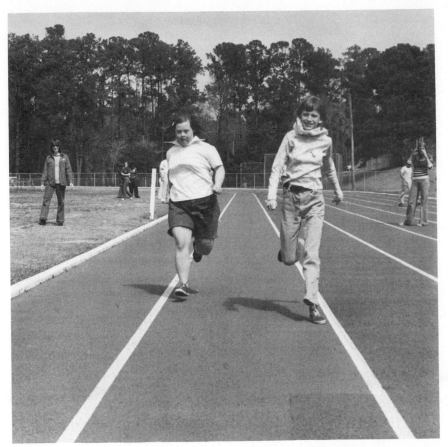

Competitive, comparative experiences are a part of living. People who are retarded need opportunities for recreational and other kinds of competitive activities under circumstances in which they realistically *can* participate and compete. (*Copyright © 1980 by Anne Campbell*.)

these persons' human qualities and strengths. It is likely that the dynamics operating in the community have applied to the nurses and that the early socializing experience for them has been one of fear, avoidance, and withdrawal.

Mental retardation is a chronic condition that cannot be cured. Progress toward defined goals occurs in small increments. The reward system for the nurse has to be redefined. Small gains, which take time and patience to validate through many intensive experiences, become important sources of role satisfaction. This is in contrast to the shorter-term interventions, which are less demanding of the self and more likely to be learned in basic nursing preparation.

The nurse can never truly identify with these adolescents or with their families. There are some aspects with which the nurse can identify, but there is a risk that the focus of these will be too narrow and will emphasize the differences rather than the similarities. Or the opposite can occur, with such a focus on positives that the special needs due to differences are denied.

Revulsion and fear in response to retarded persons are not uncommon general feelings that occur as a function of normal socialization, before actual experience. These feelings can be intensified or ameliorated during first contact with someone who has retardation. If the first experience occurs in a visit to an institution when the nurse is unprepared, the sights, odors, and sounds of the setting and the people in it can be experienced as grotesquely inhuman. Guilt-producing thoughts can occur, particularly the question, ''Why?'' Why did it happen? Why are they being saved? Nurses are socialized to be accepting. When they feel rejecting instead, they may readily feel guilty about that. When they experience guilt, it can make them angry. If they cannot channel the anger into constructive experience, they can feel depressed, overwhelmed, and shocked.

Anger can be experienced in other situations. If the parents put the child or adolescent out of the natural home, the nurse can become angry with them, especially at this time when normalization places such emphasis on providing for average experience. This anger can result in the nurse's putting undue and undeserved pressure on the family. The nurse must ask, ''Could I deal with it myself? Do I really understand what the family is experiencing?'' The honest answer is, ''I don't know.'' Nurses who experience anger can sometimes resolve it by examining the reasons for the anger.

Identification with the family produces feelings that hurt, and identification is promoted by the frequency and intensity of contact needed. Denial may occur. A nursing student became angry when she saw the staff nurse's description of the young retarded mother she was visiting. The student felt the young mother should become independent of her parents, because the student saw only what she wanted to see. In collecting planning care data, she observed the young mother's expressions of care for her infant, resented the grandmother's presence, and did not investigate why this mother's first child had been removed by the court. In this first involvement with mental retardation, and in trying to understand it, she focused so much on the positive aspects that she ignored relevant clues. Only when her faculty adviser pointed this out to her did she find out that this adolescent mother had frequent temper outbursts in which she behaved destructively and threatened the safety of the child. Independence was still an appropriate goal, but a long-term one. First the young mother had to be taught how to handle her feelings more appropriately.

Families of adolescents are often sad because they can no longer avoid the reality of maturation and the feeling of hopelessness that accompanies recognition that these adolescents will never really experience the fullest that life has to offer. There are books that will never be read, discussions about abstract subjects that will never occur, subtleties of humor that will never be appreciated, and countless other experiences that are valued by the academically oriented family in particular. The sadness and hopelessness can be felt by nurses, who may also grieve over what is lost to such adolescents. Nurses must help the family and themselves to value the qualities the adolescents *do* have, including their potential for benefiting from experiences that are developmentally within their grasp.

By the time their sons and daughters become adolescents, families have often been through a number of frustrating experiences with professionals that made them angry. Lack of follow-through, lack of recognition of the value of parent participation, false encouragement that the child would outgrow the condition, or unacceptable advice to "put the child away" all leave some bitterness and anger. Nurses may not understand why the parents are so hostile unless they find out what the parents' past experiences with nurses have been. Only then will nurses understand that the parents are projecting accumulated feelings. Accepting this anger without trying to defend the professionals who had contact with the family before is a necessary first step. Then a new, clear contract can be negotiated.

The nurse may empathize with the mother who has little time for herself and for friends because she spends so much time with the retarded child or adolescent. One nurse, empathizing with the mother, became overinvolved and tried to be the friend the mother didn't have time to find. She found a sitter and took the mother bowling. When her supervisor helped her analyze what was happening, she realized she was trying to handle the guilt she was feeling because she was so glad that the retarded adolescent was not her child. But she was doing it in a way that prevented the mother from establishing a more wholesome life for herself with long-term friendship rewards developed by herself.

Some mothers who don't have other social outlets will try to manipulate the nurse into staying for a longer time by waiting for the end of a visit to talk about something that relates directly to the focus of the visit. One mother waited until the nurse picked up her purse to say, "My husband didn't get home from work until midnight all this week." This put the nurse in conflict. She had another appointment, but she wanted to know how the mother perceived her husband's behavior. The visit went on for another hour, and the nurse felt guilty about missing her next appointment and angered by the conflict. This nurse talked with a social worker colleague about what happened. He helped her to see that the issue was one of control that could only be managed if the nurse and mother reestablished the original contract of mutual involvement for a given period of time. At the beginning of the first visit after the renegotiation, the mother greeted the nurse by showing her the lobster thermidor she had made for their lunch. The nurse said she was sorry she couldn't stay to eat it because she had other plans for lunch. From that time on the visits were focused.

When nurses have feelings that are painful, they must recognize that they are real, valid parts of their person. They must decide how they are going to handle the feelings. They have a choice between suppressing them or analyzing their source and taking action to channel them appropriately. All nurses who work with mentally retarded individuals need someone with whom they can talk about their feelings and have them accepted. Under these conditions, it is possible to understand oneself and one's actions.

Extremely rewarding feelings can occur. Many times the nurse's enthusiasm in identifying approximations toward skill development is a new experience for parents. They begin to experience their children in new ways. Deficiencies are deemphasized as strengths are perceived and appreciated. The nurse realizes how valuable his or her interventions are, and positive feelings ensue.

NURSING ROLE

As the trend toward the use of generic services increases, nurses in the community are increasingly likely to have more frequent and sustained contact with mentally retarded adolescents and their families. The multiplicity and complexity of these adolescents' needs mandates close coordination with professionals from other disciplines within each agency and with other agencies serving these individuals, as well as coordination among nurses in different settings.

The challenges to the flexibility and creativity of nurses are great. Because many of these adolescents have experienced a prolonged and often confusing childhood, the disparity between their physical appearance and their functioning increases the risk of ascribing their behavior to the condition of mental retardation. Focusing on the label rather than the person can distort thinking to such a degree that nurses may fail to recognize the existence of those human needs and behaviors that will benefit most from intervention. The social behavior and self-concept that developed primarily as a function of inadequate and insufficient previous life experiences can be changed. A major nursing contribution requires the application of the belief in the unique individuality and potential for growth of every human being. In order to help these adolescents to handle their current situation, the nurse must recognize that their previous socializing milieu was considerably different from that of other adolescents. The special learning needs of adolescents who are mentally retarded require astute observation of adolescent functioning and of adolescent and parent interaction, careful planning of intervention strategies, and considerable patience, because changes can occur very slowly. Tasks that average children accomplish at a much earlier age may have to be a focus of intervention. Basic precursor skills may need to be developed.

A *family-centered preventive counseling* approach to care is particularly relevant when the nurse is working with the adolescent who is retarded. It is critical for the nurse to focus on the entire family system, because parents, siblings, and the mentally retarded adolescent *all* can have difficulty understanding and accepting the handicapping condition.

When a nurse deals with parents who have mentally retarded children, one thing becomes clear: Parents do not wish for a child who is mentally retarded. When the child is born, emotional conflict often comes clearly into consciousness. Defenses are necessary to maintain personal integrity when the diagnosis is made:"No, not my child. This isn't happening to me." Initial denial preserves the parents' integrity. Fears about what mental retardation really means then begin to emerge. Parents often handle these fears with anger. Anger is a second healing step in the process of resolution. First it is expressed as "Why me? Why us?"; later, it is "Why him?" or "Why her?" The rate of the process of resolution of anger varies, and the treatment that parents receive from professionals is a major factor influencing the degree to which it is resolved.

As the child matures, each new phase of development and each contact with friends, strangers, relatives, and professionals has the potential for causing a reemergence of the parents' denial and anger. Some parents, by the time the child reaches adolescence, have developed healthy mechanisms for coping. Others' attempts to move in this direction are thwarted. As Gorham and colleagues have pointed out, parents of mentally retarded children repeatedly experience closed doors when seeking services. Society's message quickly becomes clear: Your child is not worthy of investment of time, energy, and money. The message may be mixed, particularly at this time of society's movement toward humanism: We recognize that your child *needs* more than other children, but he or she will get less because he or she is less worthy to society. The parents feel devalued and often *are*. They are more likely to receive services for their children during childhood than during adolescence. Vocational training and socializing recreational activities are sorely lacking for the adolescent population group.[45]

One mother has described how her anger had to be suppressed for

fear of losing a resource for her adolescent son. He was 16 and, in contrast
to his siblings, did not have access to regular summer recreation and other
developmental experiences. This summer he had been accepted in a special
school program. She arrived to pick him up after school and found he
was just waking up from a nap in the nurse's room. She was advised to
pick him up an hour earlier the next day, because he had seemed so tired
toward the end of the day. The mother felt intensely angry, because
daytime sleepiness occurred only when her son was bored or being
"treated like an object." She did not permit herself to reveal her anger,
however, because this program was the only one available.[46]

Siblings of mentally retarded individuals are often ignored by both
parents and health professionals. A quick review of professional literature
relative to the impact of the handicapped child on the family will clearly
illustrate this point. There usually is a detailed description of the emotional
reactions of parents but little or no discussion of how siblings react to the
birth of a handicapped child. Simply asking parents, "What do your other
children know about your daughter's or son's mental retardation?" will
give the nurse clues about how the parents are relating to the siblings of
their handicapped child.

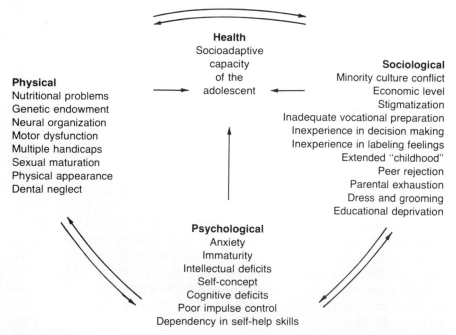

Figure 7-1   Factors influencing the health and socioadaptive capacity of the adolescent with
mental retardation. (*Modified from Sterling D. Garrard, "Mental Retardation in Adolescence,"*
Pediatric Clinics of North America, **7**[1]:*150, 1960.*)

Siblings have fears, feelings of shame and guilt, and concerns regarding peer and parental rejection, and these feelings must be handled. The siblings are at high risk for developing emotional and behavioral difficulties, which would only increase the stress on the entire family unit. Health problems of individual family members are interconnected. We have frequently found that parents are unable to consistently implement a management plan with their mentally retarded adolescent because of the demands made on their time and energy by their other children. With this in mind, it is imperative that the nurse provide service to all family members.

The primary service responsibilities of nursing in the care of adolescents with mental retardation are threefold: (1) assessment of the health and functional skills of the adolescent and family, (2) assessment of the interaction between the adolescent and significant others, and (3) intervention to facilitate optimal health and socioadaptive functioning of the family unit. The nursing process, a scientific, systematic problem-solving approach with four major subparts—assessment, planning, implementation, and evaluation—is the major tool used to meet the above nursing service responsibilities. Although each component of the nursing process is discussed separately in the following sections, it is important to remember that these four activities may overlap, repeat, and/or take place concurrently.

Assessment

Assessment is a data collection and analysis process used as a foundation for developing a management plan. During this process, the nurse should collect specific data from all available resources. Interview, observation, direct examination, and review of relevant records should be used in order to obtain accurate and complete assessment data. Strengths as well as needs should be identified. The assessment process is most effectively handled when the nurse has developed a trusting, therapeutic relationship with the mentally retarded adolescent and the family.

There are numerous variables that affect the health status of the mentally retarded adolescent. The interdependence of these variables is illustrated in Figure 7-1. The reader will quickly discern that an overwhelming number of the factors shown are influenced by the environment. Few are inherent in the individual and immune to change. That is why it is essential to do a functional assessment in the natural environments of the mentally retarded adolescent. The clinical situation is atypical in terms of the daily routine of this adolescent. It requires adaptations to new physical surroundings as well as to new people.

The functional assessment is the major vehicle used for planning and monitoring the effectiveness of nursing and other professional interventions. This assessment often provides an opportunity to demonstrate to the parent that the adolescent can learn self-care in gradual steps. Ideally, home visits to assess functioning in the various activities of daily living should be made during the time when the activities occur naturally as a part of the daily routine. Conditions at these times are more likely to be optimal for the adolescent to demonstrate the highest level of skill.

The functional assessment is a dynamic diagnostic process having two focuses: (1) the identification of the quantity and quality of the adolescent's adaptive or problem-solving strategies and (2) the identification of environmental factors that inhibit or facilitate the functioning of the adolescent. The assessment framework generally used during this process is the developmental framework. This framework focuses on developmental tasks or skills and activities that must be accomplished before the individual proceeds to the next developmental stage. It provides guidelines for the nurse to use when formulating a nursing diagnosis relative to the strengths and needs of current functioning. The developmental tasks for the adolescent have been discussed in Chapter 1 and thus will not be repeated here. The nurse, however, should review these tasks prior to doing a functional assessment.

Self-help skills, activities of daily living, social adjustment, and developmental maturation are usually the areas evaluated during a functional assessment. Some of the activities and factors the nurse should observe and/or inquire about are:

1 Parents', siblings', and adolescent's concerns
2 Eating
3 Dressing
4 Grooming
5 Toileting
6 Mobility
7 Fine and gross motor skills
8 Communication skills
9 Social skills
10 Recreational activities
11 Opportunities for making choices (and ways these opportunities are dealt with)
12 Modeling sources
13 Attention span
14 Ability to comprehend requests and verbalize understanding
15 Behaviors used to accommodate physical handicaps
16 Handling of feelings
17 General health status
18 Adolescent's management of sexual impulses and parents' responses to sexual behavior

Critical observation is essential during a functional assessment. The behaviors of the adolescent and significant others during a given task often reveal their usual patterns of interaction. Performing a part of a particular skill may be so automatic that the parent may not be aware of giving assistance. A parent may believe the adolescent is independent in dressing, but the nurse may observe the parent rebuttoning a coat instead of identifying the problem and assisting the adolescent to solve it.

The dependency message the adolescent receives may be verbal as well as active: "Here, I'll cut up your meat or you'll mess up the table." It cannot be assumed that independent functioning is present in other self-help activities when dependency is observed in one. Interviewing about toileting may reveal that a parent takes care of wiping or flushing. The parent, in describing the activity, may become aware of the degree of help he or she gives. This provides an opportunity for the nurse to suggest ways that the adolescent can manage the total task alone.

Behaviors that increase skill level in social functioning are particularly important to assess. The telephone is an important vehicle for maintaining peer contact, but often it is a terrifying obstacle to the adolescent with speech difficulties. One young man with slow speech and poor articulation was 19 years old before he tried to make the second telephone call of his life. His first call was made to a disc jockey when the youth was 12, with his parent dialing the number. The experience of having the person on the other end of the phone hang up was so traumatic that he refused to try again. It was suggested that he practice dialing a recorded message until he learned how to dial and became comfortable with the instrument. The next step was to have him practice calling family members and friends who knew of his speech impediment.

Much of the focus up to this point has been on the mentally retarded adolescent. In order to develop an effective management plan, it is important to elicit specific details about current functioning. It is equally significant, however, to determine the family's responses to their current situation. How much time and energy can they or are they willing to give to provide optimal learning experiences for this adolescent? Making family members feel guilty about their lack of involvement if they are already exhausted does nothing to help their mentally retarded adolescent. Tasks to be achieved that seem significant to the nurse may not be so significant to the family. Assess where the family is and how much they can handle. Determine what behaviors are most important for them to change at this time. Plan *with* the family, not for the family.

Planning

The planning process involves two major activities: (1) formulation of goals and (2) identification and examination of alternative interventions to achieve the goals. Contracting, or setting mutual goals, is a necessary first step in this process. Adolescent and parent involvement in goal setting clarifies the expectations of all concerned. This increases motivation to work together on the problem, increasing trust and reducing anxiety so that the adolescent and the parents are comfortably and adequately prepared for changes in their own and the nurse's behavior. The mutual determination of both long- and short-term goals also contributes to the independence of both the adolescent and the family.

The importance of involving the adolescent in the process of goal setting cannot be emphasized enough. Due to the high likelihood that the opportunity to be instrumental and self-determining in previous life experiences has been deficient or absent, special considerations are necessary. Because this is so often a new experience, there is an increased possibility that anxiety will be present. Adolescents may be anxious because they do not know why they are talking with the nurse. They may fear that the nurse will be administering a test, and the feelings accumulated from a variety of past failures may be operating. Previous contacts with nurses may have been related to illness and pain, both physical and emotional.

The process of reducing anxiety will involve considerable patience on the part of the nurse. It is helpful to begin the process when the family is together. Parental presence validates the appropriateness of the discussion and the adolescent's participation. This is most important in relation to sexuality, for often the adolescent has had strict admonitions not to talk about sex to strangers. Beginning the relationship in the presence of parents also gives the nurse an opportunity to observe the adolescent's conversational style and expressive language repertoire. During the time that the family is together, remarks concerning the adolescent should be addressed to him or her in a normal conversational tone. Only if the adolescent has difficulty hearing should the voice level be raised. Addressing the focus remarks to the adolescent in a normal tone of voice reduces the possibility of seeing the adolescent as a child not capable or worthy of contributing to his or her management in a responsible way.

This adolescent often needs a longer period of time to process what has been said and to formulate a response. The nurse should communicate a patient and positive expectancy that the adolescent will respond. During this time, the nurse should observe for cues that indicate the adolescent has understood and is working on formulating a response. Because the interval may be lengthy, the nurse may be tempted to resort to other strategies to obtain the information, such as involving the adult present or quickly rewording to obtain the information. Addressing the question or remark to the adult present discounts the value of the adolescent's contribution and places him or her in the role of dependent child. Not only is the adolescent likely to experience a feeling of rejection, but the opportunity to find out what the adolescent thinks is going to happen and how he or she feels about it is lost. Rewording a remark or question too quickly or in too many ways confuses the adolescent and interferes with both understanding and response formulation. When lack of understanding is clearly evident after an appropriate interval, the nurse should ask if the adolescent understood what was being said and should rephrase the question.

As many cues as necessary should be used in communicating with the adolescent. Use of the hands; identification of the relationship of the new word with a familiar word or activity; and use of pictures, diagrams, cards with words printed on them, and objects are all helpful. Gentle touch often communicates support and understanding.

Only one idea should be presented at a time. Words should be enunciated clearly and at a pace that can be comprehended. The language used should be that which is at the highest level that the adolescent can comprehend. Ideas should be concrete rather than abstract. "Why" questions may present difficulty.

Problems that may be encountered in communicating with the adolescent may be related to the parents' usual pattern of behavior. They may make assumptions about how the adolescent will respond and predict failure in the presence of the adolescent. They may feel that the nurse is becoming impatient while waiting for a response and may assume the role of information giver. They may never have had the experience of having the adolescent participate in health management planning and may predict lack of cooperation or inability to do so.

After the family, the adolescent, and the nurse have formulated specific management goals, these goals should be ordered from most significant to least significant. The nurse should point out that the likelihood of success is greatest when one new task or skill is worked on at a time. Again it should be emphasized that the behaviors that the family and the adolescent want to change first should be dealt with first.

There are generally various intervention strategies that can be used to achieve the stated goals. During the planning process, the pros and cons of the various options that can be used to facilitate the client's problem-solving efforts should be discussed. What the nurse sees as the most feasible alternative may not be viewed as such by the family. For instance, the nurse may believe that the adolescent can best work on self-help skills in a structured community service program. The family, on the other hand, may believe that the best alternative would be intervention in the home environment. They may allow a referral to be made to the community program but not help to get the adolescent to the center. What, then, has been accomplished? Probably frustration for all involved parties, including the nurse.

It is important, however, that the family and the nurse recognize that the nurse cannot handle all problems alone. During the planning phase, the nurse should discriminate among problems that can be handled by the nurse, problems that can be handled by the family and the adolescent, and problems that necessitate referral to other community resources, such as a clinical nurse specialist, a physical therapist, or a special education teacher. An *interdisciplinary* approach to care is particularly significant when the mentally retarded adolescent has multiple handicaps. In these situations, the nurse in the generic setting might find it especially helpful to use the clinical nurse specialist as a consultant. This nurse usually has advanced educational preparation and clinical experience that focus on both mental retardation and the interdisciplinary process. Except in institutions, specialist services are often limited to the diagnostic and management planning process. The provision of continuity of quality nursing service, that is, ongoing intervention to facilitate optimal health and socioadaptive functioning of the family unit, is frequently the responsibility of the generic agency nurse.

Implementation

Once the managment plan has been developed, the implementation process begins. When working with a mentally retarded adolescent and his or her family during this phase, the following key principles should be used:

1   Enlist the cooperation of both the adolescent and the parent in defining the particular task to be learned. The benefit to be gained in terms of mutual independence may need to be reviewed. Assurance that support will be provided if difficulty is encountered communicates acceptance of the reality of the problems that are often encountered and assures both parent and adolescent that the goal will be achieved.

2   Maintain consistency and the familiar in materials and instructions until the task is well learned; then slight variations may be introduced.

3   Structure for success:

a   Reduce stimuli to those relevant to the task, and avoid distractions.

b   Break down the task to be accomplished into its discrete components and start with the easiest, usually the terminal part of the task. The easiest part of putting on a pair of pants is pulling them up, so begin by placing the adolescent's hands on the pants to help accomplish this.

c   Define each component of a task as a whole goal.

d   Provide a concrete visible plan that includes the tasks involved and a time line for their achievement. A chart listing the separate components in sequence helps the adolescent to visualize how the parts together make a whole. Periods of practice should be identified in spaces on the same line as the task. This provides an opportunity for the adolescent to identify the completion of each practice session and helps all involved to observe the adolescent's investment in the task and progress toward the goal. Allowing the adolescent to decide whether the chart should be displayed for others to see provides an opportunity for the adolescent to be instrumental in determining who should see it and who should be provided with an opportunity to socially reinforce progress.

e Identify the best time and place for practice. The time chosen should be a period when distractions for the adolescent and the parent are minimal. The room chosen should be appropriate to the task.

f Involve the adolescent in the selection of a reward for success.

g Provide an opportunity for rehearsal. This helps the parent to demonstrate understanding of the most effective way to communicate instructions so that they are understood. The nurse learns how the parent reacts to the adolescent's response and how reward or reinforcement is communicated. Rehearsal should include anticipating feelings that might be aroused so that ways of handling them can be demonstrated and suggestions made when needed.

h Encourage modeling. Frequent modeling by adults provides an opportunity for the adolescent to see the task as related to growing up.

i Promote the development of habit patterns. Retarded people learn best when routines are maintained. Feeding, for example, includes hand washing before and tooth brushing afterward.

j Provide for repeated opportunities to learn. Retarded people need frequent repetitions to learn new behaviors.

k Reinforce successful approximations. Let both the adolescent and the family know you are pleased with the tiniest movement toward the achievement of the task. Parents and their retarded children frequently have a long experience with frustration and failure, usually because expectations are too far beyond capabilities

l Use the family's pattern of organization as their strength, and make your suggestions within the framework of the way they are organized. For instance, if the maternal grandmother lives in the home and has assumed the major responsibility for the care of the retarded adolescent, involve her in all the planning and management.

4 Plan for follow-up. Dates and lengths of time to be spent on visits should be defined. Telephone calls can be used between visits so that support is demonstrated. Frequently problems encountered are identified on the phone, between visits. Alternative strategies can then be suggested.

Perhaps an example will reinforce the validity of these principles. These concepts will be applied to the task of bathing, since this is a task involving a number of complex activities the adolescent must learn to do independently in order to gain self-respect and social acceptance. Bathing involves the following tasks:

1 Selecting a time of day when other family members are least likely to need access to the bathroom

2 Assembling the necessary materials: soap, washrag, towel, deodorant, and robe

   3   Closing and perhaps locking the bathroom door
   4   Undressing
   5   Hanging up clothing that does not need to be laundered
   6   Running the bath water
   7   Getting into the tub
   8   Washing all body parts
   9   Getting out of the tub
  10   Drying
  11   Applying deodorant
  12   Putting on the robe
  13   Cleaning the tub
  14   Hanging the washrag and towel to dry
  15   Putting soiled garments into the laundry hamper
  16   Unlocking and opening the bathroom door
  17   Going to the bedroom to dress

The components of the task that often are performed by the parent are running the bath water, applying deodorant, and cleaning up the bath area. Often these components are assumed by the parent because it is most expedient and safe for the parent to do so. Another reason may be that the parent does some of these tasks for all the children. The nurse may need to discuss with the parent the special need for this adolescent to practice all portions of the total task of bathing in the most comfortable environment, that is, the family home. Helping the adolescent learn to perform this private function in an environment outside the home is inappropriate and may not even be possible. The family's average children, even though pampered while living at home, will adapt readily to new environments. In contrast, the child who is retarded needs instruction and practice in performing *all* steps of bathing independently.

The tasks that remain to be learned so that complete independence will be achieved are then ordered in terms of their ease of accomplishment and the motivation of both the adolescent and the parent. Whichever task is selected is broken down into its smaller components. For example, if applying a roll-on deodorant is selected, the task is analyzed as follows to determine an achievable goal:

   1   Picking up the container
   2   Removing the cap
   3   Raising it to the underarm area
   4   Applying the deodorant
   5   Putting the cap back on
   6   Putting the container away

Any one of these tasks may present difficulty. An assessment will reveal which component of the task is causing the problem. Often the difficulty lies in applying a deodorant to the underarm area or in removing and replacing the cap. Observation will reveal which is easiest. It may be found that the family deodorant container is the spray type, which the adolescent, particularly one with fine motor problems, has difficulty handling, in terms of both maintaining correct pressure and controlling the area of spray. The parent may not have thought of purchasing a different type of deodorant for the adolescent's use. Alternatives should be explored. A roll-on deodorant provides the best solution in terms of ease of application and control of both the amount of deodorant applied and the area to be covered. An assessment of the adolescent's skill in using the roll-on deodorant should be done in the usual bathroom situation. If difficulties are encountered, it may be that there are too many irrelevant stimuli present, such as a variety of containers on the counter, knocks on the door, and other distractions. In this case it is appropriate to apply the principle of structuring for success. Structure for success by doing the following:

1   Develop a chart showing a series of circles.
2   Select an area that is private and where distractions are at a minimum, usually the bedroom.
3   Take only the deodorant into this area.
4   Have the parent model use of the roll-on deodorant while looking at the mirror.
5   Have the adolescent apply the deodorant while looking at the mirror, observe the movements used, and mark one circle on the chart, showing what area was covered.
6   Have the parent grasp the adolescent's hand, holding the deodorant and assisting in the application, if the underarm is not adequately covered. As the parent feels the adolescent moving correctly, the parent's hand can be removed gradually, with praise given in recognition of the increased independence.
7   Repeat the procedure. Practice should be repeated, with praise for each successful approximation, until the process is learned. This may require several sessions, with successful approximations being recorded on the chart.
8   Transfer the practice to the bathroom once the task has been mastered.
9   Repeat the same process of helping and marking the chart until the previous efficiency is achieved, if regression occurs.

In order to determine if an activity has been completely mastered, the nurse needs to continually evaluate each step in the process.

Evaluation

Evaluation is the continuous critiquing of each aspect of the nursing process and the outcome for the family, the adolescent, and the professionals

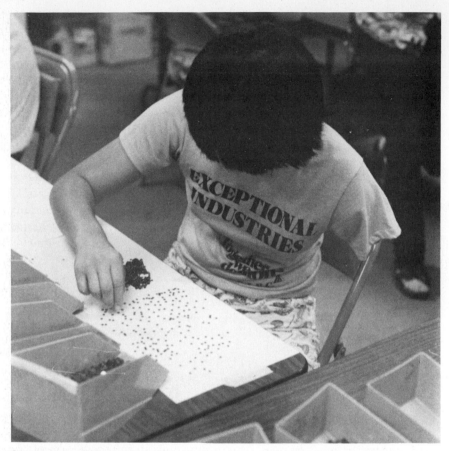

The great majority of adolescents who are retarded can learn skills (including dressing, grooming, and traveling to work) that permit them to be gainfully employed. Retarded persons can perform many required services in businesses, industries, homes, and farms, sometimes with greater care and conscientiousness than average persons. Sheltered workshops match retarded or otherwise handicapped employees' abilities with the needs of industrial or other contractors for such tasks as sorting, disassembling, and packaging. Employment promotes self-esteem, learning, experience, and at least partial economic independence. (*Copyright © 1980 by Anne Campbell.*)

and agencies involved in the management process. Although it is one of the most significant aspects of the nursing process, it is the aspect most frequently neglected. Failure to evaluate the effectiveness of client and professional interventions often prolongs the therapeutic process.

During the evaluation process, it is not sufficient only to identify that the mentally retarded adolescent and the family are participating in a management plan or have made contact with a community resource. The nurse should identify specific outcome criteria to determine if intervention strategies have been effective or ineffective. The nurse should further determine why they have been effective or ineffective. Some of the more common reasons for lack of success when working with the mentally retarded adolescent and his or her family are:

1   Lack of opportunity to practice a new task.
2   Irrelevance of an activity to the adolescent. Parents frequently may want to focus on academic skills rather than social adjustment, which is of more concern to the adolescent.
3   Discomfort in the situation. If the adolescent feels as though he or she is being tested, anxiety increases.
4   Lack of positive reinforcement.
5   Presence of undetected physical or perceptual problems.
6   Absence of approximations, with too large or complicated a step being expected at one time.
7   Inability to remember or understand the request.
8   Family exhaustion and stress.
9   Inconsistent messages from the various professionals working with the adolescent and the family.

The coordination of services among all professionals involved in the management plan cannot be overemphasized. The mentally retarded adolescent usually has contact with numerous professional disciplines and service agencies. Lack of coordination results in duplication of efforts, inefficient use of time and energies, inconsistent messages, and deficiencies in services. The interdisciplinary approach to care is most often the appropriate approach to use when working with a mentally retarded adolescent and his or her family. This approach is not effective or efficient, however, if there is a lack of coordination.

The major focus in this section has been on working with the mentally retarded adolescent in the home environment. It is not always feasible for this adolescent to remain in a home setting. Following is a discussion of the various care settings available to the mentally retarded adolescent. Whatever setting this adolescent is in, the nurse should use the nursing process to determine appropriate treatment goals and intervention strategies.

Previously discussed special considerations relative to the implementation of the nursing process with the mentally retarded adolescent and the family apply in all community care situations.

COMMUNITY PLACEMENTS

Alternatives to the natural home for the adolescent with mental retardation vary considerably at this stage in the process of deinstitutionalization.

Although the trend is optimistic, reflecting the humanitarian philosophy in practice, the degree to which ideal principles are implemented currently varies and probably will for many years to come. Variations occur not only between but also within the various settings.

Ideally, each placement meets the specific developmental needs of the individual, and movement from one setting to another should occur as needs change. Individual choice and adequate preparation and support for change for the individual and the family should be reflected in the move. Good matching of particular placement facilities to the needs of particular retarded persons and their families is most likely to occur when facilities are well known to the professionals who are making placement recommendations and when adequate quality-assurance procedures are in effect in the facilities. Wide variations currently exist in both these aspects of placement.

Other factors that may vary include: (1) funding, (2) quality of programming, (3) degree of integration into the mainstream of the community in terms of location and access to generic services, (4) staff-to-resident ratio, (5) degree of family involvement, (6) quality of health supervision, (7) number of residents, (8) similarities in ages and needs of residents, (9) degree of preparation for change, (10) consideration of resident choice in moving, and (11) length of stay within any placement.

The closest alternative to family living, in terms of length of placement, is respite care. Ideally respite care involves planned separation from the family for a short period of time to relieve the family of activities of daily living. Respite care is also used to meet emergency needs within the family or to begin training programs that will subsequently be carried out in the family home. These services can be provided by any of the other alternative residential placements but most often are provided by the institution. Not all families have used respite care prior to adolescence. Relinquishing care at any age for even a short period of time is often a painful experience for families. They can benefit considerably from nursing intervention.

Marian, a 12-year-old adolescent who was on the institution's waiting list for three years, was placed in an institution for a month so that the family could enjoy a "normal," well-deserved holiday rest, free of her disruptive behavior. In this situation, the community nurse worked closely not only with the institution personnel but also with the parents, who needed support to prepare for both the separation and the return of their daughter.[47]

Problems may be encountered if the institution requires a current evaluation to be on file and the need for care is urgent. Under these circumstances, nurses should contact the local Association for Retarded Citizens, who may have developed parent cooperatives for care.

Other alternatives to family care vary on a continuum of independence. Usually groupings of retarded persons within placement facilities reflect similar levels of independence. Moves from one level to another can occur in either direction. Successful upward mobility usually reflects adequacy in preparation for the change and support following it. Natural family contacts may occur in each placement.

Supervised apartment facilities provide for the greatest degree of independent functioning and afford the greatest access to average life experiences.

Foster homes require state licensure and provide board and room, which are paid for and monitored by state agencies. Varying degrees of dependency are accommodated in foster homes, and there may be an opportunity for family-type relationships with average children and adolescents. Ideally, no more than three residents are accommodated in one foster home, and close coordination exists among the school, the agency personnel responsible for program design, and the foster parents to ensure consistency of expectations.

Group homes are single dwellings that accommodate adolescents with varying dependency needs; usually mild to moderate dependency exists. Ideally, no more than 12 residents live in one dwelling. Programmatic needs are similar, and peer relationships are emphasized. Group homes are staffed by paid house parents and counselors and provide a homelike atmosphere with access to average community life experience.

Nursing homes are usually more sheltered environments. They also are licensed and reflect not only varying dependency needs but also variations in staff skill levels. Services are provided throughout a 24-hour period.

State institutions have historically provided terminal placement and custodial care for adolescents with all levels of dependency. Recently, these placements usually have been limited to individuals who have the highest dependency needs and who may also have multiple handicaps. Some degree of programming usually exists within the setting. When adolescents with severe to moderate dependency needs are able to do so, they frequently go into the community for education and vocational training and return to the institution for board and room.

Nurses should be cognizant of the congruency of need with the level of service available in the placement. They should be alert to the possibility of physical or mental abuse of residents, and evidence of abuse should be documented.

A major concern to be addressed, particularly when there is a discrepancy between the readiness of the adolescent and the environmental expectations of the placement facility, is the "reality shock" experienced under these circumstances. Movement from one place to another may result in temporary regression, requiring a great deal of support for the adolescent to adjust to new surroundings. When the transition occurs from the institution to the community, a major change occurs and there is a great need for preparation of the adolescent, the family, and the community.

TOWARD THE FUTURE

Society's view of the individual with mental retardation is changing in a positive direction. A major influence is recognition that the environment has great influence on the process of labeling and on these individuals' ability to attain their full developmental potential. In the future, the lives of mentally retarded adolescents will be influenced in proportion to the rate at which valid identification or labeling processes are applied and the degree to which the environment facilitates the capacities of appropriately labeled individuals to benefit from average life experiences. This section will examine current activities in both spheres.

The practice of labeling individuals as mentally retarded on the basis of performance on intelligence tests alone is increasingly being challenged in courts as a violation of the civil rights of these individuals, particularly those from minority groups. The conditions that influence the ability of these children to adapt to the increasingly complex demands of society have been addressed in considerable depth by Mercer.[48] The racial and social class biases that are built into currently used intelligence tests have been identified through analysis of the ways that individual functioning is perceived as normal or abnormal, depending on the demands of the social system in which performance is measured. Individuals who functioned as retarded in Anglo-Saxon school systems were perceived as normal in their neighborhoods, where expectations for performance were congruent with preparation for performance. The application of the concept of relativity revealed that many individuals, particularly those identified as mildly retarded, were inappropriately labeled.

The work of Mercer and her colleagues led to the development of changes in legislation in the state of California, which identified the criteria for special education placement that were consistent with the optimal performance that could be expected of a child or adolescent. Since 1971, the state has required that the following conditions must be met: (1) individual verbal or nonverbal intelligence testing must be given to each child in the primary language used in the home and in which the child has the most capacity to understand and the best fluency; (2) the child must score more than two standard deviations below the norm; (3) a credentialed school psychologist must perform a complete psychological examination including investigation of developmental factors, a school achievement record that substantiates the test results, and adaptability testing, which includes a visit to the child's home by the psychologist or by a person designated by the chief administrator of the district.[49]

California, then, has seen the establishment of a model that, if emulated in other states, would reduce inappropriate labeling and subsequent stigmatization of individuals who are capable of performing adequately in their natural environments.

An even more enlightened approach is revealed in a testing system that was subsequently developed by Mercer, "The System of Multicultural Pluralistic Assessment (SOMPA)."[50] This system identifies those factors that should be included in every school's segregating mechanism.

1   From a health perspective: screening for possible biological problems indicated by a health history; testing of vision; evaluation of hearing; and evaluation of performance on specified physical dexterity tests.

2   From a social systems perspective: viewing the child's performance in peer group roles, family roles, earner/consumer roles, community roles, nonacademic school roles, academic school roles, and self-maintenance roles.

3   From the perspective of cultural pluralism: evaluating the child in relation to others whose sociocultural background is the same; making inferences regarding the child's performance in relation to others having the same sociocultural background; and making inferences about the child's estimated learning potential.

Through the SOMPA, Mercer and her colleagues "hope to identify the non-Anglo child whose potential may be masked by the distance between the child's location in socio-cultural space and the culture of the school."[51]

When the label is appropriately applied, individuals who are mentally retarded need individualized services to help ensure their functioning at an optimal level. The individualized specialized services are most beneficial if begun early. Demonstration projects throughout the country have identified the value of early intervention programs for infants at risk and those who demonstrate developmental delay.

Early intervention programs are a relatively new phenomenon. Appropriate stimulation from infancy on can reduce developmental delay. From application of the concept of the progressive nature of development, one can assume that decreased gaps between average and retarded functioning will occur. The adolescent of the future should be better prepared to handle the tasks of adolescence at an earlier chronological age.

The future should see resolution of the current controversy around the application of the principle of normalization. Currently, application of this principle has sometimes occurred in its most literal sense; that is, some persons have assumed that exposure to average experience would, in and of itself, automatically habilitate mentally retarded individuals. Disastrous effects due to discrepancies between readiness and environmental expectation and response have occurred. Aanes and Haagenson have identified the need to view normalization as both a goal and a *process*.[52] There is "no quarrel with the goal, but to make all the means to that goal normal may indeed result in a dead end street."[53]

Mainstreaming, when implemented by putting children who are retarded directly into average classrooms without necessary specialized preparation, is one way that literal interpretation and application of the normalization principle can be detrimental. Budoff has examined one factor that might be causing some of the current failures.[54] His research revealed that even some mildly retarded children behave differently than their average peers in ways that serve to repel others. He identified the need to find ways to make the child more sensitive to the presence and social stimulus value of these behaviors and to provide programs to eliminate them.

In the future, many more processes or means of implementing normalization will be examined. Research and application of appropriate practice will resolve many of the issues currently surrounding normalization.

SUMMARY

The adolescent with mental retardation is confronted with the same developmental tasks as the average adolescent. Currently the retarded adolescent is considerably less well equipped to master the developmental tasks during the same chronological period. Not only does the psychology of past and current learning differ, but this adolescent has also often been deprived of those experiences that facilitate success earlier in life; this adolescent has had a prolonged dependent childhood. Tasks that are precursors to this stage for the average adolescent are often the focus of the retarded adolescent during this period.

As the influences of normalization and early intervention are increasingly experienced with particular attention to their learning needs, these adolescents will be better equipped to respond to the expectations of society. Application of the developmental model with an acute sensitivity to awareness of individual differences in these adolescents and their families will help the nurse to facilitate maximal achievement and adjustment for those adolescents whose milieu experiences are currently in transition.

REFERENCES

1 C. Fishman, C. Scott, and N. Betof, "A Hall of Mirrors: A Structural Approach to the Problems of the Mentally Retarded," *Mental Retardation*, 15(4):24, 1977, p. 24.

2   R. C. Scheerenberger, "Mental Retardation: Definition, Classification, and Prevalence," *Mental Retardation Abstracts*, **1**(4):432–441, 1964.
3   T. Jordan, *The Mentally Retarded*, 4th ed. Columbus, Ohio: Charles E. Merrill Publishing Co., 1976, p. 4.
4   J. W. Filler, Jr. et al., "Mental Retardation," in N. Hobbs (ed.), *Issues in the Classification of Children*, Vol. 1. San Francisco: Jossey-Bass, 1975, pp. 194–238.
5   Ibid., p. 211.
6   M. Kindred et al. (eds.), *The Mentally Retarded Citizen and the Law*. New York: The Free Press, 1976, p. xxviii.
7   Ibid., p. xxviii.
8   H. J. Grossman (ed.), *Manual on Terminology and Classification in Mental Retardation*, rev. Special Publication Series No. 2. Washington, D.C.: American Association on Mental Deficiency, 1973, p. 11.
9   President's Committee on Mental Retardation, *Mental Retardation: The Known and the Unknown*. Washington, D.C.: DHEW Publication No. (OHD) 76-21008, 1975.
10 Ibid., p. 11.
11 Ibid.
12 Grossman, op. cit., p. 11.
13 K. Nihira et al., *AAMD Adaptive Behavior Scale Manual*. Washington, D.C.: American Association on Mental Deficiency, 1975, p. 5.
14 E. E. Balthazar, *Balthazar Scales of Adaptive Behavior for the Profoundly and Severely Mentally Retarded, Section 1, Part 1, Handbook for the Professional Supervisor*. Champaign, Ill.: Research Press, 1971, p. 4.
15 E. E. Balthazar, *Balthazar Scales of Adaptive Behavior, II, Scales of Social Adaptation. A System for Program Development and Evaluation of Social Behavior Assessment among Profoundly and Severely Mentally Retarded Adults and the Younger Less Retarded*. Palo Alto, Calif.: Consulting Psychologists Press, 1973, p. 3.
16 Balthazar, 1971, op. cit., p. 3.
17 Ibid., p. 7.
18 President's Committee on Mental Retardation, 1975, op. cit. pp. 8–9.
19 *Word from Washington*, **9**(12):2–3, November-December 1978.
20 W. Wolfensberger, *The Principle of Normalization in Human Services*. Toronto: National Institute on Mental Retardation, 1972, p. 27.
21 Ibid.
22 Ibid., p. 28.
23 R. Perske, *New Directions for Parents of Persons Who Are Retarded*. New York: Abingdon Press, 1973, p. 57.
24 D. Chambers, "The Principle of the Least Restrictive Alternative: The Constitutional Issues," in M. Kindred et al. (eds.), *The Mentally Retarded Citizen and the Law*. New York: The Free Press, 1976, pp. 486–499.
25 Ibid.. p. 486.
26 S. R. Gelman, "A System of Services," in C. Cherington and G. Dybwad (eds.), *New Neighbors: The Retarded Citizen in Quest of a Home*. Washington, D.C.: President's Committee on Mental Retardation, DHEW Publication No. (OHD) 74-21004, 1974, pp. 91–103.

27 J. W. Birch, *Mainstreaming: Educable Mentally Retarded Children in Regular Class*. Reston, Va.: Council for Exceptional Children, 1974.

28 S. A. Richardson, "Mental Retardation in the Community: The Transition from Childhood to Adulthood," in P. Mittler (ed.), *Research to Practice in Mental Retardation, Volume 1, Care and Intervention*. Baltimore: University Park Press, 1977, pp. 363–369.

29 A. Pattullo, "Developing Sexuality among People Who Are Retarded," in J. Curry and K. Peppe (eds.), *Mental Retardation: Nursing Approaches to Care*. St. Louis: C. V. Mosby Co., 1978, pp. 204–223.

30 A. Pattullo, "The Early Phases of a Lifetime Preparation for Socio-Sexual Fulfillment for Vulnerable Populations Who Are Societally Stigmatized," in L. Rowitz and R. J. Meyer (eds.), *Out of the Maze: Family Life Education for Vulnerable Populations*. Chicago: U.S. Dept. of Health, Education, and Welfare, Public Health Service, Division of Health Sciences, Region V, 1974, pp. 18–26.

31 A. Pattullo, *Puberty in the Girl Who Is Retarded*. New York: National Association for Retarded Children, 1969.

32 A. Pattullo, "The Socio-Sexual Development of the Handicapped Child: A Preventative Care Approach," *Nursing Clinics of North America*, **10**(2):361–372, June 1975.

33 A. Pattullo and K. Barnard, "Teaching Menstrual Hygiene to the Mentally Retarded," *American Journal of Nursing*, **68**(12):2572–2575, December 1968.

34 J. E. Hall, "Sexuality in Mental Retardation," in R. Green (ed.), *Human Sexuality, A Health Practitioner's Text*. Baltimore: Williams and Wilkins, 1975, pp. 181–195.

35 M. Morganstern, "The Psychological Development of the Retarded," in F. de la Cruz and G. D. LaVeck (eds.), *Human Sexuality and the Mentally Retarded*. New York: Brunner/Mazel, 1973, pp. 15–19.

36 J. Mattinson, *Marriage and Mental Handicap: A Study of Subnormality in Marriage*. Pittsburgh: University of Pittsburgh Press, 1971.

37 Perske, op. cit.

38 M. L. Hardman and C. J. Drew, "The Physically Handicapped Retarded Individual: A Review," *Mental Retardation*, **15**(5):43–48, 1977.

39 S. L. Hammar and K. Barnard, "A Review of the Characteristics and Problems of 44 Non-institutionalized Adolescent Retardates," *Pediatrics*, **38**:845–857, 1966.

40 Ibid.

41 S. D. Garrard, "Mental Retardation in Adolescence," *Pediatric Clinics of North America*, **7**:147–164, 1960, p. 151.

42 K. A. Gorham et al., "Effect on Parents," in H. Hobbs (ed.), *Issues in the Classification of Children*, Vol. 2. San Francisco: Jossey-Bass, 1975, pp. 154–188.

43 Hammar and Barnard, op. cit.

44 Gorham et al., op. cit.

45 Ibid.

46 C. T. Michaelis, "Chip on My Shoulder," *The Exceptional Parent*, **4**:30–35, 1974.

47 J. B. Curry, "Nursing Intervention during Temporary Care," *Mental Retardation*, **12**(1):17–19, 1974.
48 J. R. Mercer, "Psychological Assessment and the Rights of Children," in N. Hobbs (ed.), *Issues in the Classification of Children*, Vol. 1. San Francisco: Jossey-Bass, 1975, pp. 130–158.
49 Ibid., pp. 149–150.
50 J. R. Mercer, "Cultural Diversity, Mental Retardation, and Assessment: The Case for Non-Labeling," in P. Mittler (ed.), *Research to Practice in Mental Retardation: Care and Intervention*, Vol. 1. Baltimore: University Park Press, 1977, pp. 353–362.
51 Ibid., p. 362.
52 D. Aanes and L. Haagenson, "Normalization: Attention to a Conceptual Disaster," *Mental Retardation*, **16**(1):55–56, 1978.
53 Ibid., p. 56.
54 M. Budoff, "The Mentally Retarded Child in the Mainstream of the Public School: His Relation to the School Administration, His Teachers, and His Age-Mates" in P. Mittler (ed.), *Research to Practice in Mental Retardation: Education and Training*, Vol. 2. Baltimore: University Park Press, 1977, pp. 307–313.

BIBLIOGRAPHY

Chard, M. A. and C. G. Woelk: "The Mentally Retarded Child and His Family," in G. M. Scipien et al. (eds.), *Comprehensive Pediatric Nursing*, 2d ed. New York: McGraw-Hill Book Co., 1979.
Mesibov, G. B.: "Alternatives to the Principle of Normalization," *Mental Retardation*, **14**(5):30–32, 1976.

Adolescent Sexuality

Judi Odiorne
Carol Tenerowicz

The major challenge of adolescence is to synthesize one's identity. As the young person works toward the ill-defined state called maturity, there is perhaps no other area in which he or she experiences greater exultation or perceives greater risk than in the formulation of sexual identity. Among the big questions to be met head-on during this period of the life span are: Who am I as a sexual being? What do I believe, feel, value? How shall I express myself?

The purpose of this chapter is to explore the development of sexuality as it leads to consolidation of sexual identity. The establishment of sexual identity is viewed as a lifelong process. The development of sexual identity that takes place during the adolescent years is examined in view of its interfaces with the other psychosocial tasks of adolescence. Nursing approaches for assisting young people toward establishing sexual identity are presented.

Sexuality can be viewed as an open system of four interacting and co-acting components, namely, biological sex, body image, gender identity, and sexual role behaviors.[1-4] Each component has a direct impact on the others, and any change in one dimension effects an altered state of balance within the total system. Because of the lack of definitions and the inconsistencies among definitions found in the literature, pertinent terms are defined for the purposes of this chapter. *Body image* refers to the mental representation of one's own internal and external body. Body image evolves throughout all the phases of development and includes one's own feelings and attitudes toward one's body as well as the responses of others.[5] *Gender identity* is "the conviction, established in the first 2 or 3 years of life, that one belongs to the male or to the female sex."[6] *Sexual role behaviors* include *gender behaviors*, those activities "with masculine and feminine connotations," and *sex behaviors*, those "based on a desire for sexual pleasure, ultimately for orgasm [physical sex]."[7] *Sexual identity* emerges from the successful interplay of the four dimensions of sexuality, the outcomes of the previous developmental stages, and the cultural environment. The *consolidation of sexual identity*, which occurs during the resolution of adolescence, refers to the affirmation of sexual role preference and behaviors congruent with sense of maleness or femaleness.

The adolescent, struggling with identity issues, invariably encounters sexual conflicts. The choices made in accepting and adopting sex role behaviors suitable to the self are influenced not only by the sexual norms and expectations of society, but also by the concept of self as a sexual being, male or female, which the person has acquired up to this time. To understand how adolescents resolve some of their psychosexual conflicts and attain sexual identity, it is necessary to consider the impact of childhood sexuality on personality development and life-style orientations. The adolescent is, in part, a product of earlier life experiences.

CHILDHOOD INFLUENCES ON ADOLESCENT SEXUALITY

Infancy

The process of developing sexual identity begins in utero, where the biological sex of an infant is determined by chromosomal combination and shaped by the fetal environment.[8] Male and female neonates and infants appear to exhibit differences in response as a function of their sex: Girls have "more sensitivity to stimuli" and "greater tactile and pain sensitivity"[9] than boys, and boys have stronger musculature and longer periods of restful sleep than girls.[10] In addition to these biological differences, the neonate, from the moment of birth, lives in a world that has existing expectations, attitudes, and values concerning him or her as an infant who happens to be male or female. Studies have indicated that early care-givers, nursery personnel, and parents respond to the infant on the basis of biological sex. For example, infant boys are described as more active than girls and tend to be handled more aggressively by care-givers; girls tend to be held more closely and their sounds are imitated more frequently by their mothers.[11] Many of these adult behaviors toward even young babies stem from existing notions that, constitutionally, boys are more aggressive and independent and girls are more passive and dependent. However, most authors suggest that behavioral differences between males and females, even in infancy, are the result of learning reinforced by sexual role norms of society. Thus, masculinity and femininity are fostered in the first days of life by care-givers' responses, some of which may reflect actual infant sexual differences, and some of which reflect sexual role stereotypes prevalent in society.

From birth on, the young child invests much energy in developing a sense of his or her own body and its boundaries. Bodily experiences, pleasurable and painful, are crucial to the child's learning. The infant is a sensuous, nonverbal, nonrational creature seeking bodily pleasures and dependent on physical activity for self-expression and communication. Freud hypothesized that the oral zone is the seat of libidinal drives in the infant and that consistent satisfaction of oral needs produces an inner state of well-being.

The mouth is the infant's primary source of physical and emotional nourishment, pleasure, and mode of exploration. The skin, other sense organs, and body parts serve as secondary tools in learning about self and others. Sullivan[12] believed that the infant's sense of self emerges as a result of secure and satisfying relationships with primary significant others. The infant is the recipient of love and reflected appraisals in the form of oral satisfaction, physical care, and tenderness. Infants learn about themselves as others interact with them by touching, feeding, caressing, and fondling them. Thus a child's first experience with intimacy is through physical interaction in a dependent relationship, particularly with his or her mother.[13] Infants learn to differentiate self from others and parts from wholes through exploring their own and others' bodies. Concurrently, they begin to grossly discriminate and anticipate behavior that produces experiences of satisfaction and tenderness (the "good me") from behavior that engenders degrees of anxiety (the "bad me" and "not me").[14]

Prior to the development of logical, syntaxic reasoning, the child comes to know of himself or herself and others through the processes of need satisfaction, reflected appraisals, and positive and negative reinforcement of selected behaviors. If oral and physical needs are met, if the child's body is treated with tenderness, and if body movements and explorations are supported and encouraged, the infant learns to trust others and herself or himself, to develop coping mechanisms based on predominantly "good me" or "bad me" bodily experiences, and to discriminate physical self from nonself. Thus, in infancy, the foundations are built for experiencing one's body as a source of pleasure and being able to receive and accept love. These outcomes are essential precursors to the development of mature sexuality.

The Toddler Period

During the toddler phase of development, parents alter their expectations and demands in the process of socializing the child. The expectations, values, attitudes, and sanctions that are overtly and covertly conveyed toward the child and his or her biological sex during socialization have an impact on gender awareness and body image development. The major sources of anxiety, "bad me" and shameful experiences, stem from conflicts between the desire to express a pleasurable impulse (unrestrained mobility, soiling, enuresis) or to withhold an expected response, and the need to retain the mothering one's love and approval. The child's pride in self, including gender and the sense of autonomy resulting from body mastery, is enhanced through interpersonal relationships with parenting adults; these relationships foster the gradual learning of self-control without the loss of self-esteem.

As the infant reaches toddlerhood, the focus of pleasure and tension shifts from the oral zone to the anal region. A great deal of parental (usually the mother's) attention and energy is invested in the process of toilet training. Pleasure and pain become associated with holding on and letting go, and bodily products become endowed with egocentric love and aggression. The achievement of sphincter control is the young child's first experience with being able to control self and others. It affords the child an opportunity to please, to give of himself or herself and body products, or to punish and withhold. If the child's body products and efforts to control impulses are recognized and approved by parenting adults, the child is likely to value both body and self. Conversely, if body products and body explorations are viewed as messy and dirty and significant adults react with disgust and disdain, then the child is in danger of feeling ashamed and devaluing at least this bodily area. When children meet parental expectations, they are rewarded and praised; when they do not do so, negative reactions follow. The predominance of approval or disapproval results in behavior patterns that reflect a positive or negative body image and sense of self.

Concurrent with physical maturation are increases in motor expression and mastery, cognitive growth, and verbal skills, all of which facilitate the toddler's autonomy and developing sense of gender identity. The child's unrelenting insistence that "me do," that this is "mine," and that the answer is "no," as well as the child's ambivalent or contradictory tendencies, are trying for parents as they strive for mutual regulation with their child. By the time the child is three, one thing parents can count on is the child's firm awareness of gender identity. Upon questioning or playful teasing, the three-year-old is verbally adamant that "me a boy" or "I are a girl!"

Differing expectations for males' and females' behavior and certain attitudes and beliefs about the value of the girl-child and the boy-child are conveyed and reinforced. Whether because of innate differences or because of child-rearing practices which include gender and sex role expectations, male and female youngsters continue to be treated differently. This differential treatment is reflected in the child's room decor, the choice of colors and style of clothing, and the toys provided. It is not uncommon to hear toddler boys described as physically more active, harder to toilet train and to control, or physically and verbally more aggressive and negative than their female counterparts; nor is it uncommon to hear girls described as more obedient, easier to toilet train and manage, less active, and perhaps more conforming than male children. The child learns gender expectations and behaviors not only as a result of expectations and sanctions, but also through imitating significant adults.

The outcomes of the toddler stage, with its socialization process, are extremely influential in the child's establishing a balance between love and hate, needs of others and needs of self, cooperation and stubbornness, and freedom or restriction of self-expression. The toddler's attainment of the ability to give love and the freedom to express himself or herself physically and verbally are important foundations of the development of mature sexuality.

The Preschool Period

The preschool years have been identified as a crucial time span in the development of sexual identity. It is during this period that the child confirms his or her gender identity and learns same-sex and complementary sex role behaviors. The preschooler plays out and defines capabilities and potential as a male or a female. Matteson[15] suggests that three processes culminate in the preschool years from which children learn sex role behavior: self-labeling, identification, and the acquisition of sex role stereotypes. Sexual role identification and learning for boys and girls begin to follow significantly divergent paths during the preschool years. It appears that major forces in shaping these differences are the child's discovery of (1) anatomical differences between the sexes, (2) the greater importance and prestige attributed to the father and his social role, and (3) socioculturally approved sex role behavior.

Between 2½ and 6 years of age, children become increasingly interested in their own and others' anatomy, including the genital area and its functions and sensations. Through body exploration and manipulation,

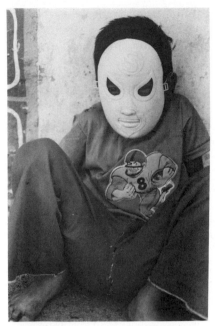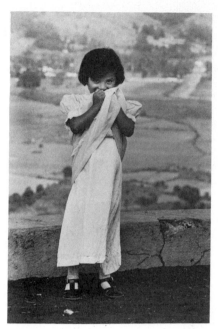

A great portion of one's sexuality is established well in advance of puberty. In most cultures, boys' and girls' sex role expectations and behaviors differ distinctly at least by the time they are preschoolers. These early influences affect adolescent and adult attitudes and behavior. (*Copyright © 1980 by George Lazar.*)

the child continues to experience the genital area as a source of body pleasure. "This discovery is probably the beginning of a lifelong association between sexual feeling and the genitals."[16] Because of the accessibility of the genitals, masturbation occurs naturally as a source of erotic pleasure and as a means of gaining comfort. The child who is sleepy, enjoying a bath, frightened, or curious may engage in self-stimulation for comfort and pleasure. Some of the child's physical interactions with others (holding, stroking, tickling, touching, and roughhousing) serve as a means of satisfying sexual curiosity and learning to feel positively about his or her own body as well as providing security, affection, and fun.

During the same period of time that the child is making an association between the genitals and pleasurable body feelings, he or she is becoming aware of the anatomical differences between males and females. The discovery that little boys and men have penises and that little girls and women do not has an impact on both sexes. This new awareness gives rise to many questions, fantasies, and behaviors. It's not uncommon to hear children ask, "Where is your penis, Mom?" "How does Heather go to the bathroom?" "How come my bone is growing?" [referring to an erection] "Where do babies come from?" "How do they get in/get out?" "Are my breasts getting bigger?" Children take the initiative in questioning and exploring the similarities and dissimilarities of the human body; at times, they take pride in displaying and exhibiting their bodies. Many of their behaviors, such as imitating the same or opposite sex, attempting to assume the role of the same-sex parent, exhibitionism, physical body exploration of self and others, and following adults into the bathroom or bedroom, are attempts to define self in relation to others. Preschoolers are dependent on audience participation and feedback in learning about themselves. What they learn becomes incorporated into their gender identity formation.

The establishment of gender identity in the preschool years is essential to emotional stability and eventual development of a healthy sense of self.[17] The consolidation of gender identity is enhanced through the process of identification with parents. Psychoanalytic theory asserts that because the preschool girl feels that her mother has deprived her of a penis and begins to recognize a mother's inferior social status, she turns her affection to the father, wishing in part to replace her mother. Loving both parents, recognizing her own limitations, and fearing retribution, the girl eventually gives up her libidinal attachment to her father and strives to be like her mother. Partly as a result of this process, the superego, or conscience, is formed as the child internalizes real and imagined parental prohibitions and restrictions. She receives reinforcement for feminine behaviors from both parents. Since the mother is the primary person engaged in child rearing, young children of both sexes initially tend to identify with the mothering one as a source of security and affection. Identifying and learning sex roles are especially difficult for girls because, although they have an immediate and available model in the home, women's roles are often perceived as relatively unappealing, and girls "eventually sense that they are expected to be persons in a very restricted world."[18] The desirable outcome is that the female child recognize her mother as a woman with self-esteem and her father as a man with respect and affection for his wife as a woman.[19]

The male child's gender identity is also influenced by identification, but the process is different from the girl's. The male child must make a shift in identification, that is, give up his primary attachment to the mothering figure and model himself after his father. This shift is fostered by the mother's admiration of her husband and cultural esteem for the male role.[20] Matteson[21] notes that sex identification of the male child is not rooted in a direct, personal, role model relationship with the father as the girl's is with her mother. It involves learning the social role of the father and men outside the home, a vague and mysterious yet esteemed role. Father absence, if only because of work, decreases opportunities for direct observation and imitation; it necessitates that the young boy spend most of his early years in female-dominated situations. As the boy learns male identity, he has to unlearn feminine identifications. Thus, in affirming his masculine identity, the boy becomes more rejecting of the feminine role. Matteson[22] suggests that boys' difficulty attendant to learning the male role and needing to reject the feminine role stems in part from the facts that boys are punished for feminine behavior more frequently than girls are for masculine behavior and that, furthermore, they most often receive those negative reactions from women. Although sexual role learning is a less personal, more complex process for boys, and their identification with the male role is less secure than girls' female role identification, the boy becomes increasingly cognizant of the value and status attributed by both males and females to the masculine role.

Who individuals feel they are or how they label themselves is primarily connected to *gender*, genetically determined sex. *Gender identity*, learning to appreciate and accept self as male or female, depends heavily on parental attitudes and behaviors and on interactions with other members of society.[23,24] The preschool child becomes progressively more a family member and less mother's baby. Even fathers previously uninvolved in infant care may interact more with their preschool sons and daughters. Fathers, males, and male roles become increasingly important and admired by both sexes. The child's primary teachers up through the preschool years (the parents) define and reinforce expected sex role behaviors for their child. Through their verbal and nonverbal behavior, parents (1) express sexual role expectations of themselves, one another, and others of the same or opposite gender and (2) convey their satisfaction or dissatisfaction with their own and others' sexual role behaviors. Children, because of their attachment to their parents, are greatly influenced by their mother and father. "Despite the importance of various biological factors, the gender assigned the child by the parents and the ensuing interactional patterns within the family can outweigh all other considerations."[25] Patterns of gender and sex role behaviors learned through imitation and identification are reinforced by prohibitions and sanctions from significant others. If the parents are overly forbidding and punitive or too encouraging and solicitous, the child may associate guilt and shame with pleasurable experiences that are in some way associated with the genitals. Parent-child interactions concerning exploratory and imitative sexual role behaviors constitute "another milestone in the sexual development of the child."[26]

The child's sense of self and his or her growing consolidation of femininity and masculinity are influenced not only by parents, but also by encounters with a wide range of socially sanctioned sex-typed behaviors and roles. In our society, many divergent gender and sexual role beliefs and expectations exist and are reflected in child-rearing practices. Yet, despite the changes presently occurring in sexual roles, it is still the case that most Americans are fully acculturated into stereotyped sex role behaviors.[27] Regardless of numerous individual differences in home background, parental roles, and sex role teaching, young children tend to maintain stereotypic male and female role conceptions.[28] "Children agree earliest and most completely that fathers are bigger and stronger than mothers, next that they are smarter than mothers, and next that they have more social power or are the boss in the family."[29] Even in families where mothers' and fathers' sex roles are least differentiated, mothers are expected to have and are perceived as having a greater nurturing role with children. Children of 5 and 6 years begin to separate socially according to gender, boys wanting little to do with "yuckey" and inferior girls and desiring associations with socially preferred males. From 5 years on, girls' "preferential evaluation of their own sex continues to decline."[30]

The consistency in children's sex role stereotypes may be explained by the fact that they learn about sex roles very early in life not only from parents, but also through their own observations and interactions with siblings, peers, and other adults. The preschool child's discovery of what it means to be a male or female is also congruent with his or her preoperational mode of thinking. The child knows who he or she *is* by gender, but limited cognitive comprehension prevents the child from accurately conceptualizing what he or she may or may not *become*.[31] It is not uncommon for children this age to fantasize (or fear) that their gender will change when they grow up. Thus, the preschooler's conception of maleness and femaleness includes highly intuitive, egocentric, value-laden, broad generalizations of sex role stereotypes.

In general, the expected outcome of the preschool or Oedipal phase of development is that the child firmly accepts his or her gender identity and sex role as conveyed by parents and their value orientations. Throughout this developmental stage, the child is learning to (1) appreciate his or her male or female body as good and as a useful tool in relating with others, (2) relate comfortably with members of the opposite sex, (3) acquire and compare sex-typed behaviors, and (4) develop patterns of behavior based on sex role stereotypes. It is during the preschool years that foundations for the integration of one's gender and sex roles, the fulfillment and pleasure through genital activities, and the capacity for mutually satisfying relationships with members of the same and opposite sex are begun.

The School-Age Period

The school-age child, in moving out from the home into the school and community, confronts new expectations, acquires different values, makes new friends, and develops an expanding, more realistic view of himself or herself and the social world. His or her sense of sexual identity is reinforced and/or altered by changes in body image, new conceptions of masculine and feminine social roles, and experimentation with sex role behaviors among peers. Although no new libidinal zone becomes preeminent at this time, the school-age child is not sexually latent. There is little evidence that the child experiences a diminution in the sexual drive, the impulse to masturbate, or sexual curiosity.[32] What probably happens is that energy is invested in a series of new skills and people and that sexual activities and inquiries are largely confined to peers.

One of the developmental tasks confronting the school-age child is that of "adjusting his changing body image and self-concept to come to terms with the masculine or feminine social role."[33] Children's self-concepts derive from reflected appraisals of significant others, task mastery, and self-evaluation. They begin to see themselves through the eyes of peer group and special friend(s). The peer group standards and values, such as honesty, ability to compromise, loyalty, bravery, athletic prowess, and responsibility, become criteria for acceptance or rejection, both by the group and by oneself.

The school-age child's body is central to developmental task mastery, including sense of industry. The acquisition of physical and cognitive skills facilitates the child's competence in play, work, and social interactions and contributes to acceptance by peers. If cognitive and physical resources fail, the child is in danger of developing a sense of inferiority. Activities, group behaviors, and values differ for boys and girls; boys are generally more active physically, more competitive, and oriented to a large group or gang, and girls engage more in quiet activities in smaller groups closer to home.[34,35] Thus, gender role patterning continues as the girl invests her energy in interpersonal relationships and the boy concerns himself with competition and winning. Furthermore, the 6- to 11-year-old is made acutely aware of his or her body by the attention given to physical characteristics, size, and capabilities during school and in play activities. Children compare themselves with and are compared by peers, teachers, and family. This can strengthen previous positive self-regard or it can present some difficulties. The boy may behave aggressively during school in an effort to become an important member of his peer group and, consequently, may receive negative reactions from his teacher. The girl may act quiet and passive in order to be accepted by the teacher, but, as a result, may never understand the lesson being taught. Whether one is perceived and responded to as the strongest, smartest, clumsiest, prettiest, or dumbest influences the child's self-regard and sense of masculinity or femininity.

Entry into the school-age period is marked by the need for peers of the same sex. Through peer interactions, the child learns to win and lose, to give and take in reciprocal relationships, and to form an increasingly realistic evaluation of self. Being accepted as a part of the group engenders a sense of belonging that fosters the child's identification with society and a commitment to its values.[36]

The same-sex peer group affords the child an arena to test out, reinforce, or incorporate sexual role concepts and behaviors. Frequently, the peer group is viewed as an extension of self, inasmuch as the members hold very similar concepts of sexual roles. "For some children, peer experiences strengthen patterns of dominance, social spontaneity and positive self-evaluation. For others, peer rejection and perception of marked deviation from peer-valued attributes lead to social anxiety, social submission, and a sense of ineffectiveness."[37] The school-ager's beliefs about what constitutes a girl or boy and how each should behave, although expanding, are still bound by narrow perceptions and moral restraint.

In general, the peer group provides a safe and secure environment for the sharing of sexual curiosities and explorations. Discussions of sexual matters reflect not only the youngster's knowledge and feelings but also his or her misinformation, misperceptions, and fantasy. Sexual role behaviors may include telling jokes, using sexual terms, exhibitionism, and group sexual experimentation. Peer group humor frequently involves bodily and sexual referents, some of which reflect anxieties in these areas. Sexual terms and gestures may be used to degrade another, to achieve a sense of importance, or to express emotion. To the child, the meanings of these words and symbols are often distorted and partially understood. Individuals in peer groups may enjoy group showers and the opportunity to show off or compare body parts. Group sexual experimentation is more common among boys than among girls. The same-sex peer group, through establishment of norms and taboos, helps to solidify the child's sexual identity and provides a comfortable place to experiment with sexual role behaviors.

Preadolescence

One of the most significant events in the life of the preadolescent is having a special friend or "chum."[38–40] This friendship is the child's first intense interpersonal attachment outside of the home. The chumship coincides with the developing capacity for mature love, i.e., the ability to place one's self in another's position, to hold another's happiness and worthwhileness in priority, and to engage in reciprocal caring. The need for interpersonal intimacy or closeness is met through this very special relationship and provides experiences of consensual validation of self-worth.[41] Within the same-sex relationship, each child shares inner feelings, ideas, doubts, and later sexual concerns. Together they discuss and confirm what they vaguely know or suspect has sexual significance. Despite the uncertainties, this type of friendship, built on mutual regard and support, is a most effective vehicle for acquiring greater sexual knowledge and assuredness.[42] The preadolescent learns more about himself or herself, but, most important, learns to accept that self with both strengths and limitations and then to accept others. Not only does the child affirm gender identity, but this chum relationship serves as a basis for future intimate relationships with both sexes. Many of the personality qualities and motives and patterns of sex role behavior are essentially formed by the end of latency.[43] Manaster,[44] in referring to gender identity, states that it "is essentially fixed prior to adolescence." One of the most striking findings in the Kagan and Moss[45] study was that sex role identification and patterns of sexual behavior in adulthood were related to reasonably analogous tendencies during the period from 6 to 10 years of age.

Thus, during the school-age period, the child sets out to master skills associated with maleness or femaleness and acquires relatively stable sex-typed attitudes and behaviors. These aspects of development are accomplished not only through family experiences, but also as a result of expanding relationships with new peers and adults and access to sexually related beliefs and behaviors through mass media. The extent to which each child perceives himself or herself as possessing attributes of his or her sex, being like male or female friends, and receiving approval for such characteristics and behaviors influences the development of the child's self-concept. But even those youngsters who approach adolescence with a healthy sense of self experience anxiety, doubts, fears, and ambivalence associated with the changes ushered in by puberty.

THE DEVELOPMENT OF SEXUALITY THROUGHOUT ADOLESCENCE

One of the primary tasks that each adolescent confronts in striving for personal identity is that of consolidating his or her sexual identity. Sexual identity refers to an individual's inner feelings and self-perception of maleness and femaleness which have continuity over time.[46,47] The problem is not so much one of discovering male or female roles, but rather one of determining sex role preferences. Each individual adolescent is faced with choosing and accepting his or her particular style of being a man or woman.[48] To this end, the adolescent reevaluates old and new gender behaviors and experiments with sex behaviors not previously experienced. The adolescent sexual crisis is resolved by the young person's learning to integrate sexual urges with previously learned values and behaviors, to experiment with alternative modes of sexual expression, to affirm his or her sexual role preferences and behaviors, to accept that the body is always changing, and to strengthen the capacity for intimacy with another human being.[49-51]

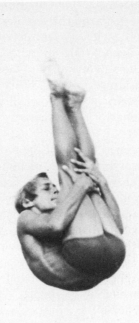

Feelings about one's own physical appearance and physical abilities are closely linked to self-esteem and to one's expectations about being acceptable to others. (*Copyright* © *1980 by Anne Campbell*.)

Physical Changes

It is the sexual maturation of puberty which signals the youngster's exit from childhood and entrance into adolescence. Genital sexuality differs markedly from childhood sexuality in that:

> Prepubertal sexuality concerns erotic and sensuous aspects of affectional attachments, including the influence of stimulation of erogenous zones, upon general attitudes, thoughts and behaviors, but it is not drive-impelled in the same sense as adolescent and adult sexuality; it does not involve increased hormonal secretions, a need to discharge sperm and semen, shifts in the menstrual cycle, or the increased erogenous sensitivity that follows the maturation of sexual organs at puberty.[52]

The physical body changes, the maturation of the reproductive organs, and the new experiences of sexual excitement and drive have a pervasive impact on the adolescent and those with whom he or she interacts. Not only is the body changing, but the "kid" in the body is changing. These multiple, interrelated changes intensify the young person's focus on self; they also generate new responses and reactions both in the adolescent and in other people.

The most obvious signs that a youngster is approaching physical maturity are changes in body size and shape and in the primary and secondary sexual characteristics. When the young adolescent or preadolescent stands in front of a mirror, he or she sees a change in body. The girl observes breast enlargement, longer legs, rounding hips, and growth of pubic and axillary hair. Not so apparent or often examined are her sex organs. Although young girls are often preoccupied with their breast development, few of them know and understand their external genital anatomy.[53] The boy sees changes in scrotal skin, testes, penis, muscle mass, and body hair. Because of the external, visible nature of his sexual anatomy, there is a tendency for boys to explore these body parts. Youngsters of each sex are aware of bodily proportions, size, and weight; they may become concerned with facial blemishes and body odor. If earlier developmental experiences have given the adolescent a good feeling about himself or herself and his or her physical body, the new changes will not be as difficult to adjust to as they are if the adolescent enters this period "feeling negative about himself or his body."[54] In either case, the body becomes a source of worries and newfound pleasures, of self-consciousness and pride.

Adolescents of both sexes experience an event of psychological and physical importance which connotes entry into physical adulthood. For the girl, this event is the menarche. The average girl begins menstruation at 12.6 years, approximately 2 years after the peak rate of growth occurs.[55] Lidz states, "It is usually the onset of menstruation rather than the profound change in her appearance that is most disturbing or satisfying to the girl."[56] Reactions range from fear and embarrassment to the joy of experiencing "womanhood." The overt sign of a boy's entering puberty, comparable to the menarche in girls, is ejaculation, which usually occurs during the twelfth or thirteenth year.[57] The capacity to ejaculate is directly linked to the experiencing of sexual pleasure and generally precedes the peak growth spurt in boys by approximately 2 years.[58] "Thus boys may begin to deal with new sexual feelings prior to experiencing changes in their body as a whole, while girls must deal first with a new body image."[59]

Fantasies

The fantasies and erotic impulses which the young person experiences during this time are new, frightening, irresistible, pleasurable, and uncomfortable. Fantasies, although not an overt sexual role behavior, are prominent in the adolescent's sexual development. The young man's sexual fantasies are most frequently erotic, including scenes of nude women or involving sexual activities. These fantasies occur during daydreams and nocturnal wet dreams and frequently accompany masturbation. "Males are eager to become physically involved for the purpose of having sex; they want to experiment and explore."[60] A common theme of the young woman's fantasies is romance, rather than eroticism. She may daydream about love stories, romantic moments, or being married, which may or may not include some sexual activities.[61,62] These fantasies occur during daydreaming and at night and frequently accompany listening to music, watching a movie, or reading a novel. The difference in the nature of males' and females' fantasies is possibly explained by differences in gender stereotypes, societal expectations, or the intensity of sexual urges.

Fantasies are a natural, usually private, component of sexual development which help prepare the adolescent for sexual activities. They tend, however, to generate a mixture of pleasure and distress. Fantasies provide a means for attaining temporary satisfaction and wish fulfillment and for expressing forbidden wishes. On the other hand, the content of sexual fantasies can cause the adolescent painful worries and doubts regarding his or her normalcy. Fantasies that involve socially unacceptable behaviors, such as group sex, being forced to submit, violent sex acts, homosexuality, incest, and prostitution, may evoke anxiety, guilt, and a lowering of self-esteem. Money[63] indicates that the adolescent may also experience conflict between the *ideal* of gender identity that he or she views as normal and the *actual* (conventional or nonconventional) image revealed through fantasies and dreams. He also suggests that this inconsistency between ideal gender identity and erotic imagery may account for much of the adolescent's "difficult" behavior. Thus, it may help the adolescent to know that fantasies serve a useful function, that socially unacceptable content is common, and that fantasies are thoughts which are infrequently acted out.

Masturbation

The young adolescent has no past experience with which to label or understand his or her current sexual urges and desires. Thus, these new feelings are often misunderstood and conflict with earlier teachings. Boys and girls alike may experience genital sensations and orgasm from nonsexual activities and objects that inadvertently stimulate the genitals, such as rubbing against an animate or inaminate object, dancing, engaging in sports, and bike riding. The penis of the young boy is especially vulnerable to chance stimulation resulting in spontaneous erection. Pleasurable genital sensations in both sexes frequently lead to self-stimulation and masturbation.[64]

Masturbation is a normative sex behavior in adolescence.[65-67] Definitions of masturbation vary from deliberate activities of self-arousal that culminate in orgasm to masturbatory-like acts that give sensual pleasure. A common theme reflected in the literature is that masturbation is an erotic activity involving voluntary self-stimulation.[68] Although children prior to puberty have discovered genital pleasure, voluntary, drive-impelled masturbation becomes a common sex practice during adolescence.

There are potential benefits to adolescent masturbation. It is an easily accessible avenue for pleasurable experiences; it can teach the adolescent, particularly the girl, how to achieve orgasm;[69] it affords the girl an opportunity to become familiar with her body and reactions so that later she might teach someone else how to please her sexually;[70] it can help the boy learn to delay orgasm so that, during intercourse, he will be able to wait until his partner is ready.[71] Masturbation can offer the adolescent a variety of sexual experiences, including tension release, without invoking harm and risk to self or others. It is also a mode for fantasizing and rehearsing future sexual behavior. "Psychiatrists regard masturbation as normal for adolescent development and even necessary for the control and integration of sexual urges and for mastery of one's sexual capacity."[72]

Among adolescents, there exist several differences in the ways boys and girls experience and learn about masturbation. Masturbation and the striving for orgasm are more common in male than female adolescents. At the time of first ejaculation, most boys have begun masturbating; only about 15 percent of girls have masturbated at menarche.[73] By age 15, 80 percent to virtually all adolescent boys have masturbated, whereas approximately 20 to 25 percent of girls have done so.[74,75] The lower percentage of adolescent girls masturbating as compared to boys may be related to girls' less frequent discussions of sexual behavior among same-sex peers; the location of the clitoris, which reduces chance stimulation; boys' greater buildup of sexual tension during periods of sexual inactivity; and/or social taboos that do not encourage or expect sexual behavior in girls.[76-78]

Boys masturbate not only sooner but also more often than girls. Girls have the biological and emotional sexual equipment for self-induced orgasm, but most do not use it as regularly as boys. Since there is no physiological basis for these differences, it is assumed that they emerge from cultural attitudes and expectations.[79,80] Young adolescent boys are preoccupied with sexual excitement and orgasm; girls are more preoccupied with romance and "love." The need for sexual release of biological tension is often of greater importance than the object of that release for both sexes, but especially for boys. It is as difficult for adolescent girls to understand that boys have feelings of great sexual urgency as it is for adolescent boys to comprehend why it is that girls can take or leave sex so easily.[81] Perhaps because of a combination of forces, including the external location of the penis, the increase of hormonal secretions, and masculine expectations and stereotypes, adolescent boys engage in group discussions about masturbation as well as in group masturbatory experimentation. Whereas boys learn about masturbation from other boys, most girls discover it for themselves, often accidentally or from reading.[82] The sexes also differ in their thoughts during masturbation. Although there is little research in this area, it appears that the differences in the nature of their fantasies are consistent with their differing sex attitudes and orientation to the other sex. In boys, masturbation is generally accompanied by fantasies that emphasize eroticism, such as naked women or intercourse with one or more females. A number of girls think only about the sensation itself; for those who do fantasize, the emphasis is on romantic and more realistic experiences, such as falling in love, holding, and kissing.

Even though masturbation is gaining acceptance as a normal and useful sex behavior for adolescents, society generally maintains values, beliefs, and myths that oppose it. Many people believe that masturbation and, in fact, any sexual behavior that does not have procreation as its purpose is morally wrong; that masturbation is a psychologically immature, undesirable sexual act; or that physical harm will result. Adolescents influenced by these sociosexual taboos may have difficulty deriving pleasure from masturbation and experience guilt and anxiety from the activity or from their associated fantasies. Although ignorance of one's body, superstitions, and social taboos foster discomfort and guilt feelings among many adolescents, Sorensen[83] found that 51 percent of all masturbating adolescents rarely or never express feelings of anxiety or guilt about their masturbation. However, Sorensen reports that adolescents in general express more defensiveness and greater need for privacy about masturbation than about other sex practices discussed in his study. He proposes that self-esteem, embarrassment, and personal disgust constitute the major inhibiting factors to discussion of this topic among adolescents.[84] The decision to engage or not to engage in any sexual act, including masturbation, and the level of comfort and satisfaction with one's decision depend upon (1) the degree to which the behavior is congruent with one's value system and with the sexual norms of one's significant others and (2) one's understanding of the practice. Many adolescents need adult assistance in sorting through their own religious and moral values, in understanding and evaluating societal views on masturbation, and in comprehending factual information about such matters as the harmlessness, normativeness, and advantages of masturbation.[85]

Psychosocial Aspects of Adolescent Sexuality

Adolescent behavior reflects the composite of physical, psychological, cognitive, and social changes with which the adolescent must cope. Unpredictable and contradictory behaviors are distressful not only to the youngsters themselves, but also to adults. As a learner of new experiences related to his or her unfolding sexuality, the adolescent is in a vulnerable position. He or she is curious and wants to explore and test out new sexual ideas, fantasies, and behaviors; yet, the freedom to do so is often sharply curtailed by external and internal pressures to control himself or herself. From childhood experiences and relationships, the adolescent has acquired many of the necessary tools with which to tackle sex-related developmental tasks yet is unsure of his or her changing body and sense of male or female self. The adolescent recognizes the overall expectations of others and self for increasingly independent decision making and behavior but is confronted with incongruent messages and personal ambivalence. These interpersonal and intrapersonal dilemmas surrounding developing sexuality are manifested in a variety of often misunderstood behaviors.

The adolescent is self-focused. Developmentally, the adolescent is in the process of finding (which includes the fear of losing) himself or herself. This self-centeredness is evidenced by preoccupation with physical appearance and behavior and by self-consciousness. The adolescent may spend hours in front of a mirror admiring or lamenting his or her reflection. Likewise, much time and energy may be invested in getting ready for social occasions, that is, in selecting attire and experimenting with extremes in dress. Adolescents also expect others to be as absorbed in their physical self as they are and thus anticipate both criticism and admiration.[86] Even the slightest well-intended criticism about their ap-

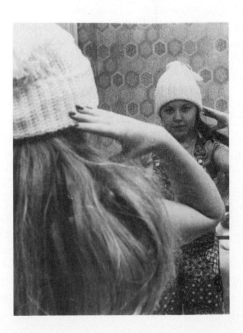

Adolescents, especially young ones, are highly attentive to details of their appearance and believe that others also inspect them with great scrutiny. (*Copyright* © *1980 by Patricia Yaros*.)

pearance, their clothing, or their idols, for example, can be interpreted as a major blow to their self-esteem and sense of masculinity or femininity. Compliments overemphasizing areas of bodily concern may also cause uneasiness. Genuine praise for physical attributes can enhance body image and self-esteem. New experiences, including bodily changes, unfamiliar sensations, and fantasies, cause the adolescent to feel discomfort and self-consciousness. Although the unevenness and rapidity of physical growth cause awkwardness in the adolescent, Matteson proposes that indecisiveness and lack of confidence in learning to use the changing body, rather than neuromuscular or physical inability, may account for the uncoordinated, clumsy movements. Feelings of self-consciousness are also accentuated by comparisons with others as the adolescent compares herself or himself with and is compared by peers and the larger society. In our culture, physical attractiveness, fitness, and skills are highly valued criteria for social acceptability and are especially valued among *young* adolescents, who tend to stereotype rather than to value individual differences. The stereotypes become consistent components of the adolescent's ideal body image.[87]

As adolescents compare their own body to their ideal body image, they may become highly self-critical and hypersensitive to positive and negative reactions from others, particularly parents. The greater the disparity between actual and ideal body image, the more likely the adolescent is to devalue body and self and to discredit even positive responses from others. Adolescents' fears of being exposed and devalued, and their growing sense that certain body parts and expressions have negative sexual significance to adults, may create strains in adolescent-adult relationships. These dynamics also help to explain why adolescents may be so insistent with parents about their privacy and modesty. Unexpected intrusions, displays of adult nudity, sexually tinged conversations, and adult references to the adolescent's sexual maturation can produce anger, tears, embarrassment, and diminished self-esteem. Some of these behaviors continue to exist along with contradictory episodes of seductiveness, voyeurism, and apparent disinterest in parental sexuality. Bryt[88] suggests that parental (adult) tolerance and respect be given these situations to prevent emotional upset and to help the adolescent develop consideration for others.

Peer Activities   In the process of establishing self-definition, types of relationships desired, and sex role orientation, the adolescent reaches out to a range of personality and behavior models. Parents and adults have a significant role in adolescent sexual development; they do not always exercise it adequately, and occasionally they abuse it. The adolescent depends on adults' guidance and support in solving problems and making choices at a time when he or she desires greater independence from adults and is expected to assume increased responsibility for his or her actions and associations. Thus, as adult standards and advice are deemed insufficient or intolerable, the adolescent turns to those most like himself or herself, the immediate peer group and the larger youth culture. In general, the peer group affords the adolescent opportunities to compare with a reference group in developing a positive body image, to continue to clarify and validate concepts of masculinity or femininity, to share sexual information and experiences, to experiment with sexual behaviors, and to develop more intense sociosexual relationships. The peer group offers security and direction by providing the adolescent a sense of belongingness, norms for acceptable sexual behavior, and a resource group.

During the first half of adolescence there may be a change from the same-sex peer group that existed during late school-age to a new group of same-sex friends. This shift may result from changes in interest and differences in rate of physical maturation, as well as from assignment to new schools or school groups. For both boys and girls, peer groups of the same sex seem to take precedence over heterosexual attachments at this age.[89] Moving into the proper group, as a step toward independence from the family and toward finding oneself, is more important than forming love relationships and finding heterosexual outlets.[90] Even though heterosexual interest may not be the primary focus of peer interactions, young adolescents share sexual information and further develop their sexual role.

The adolescent girl receives some sexual information (usually regarding menstruation) from her family and school, but she learns more from reading and talking with her girlfriends. The same-sex peer group frequently continues to support the previously learned social stereotypes of female sexuality. Matteson[91] writes that social learning for girls has stressed the acceptance of emotions and their interpersonal expression, so that, when sexual feelings emerge, they are easily interpreted as an increase in emotionality and a desire for romance. He points out that the cultural double standard discourages the acceptance of purely genital sexuality in women. The female peer group during early adolescence tends to share this romantic viewpoint and to reinforce it.

The adolescent boy generally receives less sexual information from his family than the girl does. Matteson[92] discusses an interesting point regarding this lack of communication. He suggests that possibly the family is more comfortable about menstruation than about first ejaculation, because they can desexualize the former as a biological event whereas the latter is clearly seen as a sexual experience. So the boy is supported by and largely dependent upon sexual information gained from his peers, who are interested in sexual matters and feelings. Boys tend to discuss sexual acts and erotic fantasies in the gym locker room or wherever the group gathers. And, in their discussions, an image and role set for the behaviors of a "man" as previously learned and influenced by society are reinforced. The boy feels that his masculinity hinges on being superior to others and being goal-directed.[93] Goal direction often refers to obtaining sexual pleasure and release, or to culminating sexual contact with coitus.

Early adolescent sexual awakening coincides with the developmental task of establishing same-sex friendships. Early adolescents frequently have a best friend whom they love as well as they love themselves. This is a person similar to himself or herself with whom the adolescent shares his or her happy, exciting experiences, secrets, dreams, fears, and traumas. In the context of such an intimate relationship, it is not difficult to understand why the young person may experience sexual feelings toward such a friend.[94,95] Although homosexual or homoerotic activities may occur (more frequently in boys than in girls), these experiences rarely foretell the behavior patterns and psychological relationships of adult homosexuals.[96] Such experiences, not to be confused with preferential homosexuality, constitute one of the means by which young people in our culture can juggle "successfully the urges and prohibitions and expectations thrust upon one at adolescence"[97] prior to heterosexual maturation.

The early adolescent may also experience "crushes." Several members of the peer group may participate in a group crush on the same person. The object of these infatuations may be a member of either sex, usually someone older, such as a teacher, rock star, or sibling of a friend. This tendency to have strong romantic or sexual feelings for an older person is a natural occurrence. Usually, the object of the crush does not reciprocate, and the adolescent resolves his or her unrequited love through new attachments to age-mates. However, there exists the potential danger of heterosexual or homosexual seduction by an older person. Generally, crushes serve to help the adolescent move away from the family, formulate ideal role images, and prepare for later heterosexual relationships.[98]

The need for belonging is one force which drives the adolescent toward an association with fellow age-mates or the peer group. "The need to belong implies a general sense of membership in, or participation with, another person or outside group."[99] This need motivates adolescents toward each other, gives them opportunities to learn how to cope with group members as well as themselves, and gives them a feeling of membership and social value.[100] Mitchell[101] suggests a relationship between the need for belonging and adolescent sexuality. The search for belonging, which urges one adolescent toward another, often results in a relationship where compatibility, affiliation, and openness facilitate "the onset of sexual behavior."[102] Mitchell further suggests that the need for belonging

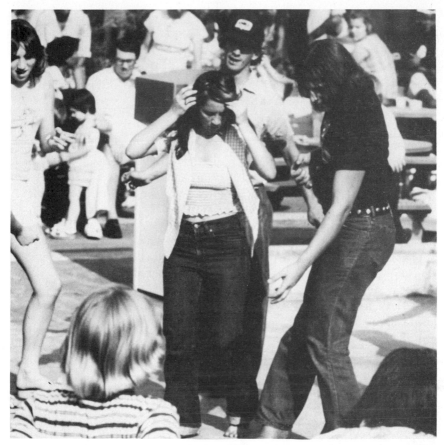

Sex role learning entails exposing oneself to peer critique and feedback and is an often stressful part of adolescent psychosocial development. (*Copyright © 1980 by Patricia Yaros*.)

influences the female to consent to sexual demands by the male because her sense of affiliation is threatened if she refuses.

Transition to a Couple Relationship The same-sex peer group helps the adolescent feel more secure in her or his own sexual identity, and this lays the groundwork for heterosexuality. As adolescents move along, mingling of male and female peer groups starts at school activities or local gathering spots. The adolescent can venture out to the opposite sex with the security of having the same-sex peer group present. Group parties, social events, and sports activities help make the transition a little more comfortable. Gradually, small group parties and pairing-off occur as the young people become more comfortable and confident with themselves, their urges, and their social skills, as well as with the others' behavior.

Successful social experiences with peers of both sexes during middle adolescence assist the young person in correcting the self-assessment uncertainties characteristic of early adolescence and help to form a new basis for an expanding sense of self.[103]

Double dating and single dating also provide an opportunity to get to know members of the opposite sex and to test out one's own self through the relationship. "'Dating' is a system whereby the adolescent may enjoy himself in heterosexual relationships while learning his strengths, weaknesses, and coping strategies in social situations and whereby he determines his preferences for choice of qualities in a mate."[104] Through dating, the adolescent can learn and experiment with social and sexual behaviors and continue to develop an understanding of self.

Petting is one of the earlier sex behaviors that occurs during the dating process. This behavior is the usual mode of entry into sexual activity[105] and is one of the most acceptable kinds of sexual behavior for the girl.[106] Petting involves a series of behaviors such as embracing, kissing, and fondling the body with the hand. The adolescent may continue along in this series of behaviors, advancing toward intercourse, or may stop at any point, depending upon his or her readiness and need for further sexual expression and/or experimentation. Petting entails sexual pleasure as well as relationship qualities. Through petting, adolescents can explore their own feelings, learn to gain control or direct their impulses, and learn about each other's body and each other's sexual responses.[107,108] Petting is a means of communicating affection, interest, and appreciation of another. It also provides the adolescent an encounter with another where feelings can be shared, the beginnings of heterosexual intimacy can be experienced, experimentation of feminine and masculine role behaviors can occur, and social rules and customs can be learned.[109]

Sexual Intimacy   Because of these earlier social-sexual activities, the movement into sexual intimacy later in adolescence might be expected to be natural and developmentally simple. Yet the sexual attitudes that the boy and girl bring to the relationship can make this new experience difficult. Earlier sexual repressions, acceptance of one's body, understanding of self, fantasized ideas about relationships, social skills, and sexual attitudes and behaviors are factors that influence the comfort and ease with which young people achieve both the physical and emotional components of an overtly sexual relationship.

In attempting to relate to the opposite sex, the adolescent is confronted with the different standards that society holds for boys and girls, men and women. Alternatives to the "double standard" phenomenon are discussed and analyzed frequently by current-day adolescents; this is still largely a theoretical exercise and causes conflict for many girls and boys. Although a girl may want to take the initiative in asking a boy out or show affection first through a physical means, she is afraid that the boy will reject her or might not appreciate her honesty and approach.[110] Even though the girl may wish to engage in intercourse, she must consider the repercussions of condemnation from the boy or other persons. On the other hand, the boy may enjoy an invitation for a date and for intercourse but find he has difficulty continuing to care for the girl because she is no longer "sacred" or "clean."[111] Sexual attitudes and traditional roles appear to be changing, at least on a cognitive level, but the practice of these insights is more difficult. It appears that men are accepting more changes in women and that men and women are moving toward the same standard of *sex with affection*[112] (i.e., the acceptance of sexual activity within the context of an affectional relationship). There appears to be a decline, not a fall, of the double standard;[113] hence, the adolescent must continue to negotiate individual standards with those of the opposite sex and the larger society.

The young male and female may well approach the heterosexual experience with different attitudes as a result of the background differences which have been discussed previously. The female enters the relationship looking for emotional and romantic experiences, accepting some physical expressions, but hesitant about genital contact.[114] The male's focus in the heterosexual relationship is more directed toward physical sex and proving his masculinity. Matteson[115] writes that, as male sexual identity becomes confirmed, security to "lose himself in another person and thus to accept the personhood of the woman" can follow. In contrast, girls generally accept the socioemotional aspects of love first, and later accept the sexual act within the framework of an intimate relationship. Somehow the boy and girl must negotiate these differences. Each has something to share and something to learn toward integration of the physical and emotional dimensions inherent in a sexual relationship.

The extent to which sex behaviors are a part of the heterosexual relationship is a decision made by the adolescent partners. Whether or not to engage in petting, mutual stimulation, or intercourse is a private matter that must be decided between the two adolescents. To make the decision successfully, both male and female must be cognizant of acceptable and unacceptable sex behaviors to themselves as well as to their partner and must be capable of making a conscious choice with minimal conflict. As in any decision, there are internal and external forces which affect the outcome. The stability or fragility of the young person's sense of self, the acceptance or rejection by the partner and/or society, and the congruity or incongruity with peer group and societal norms can make this decision comfortable or painful for the adolescent.

Intercourse is a natural mode of heterosexual expression and experimentation for the adolescent. Sorensen[116] reports that 52 percent of all American adolescents between the ages of 13 and 19 have had sexual intercourse; 59 percent of the boys and 45 percent of the girls reported having coitus at least once. Whether these percentages are high and whether premarital intercourse has increased over the years are debatable and perhaps irrelevant questions. What is important is to recognize that intercourse is an optional behavior for sexual expression. The experience of intercourse affords the adolescent opportunities for release of sexual tensions; experimentation in sexual activities; learning about sexual responses; decision making and independent action; communicating love and affection; and the sharing of fun, pleasure, and intimacy. Whether this sexual activity is a result of an ongoing relationship or of a brief encounter, whether it is planned or spontaneous, whether it is for love or for pleasure, the adolescents learn something more about themselves and their partner.

The adolescent may be motivated to engage in intercourse as a reaction to psychological stress, various intrapsychic needs, parental authority, and so on. He or she may be influenced by peer group pressures and mass media. Films, magazines, frank discussions of sex, and pornography can motivate the young person to be curious about and to engage in intercourse. Sex role standards which stress sexual capacity and prowess and goal-directed sexual activity urge the young male toward intercourse as a proof of masculinity. Standards suggesting that a girl is responsible for arousing and gratifying a boy or that intercourse is a symbol of love can influence the girl. Although there appears to be increasing acceptance of intercourse among adolescents, some differences exist in initial reactions to this sexual experience among boys and girls. Sorensen reports these findings:

> A much higher proportion of boys than girls were positive, optimistic, and generally affirmative in their immediate reactions to first intercourse; a much higher proportion of girls than boys were generally negative, pessimistic, and fearful in their immediate reactions to first intercourse.[117]

Perhaps the difference in sex role standards with the concomitant familial and societal sanctions helps to explain these findings. Of those adolescents questioned, 54 percent of the girls and 67 percent of the boys responded that, in retrospect, they were glad they had this first intercourse experience.[118]

The above reactions need to be considered as well as other problems that may follow from intercourse, such as disapproval and punishment from peers and parents, and health and social problems, such as venereal disease and pregnancy. Adolescents, typically present-oriented, infrequently consider the consequences of intercourse. For example, Sorensen[119] reports that 55 percent of the adolescents did not use birth control methods during their first intercourse experience.

> It is true that adolescents are making some mistakes; they may opt for intercourse before they are ready; they may mistake genital sex for sexual love; they may often ignore love in favor of genital satisfaction. But in general they are trying to become whole and feeling people.[120]

The degree to which intercourse is a healthy, growth-promoting experience depends on the adolescent's motivations, attitudes, values, and acceptance of sexuality; prevalent sex role standards; societal prohibitions and sanctions; and the congruity of these elements. The more the above elements are incongruent and partners act irresponsibly or seek intercourse because of maladaptive responses to intrapsychic difficulties, the more the adolescent is likely to experience unhealthy outcomes.

The need for intimacy is a force which may drive one toward or bind one in a sexual relationship. "Although definitions of 'intimacy' vary, most of them include the need for close personal relationships with another person, the need for intense closeness and involvement with something meaningful."[121] During adolescence, when the young person is experiencing various conflicts and becoming more independent of the family and seeking his or her identity, it is not surprising that he or she would seek a secure, trusting, continuous, close relationship. "With the partial disintegration of the peer group as well as the tendency toward heterosexual pairing-up, the intimacy need becomes even more accentuated."[122]

The energy invested in meeting this need is unparalleled. Parents frequently become disturbed over the choice of the companion and the intensity and priority of the relationship that is displayed by their son or daughter. When the adolescent's demand and need for an intimate relationship is denigrated by adults, problems can result. For the adolescent this relationship is honored, valued, and necessary.

Intimacy, with all its relationship components, also involves such physical behaviors as fondling, embracing, and touching and such sexual behaviors as petting and coitus. Intimacy can lead to sexual involvement; and sexual behavior for the purpose of pleasure can facilitate intimacy by providing an atmosphere of openness.[123] Sexual intimacy expresses mutuality of interest, satisfaction, and pleasure without elements of self-sacrifice, disrespect, and exploitation.[124]

The emotional relationship aspects of intimacy, as well as the sexual and nonsexual behaviors, are indicators of the strength of the commitment of two young adults. The close personal relationship is a commitment in time and space. Adolescents need relationships in order to learn "without having to commit themselves irrevocably"[125] and without having that relationship devalued for a lack of permanency. To the adolescent, the experience in itself is meaningful and growth-promoting.

NURSING SUPPORTS FOR ADOLESCENTS' DEVELOPING SEXUALITY

Throughout adolescence needs emerge which have a direct or indirect impact on one's sexuality. Specific developmental needs are common to all adolescents, yet the manner in which the needs are expressed and the degree to which they are met or engender conflicts differ with each young person. In the nursing care of adolescents, the clarification of existing needs and the selection of priorities and approaches are best undertaken by the nurse and adolescent working together. The following brief examples are intended to exemplify nursing approaches congruent with the adolescent's sexual needs.

Need to Understand One's Own Body

Factual information is necessary and perhaps best received through a relationship that conveys respect and acceptance and an environment that provides opportunities to explore teaching aids. In addition to individual or group discussions regarding anatomy and physiology, menstruation, the birth process, and venereal disease, young people need to explore and validate standards of sex behavior, learn about sexual response cycles, and resolve concerns about the normality of homosexual desires, fantasies, and body comparisons. The nurse is in a position to anticipate the adolescent's concerns and may initiate discussion on a specific topic or provide resource materials which enable the adolescent to pursue his or her own questions and answers. For example, if the nurse in caring for a young adolescent boy observes breast enlargement, it is helpful to say matter-of-factly that this often occurs in boys his age and to explain the physiological reasons and their outcomes. Adolescents in hospitals, as well as in other settings, have a need for privacy and time alone to process information and increase their understanding of their own bodies.

Need to Explore and Experiment with One's Own Body

The adolescent engages in self-exploratory behaviors. In the delivery of nursing care, numerous opportunities exist to facilitate adolescents' discovery of their own body parts and sensations. Approaches that communicate to the young person that it is appropriate, acceptable, and helpful to look at and touch one's own body may encourage self-acceptance. For example, in the process of catheterizing a teenage girl, the nurse unavoidably expresses certain attitudes toward the young person and her body. The manner in which she touches the client, the ease or discomfort expressed nonverbally, and the presence or lack of verbal interaction create an atmosphere of comfort or anxiety. The nurse's actions should be accompanied by explanations regarding the procedure, why it is necessary, and what is to be expected, including the sensations the patient will experience. The intent is to alleviate fear and anxiety and increase the young person's knowledge of her body and bodily functions. The interaction may motivate further questions and explorations on the part of the adolescent.

The situation in which a nurse walks in on a masturbating adolescent is one that frequently causes distress. The tendency to rush out in embarrassment and to avoid returning or to tell the adolescent to stop negates the youngster's normal need for body pleasure, exploration, and security and may also reinforce guilt and self-devaluation. The nurse's allowing for privacy and indicating that she or he will return shortly may not alleviate the youngster's initial embarrassment but can convey understanding. Recognizing that masturbation is one of the most private and difficult-to-discuss sex behaviors, the nurse needs to assess the adolescent's need and readiness for any continued discussion.

Need to Experiment with Sexual Role Behaviors

The adolescent's natural experimentation with sexual role behaviors can be misunderstood by the nurse. Frequently, nurses tend to focus on the surface behavior and overlook the underlying needs and motives of the young person. An adolescent girl, in her attempt to appear feminine and attractive to others, may dress and act seductively and thereby elicit negative reactions. For example, the young girl's half-buttoned or semi-transparent nightgown may be viewed only as an attempt to seduce. However, it may be an expression of her seeking to validate her femininity, i.e., to affirm that she is pretty or has an attractive figure; it may indicate a wish to attract or draw people toward her for security and comfort. The adolescent may need verbal recognition of her feminine qualities, attractiveness, and likeableness and may at the same time need assistance from the nurse in recognizing the consequences of the behavior. The nurse can aid the adolescent in exploring alternative modes of expression leading to need satisfaction and self-esteem.

Similarly, the young man who actively flirts with the nurse, talks suggestively, or boasts about his sexual conquests may simply be attempting to validate his masculinity. However, this behavior is frequently met with anxious and angry retorts. Responses which provide limits or guidelines without hurting his pride or devaluing his sense of manliness are more likely to assist him in learning behaviors conducive to effective, mature male-female interactions.

Need for Peer Relationships

Health care settings, especially hospitals, by virtue of their organization and physical structure, impose barriers to maintaining outside peer support systems and to developing new peer relationships and group interactions. Yet adolescents need peers, both individuals and groups, to share their ideas and concerns, to explore alternative solutions to problems, and for mutual support. It sometimes takes a great deal of skill, energy, and creativity to design an environment conducive to informal peer group interactions and formal group learning experiences. Both types of group interactions, whether initiated by the young people or the nurse, can enhance interpersonal and social skills and facilitate adolescents' sharing of sexual concerns and learning from one another. Nurses must find ways of encouraging mobile and nonmobile adolescents to meet and interact with one another, arranging schedules that accommodate group activities, initiating group sessions with physical and mental health focuses, and allowing for peer visits.

Numerous adolescent sexual behaviors occur in health settings. Leeway must be provided for healthy modes of sexual expression. Displays of physical affection, such as holding hands, placing arms around one another, or kissing, may be allowed or discouraged, depending on the timing of the interaction, the discretion of the couple, and the needs of others. Some forms of sexual expression may require immediate limits; others may be more effectively dealt with through individual discussions at a later time or through group problem solving.

Need for Developing and Maintaining Heterosexual Relationships

Through observations and interactions, the nurse may learn that some young people move easily into new heterosexual peer groups and seem to have the capacity to participate in activities with persons of both sexes, while others exhibit difficulties. It is important to ascertain whether difficulties are related primarily to illness and hospitalization or whether they are previously established patterns of behavior. The nurse, in general conversation while providing care, can often provide reassurance and anticipatory guidance.

One 14-year-old female refused to go to the teen lounge on any occasion although she easily interacted with her three roommates. The nurse, after encouraging her to join her peers in the lounge, asked if she was concerned about her appearance and the fact that several of the patients were young men. As they talked, it became evident that the girl was sensitive about the bulkiness of her chest bandages, felt that the boys would be staring at her, and was worried about what to say. The nurse listened and responded sensitively, determined that this adolescent really wanted to go to the lounge but was afraid, and helped her to decide on wearing pajamas and a robe that would decrease the bulky appearance of her breasts; and together they devised a plan for entry into the social situation. The plan involved sequential steps, whereby the girl first went to the lounge with the nurse at a time when the boys were not present. In the subsequent visits, the girl was present in the room prior to the arrival of her peer group. She gradually became able to enter the lounge with her age-mates. During this process, which took over two days, questions regarding boy-girl relationships and concerns related to her body image were explored as a part of nursing care.

In caring for hospitalized or ambulatory adolescent clients, the nurse is frequently challenged to design opportunities and to plan for options that allow for the support that comes from boyfriend-girlfriend interactions. It is important to find ways to provide for these normal adolescent needs. With the help of adolescents themselves, nurses can devise visitation policies which support attainment of developmental tasks and, at the same time, provide responsible guidance and protect the rights of all involved.

Need for Adult Guidance and Assistance

The nurse's role includes being astute to cues that an adolescent wants certain information or wishes to talk about a particular issue but is having difficulty in articulating the request. Sometimes this difficulty is reflected in comments such as the following: "Can I talk with you later. . . ?" "Oh, never mind, it was nothing." "I was just wondering . . . but it's too silly." "You'll be mad if I ask you." An initial response similar to "You may feel silly and uncomfortable, but it doesn't mean that your question is a silly one" or "Perhaps, but it is something you've been wondering about and wanting to discuss, no?" may encourage the adolescent to continue. As the young person begins to verbalize vague bits and pieces, the nurse may become able to formulate questions close to his or her underlying concern, for example, "Are you wondering whether or not the surgery will interfere with sexual relations?" Or "Sometimes people your age are concerned about . . . . Is that what you're getting at?" This type of response allows the adolescent the options of saying no and dropping the subject or of pursuing it.

In caring for a dying 15-year-old boy whom she had known for many months, a particular nurse was asked, "Can I talk with you later?" When she returned, he insisted it was nothing, yet he continued to approach his question over three consecutive days. She verbalized his apparent struggle but did not lose patience with his repeated and uncompleted requests or push him to talk. Finally, on the fourth day, he responded to her encouragement with, "Have you ever had intercourse?" The nurse replied, "Why do you ask?" With much hesitation, he looked toward her and asked, "What does intercourse feel like?'' Before she could say anything, he blurted out almost apologetically, ''It's the one thing that I don't know and I really want to know, and you're the only person I can ask.'' As she sat beside him, the nurse responded, ''Matt, you've been wondering about intercourse and picturing it in your mind; what do you think it feels like?'' ''I don't know, I never did it.'' ''But you do have some ideas, right?'' Matt looked at her and offered, ''It must be a beautiful feeling to love someone that much and to be that close to that person.'' The nurse affirmed his point of view by stating, ''For many people, that's exactly what the experience is like.'' Matt seemed satisfied, was silent for a few moments, and then continued to seek clarification and answers for the many questions he had been asking himself for a long time.

CONCLUSION

In assisting the adolescent in his or her sexual development, the nurse has two predominant roles: teaching and guidance. To function competently in these roles requires being able to listen to the expressed concerns; ''hear'' the underlying messages; provide support, information, and anticipatory guidance; and use a collaborative problem-solving approach in helping the adolescent to arrive at decisions. The adolescent's need is for help to identify and clarify problem issues, determine alternative courses of action and points of view, weigh the advantages and disadvantages of each, and arrive at decisions he or she can live with comfortably. Attempts to impose beliefs and actions based on our value system and needs are doomed to failure, certainly once the youngster has left our setting. Adolescents are bound to make choices and decisions we do not agree with and do not like or that we know have potential dangers. We can and should share the beliefs, concerns, and knowledge of dangers that we have, but, ultimately, the adolescent must make and live with his or her commitments. If we can assist adolescents to acquire and use a problem-solving approach, then they will have a useful tool they can carry with them.

Adolescents express manifold questions, compelling concerns, and wonderment about their own sexuality and sexual experiences. Theories of human development and sexuality enable health professionals to develop a paradigm for understanding the direction and process of healthy sexual maturation. In addition, the nurse's personal point of view influences the assessments and interventions made in the effort to facilitate the adolescent's progress toward sexual identity and maturation. However, the young person himself or herself is the prime mover in knowing where he or she is, where he or she wants to go, and with whom he or she wishes to engage. To avoid viewing adolescence and adolescent sexuality as a ''dangerous abbreviation,''[126] it is imperative to understand the dynamics and range of normal adolescent sexual behaviors. It is also essential that nurses recognize their own sexual attitudes and continue to validate their competencies to provide comprehensive care for adolescents, who are—among other things—sexual beings.

REFERENCES

1 M. Diamond, "Biological Foundations of Social Development," in F. A. Beach (ed.), *Human Sexuality in Four Perspectives*. Baltimore: Johns Hopkins University Press, 1977.
2 H. I. Lief, "Introduction to Sexuality," in B. J. Sadock, H. I. Kaplan, and A. M. Freedman (eds.), *The Sexual Experience*. Baltimore: Williams and Wilkins Co., 1976.
3 D. R. Matteson, *Adolescence Today: Sex Roles and the Search for Identity*. Homewood, Ill.: The Dorsey Press, 1975.
4 J. Money and A. A. Ehrhardt, *Man & Woman, Boy & Girl*. New York: A Mentor Book, New American Library, 1974.
5 R. Murray and J. Zentner, *Nursing Assessment and Health Promotion through the Life Span*. Englewood Cliffs, N.J.: Prentice-Hall, 1975.
6 R. Stoller, "Gender Identity," in B. J. Sadock, H. I. Kaplan, and A. M. Freedman (eds.), *The Sexual Experience*. Baltimore: Williams and Wilkins Co., 1976, p. 185.
7 Lief, op. cit., p. 5.
8 Ibid., p. 4.
9 J. Bardwick, *Psychology of Women: A Study of Bio-Cultural Conflicts*. New York: Harper & Row, 1971, p. 93.
10 Diamond, op. cit., pp. 45–48.
11 H. A. Moss, "Sex, Age and State as Determinants of Mother-Infant Interaction," *Merrill-Palmer Quarterly*, 13:19–39, 1967.
12 H. S. Sullivan, *The Inter-Personal Theory of Psychiatry*. New York: W. W. Norton & Co., 1953.
13 J. J. Mitchell, "Some Psychological Dimensions of Adolescent Sexuality," *Adolescence*, 7:447–458, 1972.
14 Sullivan, op. cit.
15 Matteson, op. cit.
16 D. Offer and W. Simon, "Stages of Sexual Development," in B. J. Sadock, H. I. Kaplan, and A. M. Freedman (eds.), *The Sexual Experience*. Baltimore: Williams and Wilkins Co., 1976, p. 133.
17 T. Lidz, *The Person: His Development throughout the Life Cycle*. New York: Basic Books, 1968, p. 208.
18 Matteson, op. cit., p. 80.
19 Lidz, op. cit., p. 214.
20 Ibid., p. 216.
21 Matteson, op. cit.
22 Ibid.
23 Lidz, op. cit.
24 Matteson, op. cit.
25 Lidz, op. cit., p. 209.

26 Offer and Simon, op. cit., p. 133.

27 Matteson, op. cit., p. 47.

28 Ibid., p. 15.

29 Ibid., p. 24.

30 Ibid., p. 80.

31 Lidz, op. cit., p. 213.

32 Ibid., p. 226.

33 Murray and Zentner, op. cit., p. 152.

34 Diamond, op. cit.

35 Lidz, op. cit.

36 Ibid., pp. 265–266.

37 J. Kagan and H. A. Moss, *Birth to Maturity: A Study in Psychological Development*. New York: John Wiley and Sons, 1962, p. 272.

38 A. Bryt, "Adolescent Sex Crises," *Medical Aspects of Human Sexuality*, **10**:8–34, 1976.

39 Lidz, op. cit.

40 Sullivan, op. cit.

41 Ibid., p. 246.

42 Bryt, op. cit., p. 15.

43 Bardwick, op. cit.

44 G. J. Manaster, *Adolescent Development and the Life Tasks*. Boston: Allyn and Bacon, 1977, p. 72.

45 Kagan and Moss, op. cit., p. 266.

46 Matteson, op. cit.

47 Lief, op. cit., p. 4.

48 Matteson, op. cit., p. 145.

49 Bryt, op. cit.

50 Manaster, op. cit.

51 Matteson, op. cit.

52 Lidz, op. cit., p. 301.

53 W. B. Pomeroy, *Girls & Sex*. New York: Dell Publishing Co., 1969, p. 40.

54 Murray and Zentner, op. cit., p. 173.

55 Matteson, op. cit., p. 124.

56 Lidz, op. cit., p. 307.

57 Matteson, op. cit., p. 125.

58 Offer and Simon, op. cit., p. 135.

59 Matteson, op. cit., p. 125.

60 G. D. Jensen, "Adolescent Sexuality," in B. J. Sadock, H. I. Kaplan, and A. M. Freedman (eds.), *The Sexual Experience*. Baltimore: Williams and Wilkins Co., 1976, p. 145.

61 Jensen, op. cit.

62 H. A. Katchadourian and D. T. Lunde, *Fundamentals of Human Sexuality*. New York: Holt, Rinehart and Winston, 1972.

63 Money and Ehrhardt, op. cit., p. 193.

64 Jensen, op. cit., p. 143.

65 Jensen, op. cit.

66 W. B. Pomeroy, *Boys & Sex*. New York: Dell Publishing Co., 1968.

67 R. C. Sorensen, *Adolescent Sexuality in Contemporary America: Personal Values and Sexual Behavior Ages 13–19*. New York: World Publishing Co. 1973.
68 Katchadourian and Lunde, op. cit., p. 219.
69 Jensen, op. cit.
70 Katchadourian and Lunde, op. cit.
71 Pomeroy, 1968, op. cit.
72 Jensen, op. cit., p. 144.
73 Katchadourian and Lunde, op. cit., p. 224.
74 Offer and Simon, op. cit.
75 Pomeroy, 1969, op. cit.
76 Jensen, op. cit.
77 Katchadourian and Lunde, op. cit.
78 Pomeroy, 1969, op. cit.
79 Bryt, op. cit., p. 24.
80 Jensen, op. cit., p. 143.
81 Pomeroy, 1969, op. cit., p. 141.
82 Katchadourian and Lunde, op. cit., p. 224.
83 Sorensen, op. cit., p. 145.
84 Ibid., p. 144.
85 Jensen, op. cit., p. 144.
86 D. Elkind, *Children and Adolescents*. New York: Oxford University Press, 1970.
87 Matteson, op. cit.
88 Bryt, op. cit., p. 15.
89 Lidz, op. cit., p. 332.
90 Ibid., p. 332.
91 Matteson, op. cit., p. 148.
92 Ibid., p. 150.
93 Ibid., p. 156.
94 Ibid., op. cit.
95 Sullivan, op. cit.
96 Jensen, op. cit.
97 W. J. Gadpaille, "A Consideration of Two Concepts of Normality as It Applies to Adolescent Sexuality," *Journal of the American Academy of Child Psychiatry*, **15**:679–691 (p. 687), 1976.
98 Lidz, op. cit.
99 Mitchell, op. cit., p. 450.
100 Mitchell, op. cit.
101 Ibid., p. 451.
102 Ibid.
103 Bryt, op. cit., p. 32.
104 Manaster, op. cit., p. 146.
105 Offer and Simon, op. cit.
106 Pomeroy, 1969, op. cit.
107 Lidz, op. cit.
108 Katchadourian and Lunde, op. cit.

109   Ibid., p. 184.
110   M. Hultén, "Sex Education: Lowering the Taboos," *World Health*, December 1976, 22–25 (p. 23).
111   Hultén, op. cit., p. 23.
112   E. O. Smigel and R. Seiden, "The Decline and Fall of the Double Standard," in H. D. Thornburg (ed.), *Contemporary Adolescence: Readings*. Belmont, Calif.: Wadsworth Publishing Co., 1973, p. 84.
113   Ibid., p. 85.
114   Matteson, op. cit., p. 155.
115   Ibid., p. 159.
116   Sorensen, op. cit.
117   Ibid., p. 214.
118   Sorensen, op. cit.
119   Ibid.
120   Ibid., p. 375.
121   Mitchell, op. cit., p. 448.
122   Ibid.
123   Mitchell, op. cit., p. 449.
124   Bryt, op. cit.
125   G. Konopka, "Requirements for Healthy Development of Adolescent Youth," *Adolescence*, **8**:291–315 (p. 304), 1973.
126   F. Redl, Seminar on adolescence presented at the University of Michigan Fresh Air Camp, 1965.

BIBLIOGRAPHY

Erickson, E. H.: *Childhood and Society*. New York: W. W. Norton & Co., 1963.
Jeanneret, O.: "That Awkward Age," *World Health*, December 1976, 4–11.
Kagan, J.: *Change and Continuity in Infancy*. New York: John Wiley & Sons, 1971.

Chapter 9

The Adolescent at Risk: Crisis, the Delicate Balance

Rae Sedgwick
Susan Hildebrand

For clinicians who work with families and children, it is impossible to talk about adolescents at risk without also talking about families at risk. The family, however defined, probably exerts more influence over the individual and his or her development than does any other social force with which the individual comes into contact over the span of a lifetime. The family as a significant source of values, beliefs, and personal practices supplies the character traits from which the individual draws in the process of putting together lifetime behavior patterns. If the family is weak, nonsupportive, or in opposition to the mainstream of society, the individual will experience difficulty in personal development and interpersonal functioning.

THE FAMILY AS A SETTING FOR RISK OR STABILITY

The growing child within the family learns to relate to the overall society in the same manner in which the family relates, whether successfully or not. The family relates to its members in accordance with the way the society relates to the family. It becomes readily apparent that the individual, the family, and the larger society are interwoven very closely: What affects one affects the others.

It has been said that we live in a "throw-away" society: plastic cups, disposable dishes, transitory relationships. If you don't like something, throw it away and get a new one. This philosophy permeates a swiftly moving, highly technological society which crowds the family and in many ways works counter to its function as the pervading socializing force in the lives of its members. Many of the family's historical functions—education, religious training, skill development, and social adaptation—have been delegated to schools, churches, and colleges. The contemporary functions of the family are less well defined than family functions were in the past.

Three decades ago, when people had children they had some idea of the kind of person their child might become and they held some rather firm notions about what kind of role that child might play in the future of society. Fathers handed down to sons; mothers handed down to daughters; and the vocations and social roles that children might eventually occupy were fairly well predicted by what their parents had done in the past. Psychological and social security grew from the predictability of the future; people knew what to expect and, generally, how to prepare their children.

Today when a child is born, the parents have no way to predict what kind of person the individual will become or what kind of work or life-style may be available. Social changes and technological and scientific developments proceed with a rapidity that makes it next to impossible to predict what the outcome will be by the time that child grows up. Furthermore, support for those experiencing such uncertainty is more lacking today than in the past.

The mobility of families makes it difficult for immediate family members to rely on one another for advice and support. Gone is the day when grandparents were ever near for consultation and encouragement; gone is the day when the knowledge of parenting was handed down from mother to daughter, and business advice was passed from father to son; gone is the day when social roles were neatly defined and responsibilities neatly packaged. Here is the day when daughter may be taking over father's business, son may work so that mother can go back to school, and parents as well as their children experiment with open relationships and mind-altering drugs. It is in fact a new day, with which we have very little experience either as adults or professionals.

Place into this fluid social environment an adolescent bright with ambition, burning with curiosity, experiencing an upsurge of sexual drive, and reaching with increasing intensity toward an unknown future. That adolescent is, for a number of reasons, in a delicate, precarious balance.

DEVELOPMENTAL CRISES

A *crisis* is a situation that calls for action or adaptation but for which one's customary, previously effective modes of response are inadequate. Crises are commonly classified as developmental (maturational) or situational. *Developmental crises* are those that arise as a result of developmental change: They are more or less universal situations that occur predictably at various points along the life continuum. Puberty, marriage, and retirement are examples of developmental crises. *Situational crises*, which are discussed in a later section of this chapter, are crises that arise because of some more unpredictable event such as illness, divorce, natural disaster, and the like.

The adolescent is in the process of becoming, of changing, no longer a child but not yet an adult. Experiencing adult desires but ill-equipped with only partially developed adult judgment, the adolescent is often confronted with decisions whose outcomes sway in the balance between the extremes of conservative action (or inaction) and liberal acting out. Adults, sometimes confused by the adultlike appearance, language, and body size of the adolescent, fail to provide the guidance and consultation necessary for appropriate, constructive actions. If the family background has provided the adolescent with a set of skills that involve testing within reason, experimenting within bounds, seeking help where there is doubt or confusion, and experiencing within a given responsibility, the young person has a better chance of getting through these tumultuous years with fewer scars.

Families who do not provide the individual with a set of social and psychological traits—self-esteem, a personal sense of competence in spite of social or academic failures, unconditional regard for other people, and a belief in living that extends beyond the self—do not provide the tools necessary to circumvent the doubting, testing, and challenges of the adolescent years or adulthood.

Doubting, testing, and challenging are inevitable developmental experiences of adolescence, for it is during these years that young people begin the lifelong process of searching for meaning in life and in living and for their personal place in the world. Prior to adolescence children ask, about events around them, "Why?" The answers that satisfy are those that deal largely with the world *around* the child. When the individual reaches adolescence, however, questions begin to be more self-oriented: "What part do I play in all these things going on around me? Am I an important member of my family? Am I loved? What is most important to me?"

As the adolescent seeks to answer these questions, the peer group begins to exert a new influence: Friends gradually move into roles that include new kinds of testing, competition, and experimentation. The adolescent begins a struggle between loyalty to peers and loyalty to family. For a brief span of years, peers reach new heights of importance, almost to the exclusion of family. Perhaps it is because adolescents are newly aware of themselves and their fledgling identities that they seek refuge in their circle of friends. In their confusion and internal chaos, adolescents seek to compare and contrast themselves to others who are having similar thoughts, feelings, and experiences. When forced to choose between family and friends, the adolescent more often than not chooses friends, out of blind loyalty, devotion, mutual need, frequency of contact, and the developmental need to be emancipated from parents. If adults attempt to curtail adolescents' opportunities for contrasting and comparing themselves to peers, adolescents may become deceptive in order to meet their pressing needs for peer group affiliation and socialization; that is, they may lie in order to be in contact with friends. Under these circumstances, adolescents may not make sound choices, but they will make choices, and for them that in itself is vitally important.

The desire and need to be with peers is often a source of conflict between parent and adolescent. This is particularly so when the family is different from the surrounding social environment or maintains strict, inflexible religious or social beliefs.

> Lyn Johnson is the firstborn child of parents who hold very strong religious beliefs and who make stringent demands for church attendance and participation. There are few young people in the church, and Lyn's primary source of social stimulation is older people. Lyn's strong desire to attend school functions and socialize with peers is repeatedly refused by her parents. One attempt to sneak out for a school play is met with a physical beating, which is detected by the school nurse.
>
> During discussions with Lyn, the school nurse learns that Lyn knows very little about herself as a young woman and even less about herself as a member of a changing world. The school nurse also learns about Lyn's desire to ``be like the other kids.'' In order to help her learn about herself, including aspects of menstruation, self-examination of breasts, sexuality, and dating, the school nurse initiates the formation of a discussion group of five or six other freshman girls. Through these discussions, which occur during school hours, Lyn is able to learn more about herself and begins to experience herself in relation to her peers without censure from her parents.

Lyn Johnson's parents may never change. Lyn at least will have the chance to explore alternative beliefs, experience herself as a healthy, developing adolescent, and find out that help is available (legal as well as medical) to children who are abused by parents.

Adolescents with parents whose religious beliefs or social practices differ greatly from those of others around them are definitely adolescents at risk. Most adolescents need an underlying belief system to hold onto during the times of doubting and struggle. They will, in fact, challenge, test, and demand explanation from their parents regarding beliefs, values, and practices. Adolescents whose parents respond with violence, lack of support, or punishment do not know where to turn. Such teenagers may even question their own right to ask questions and to explore the world around them. Not every adolescent is as lucky as Lyn Johnson in finding an adult who can help in the growing process in spite of the constraints placed on that growth by well-meaning parents.

Adolescents spend a great deal of time comparing themselves to others, particularly peers. If in that comparison the adolescent finds stark differences, doubt of self or others results. Self-doubt is a common experience for the average teenager. When something goes wrong—poor grades, for example—adolescents do a lot of verbal blaming of others. But they also question themselves. The adolescent then looks for someone who will give the message that he or she is "okay," that he or she is important, and that it is all right to make mistakes. The adolescent who is unable to make mistakes, who is expected by parents to be perfect, is someone who at one time or another generally gets into trouble.

One of the more frequent complaints of troubled adolescents is, "My parents want me to be perfect." Perhaps there is an inner drive of the teenager to try to be perfect; perhaps society pressures adolescents to be perfect; and perhaps families do place inordinate demands on struggling teenagers. Whatever the source, most adolescents get the notion at one time or another that someone expects perfection of them. Sensing their humanness and their imperfections, these adolescents strike out, often in confusion and frustration.

Many teenagers set out, for reasons unknown to themselves, to prove their parents right; they become star athletes, achieve high academic honors, win a lead in the school play, or take first chair in the band. But others reach beyond their grasp and feel a sense of failure. Maybe they bring home a B instead of an A; perhaps they win third chair rather than first; maybe they don't even get a minor part in the play. The sense of failure may grow to distorted dimensions. What happens next depends on the parents' response as well as the kind of inner sense of competence the adolescent has built over the preceding years.

Those adolescents who have grown up with a sense of belonging and a sense of unconditional importance to others weather these storms of disappointment, although their distress can be severe. However, for those who have not acquired that sense of essential importance and connectedness to someone else, trouble in some form commonly results. These youngsters are particularly at risk for shoplifting and pregnancy.

> Tom Allen is the third child of a lower-middle-income family of two parents and five children. At the time of conception, Tom's mother did not want

another child; this unwillingness stuck with her all during pregnancy as well as during Tom's growing years. Although she never spoke to Tom about her feelings and maintains that she and his father never showed preferences among their children, Tom grew up with feelings of not being wanted and of not belonging. When he questioned his parents about their feelings, they denied his intuition about his place in the family. Tom was active in the Boy Scouts and in his church, got good grades in school, and was well liked in the community. One bright spring day he was brought to my office for evaluation: He had been picked up for shoplifting. During that evaluation period Tom disclosed his longtime feelings of not being wanted. He stated that he shoplifted to get his father to prove to Tom that he liked him no matter what Tom did, right or wrong. The father, however, turned Tom over to the police for questioning and stated that the boy could either pay for the damages or go to jail; he didn't care one way or the other. Tom's intuition about his parents was, unfortunately, quite accurate. Although therapy helped relieve the situation, Tom will never be the fully accepted member of his family that he wants to become. His parents are geared to reject him no matter what he tries.

Tom's case is a clear example of how long-standing family problems come to rest on the family members. The parents feel they were trapped by an early marriage, cannot achieve the economic status they desire because of lack of education and skill, and have five children who surpass the parents in intelligence. In order to act out their frustrations, the parents have unwittingly selected one of their children as the "scapegoat." While they verbalize understanding of what they have done, they seem powerless to effect much change in their daily actions.

While the clinician can provide positive support for the individual, treat the person with respect, and give the person some sense of overall importance and uniqueness, without the parents' regard and approval there is a point beyond which the individual cannot grow—particularly in relationships with significant others. There is no substitute for parental love and approval. One's relationship with parents, negative or positive, seems strongly to color the way future relationships are handled or worked out over time.

It is important to recognize that communication need not be verbal in order to influence another in a significant and powerful way. While Tom's parents never openly expressed their feelings about Tom, he picked up and acted on their unspoken message. If the parents had thought about and worked on their feelings and relationship with each other, there might have been an opportunity to alter the direction that Tom's life seems to have taken.

In Tom's case, as in most, it is easy in retrospect to see that the episode that clearly showed that he was troubled (the shoplifting arrest) was really not an abrupt departure from earlier behavior but was an outflow from the preceding pattern. Tom's shoplifting, for example, was preceded by a series of small, seemingly insignificant acts, which, although they did not risk the censure of law or school officials, also failed to gain Tom the needed attention from his parents. For a while he had demonstrated highly successful behavior—good grades, music, Scouts—and when these failed to gain him the needed spot within the family, he turned to less acceptable forms of love-getting behavior. With his family, that too failed.

SITUATIONAL CRISES

There are families whose members are not good for one another. There are people who probably should never have been parents—not without formal training, at least. Adults who themselves have had inadequate parenting and insufficient love in their own childhood and adolescence generally do not become healthy, effective parents. Their children are then extremely high risks, both socially (as in the case of shoplifting, stealing, or teenage pregnancy) and psychologically (as in the case of pregnancy or suicide).

Teenage pregnancy, seemingly on the increase, may be a form of striking out against insufficient parenting and the adolescent's belief that perfection is required. Seeking love and recognition, which do not come unconditionally from the parents, the unskilled and oftentimes uninformed young woman is caught in a "Catch 22." Wanting love and closeness, fighting against parental coldness and high expectations, having insufficient information about her body and perhaps experiencing unexpected sexual urges, she often finds herself in a predicament that is beyond her ability to handle. Needing to turn to parents or other adults because of her pregnancy but not being able to for fear of rejection or disapproval, the pregnant teenager may think about running away or killing herself. Such a drastic choice among alternatives points out the seriousness with which the pregnant teenager faces the consequences of her actions.

Ann Wilson is the 16-year-old eldest daughter of well-to-do, college-educated parents. Ann's parents married at an early age, moved several hundred miles from their own parents, and began the long and arduous journey up the economic and social ladders. Twice during Ann's growing up, the family moved to a better neighborhood and a finer house; finally, in Ann's second year of junior high school, the family (which by then included a younger brother) moved to a secluded country club estate. Three years later, Ann discovered that she was pregnant. The father of the baby was a boy who attended school with Ann and whom she had dated for well over a year.

Ann's reaction to finding out she was pregnant was to take an overdose of pills. She felt "ashamed and dirty," but more than anything she knew how much she had "hurt and let my parents down." She gave little thought to the impact of the experience on herself and had little hope of being able to obtain her parents' forgiveness for the "terrible thing" she had done. While she verbalized the knowledge that sexual intercourse carried with it the potential of pregnancy, Ann thought it "would never happen" to her.

There are a number of ways to explain why Ann got pregnant, none of which change the fact of the pregnancy or the events that followed. What seems more instructive is to examine Ann's and her parents' responses to the pregnancy. For Ann's father, it was "expected," as he had been observant of the relationship between Ann and her boyfriend. The father was angry at the mother for having refused to heed his advice to "do something" with the girl. The father viewed Ann as "helpless and easily influenced" and as "led into such acts" by the "irresponsible boy" that "got her pregnant."

The mother felt "wounded" by the pregnancy and "fooled" by the two "young kids" she had trusted not to "fool around." She saw Ann as "advanced for her age," a "source of friction" between herself and her husband, and a source of "public embarrassment." The mother was "disappointed" with Ann, "angry at the stupid boy," and "frustrated" with her husband, who was knowledgeable and "authoritarian" enough to have done something about it before it happened.

The fact that Ann was potentially suicidal was an indication of "personal failure" to the father, "unbelievable" to the mother, and "fearful" to Ann. More than anything else, Ann feared rejection and mistrust by her parents, even after the birth and adoption. Her fears made her "perform" in an almost manic nature on the cheerleading squad, in the band, on the drill team, and in the classroom. As she pulled closer to her parents, they pushed her farther away in a seeming attempt to make her "pay for her mistakes." She was a source of public embarrassment, feelings of personal failure, and tension for the parents. Because of the parents' overwhelmingly judgmental attitudes, it was difficult to help the young woman attain a sense of self-respect or self-forgiveness.

What Ann had feared most all during her childhood, rejection by her parents, finally came to fruition with the birth of her child. At no time did the parents ever tell Ann that Ann's mother had been pregnant with Ann at the time of their marriage or that the pregnancy and the fear of parental disapproval was their primary reason for having moved away from their parents and for the aggressive attitude that Ann's father took in order to prove his worth to himself and to his parents. Ann could be helped only to the extent that her parents were willing to look at themselves and at Ann in relation to their own experience.

The overwhelming impact of the family, particularly of parents on children and on each other, is seen again in this family, as in Tom's. Unresolved or mishandled situations, such as the unexpected pregnancy

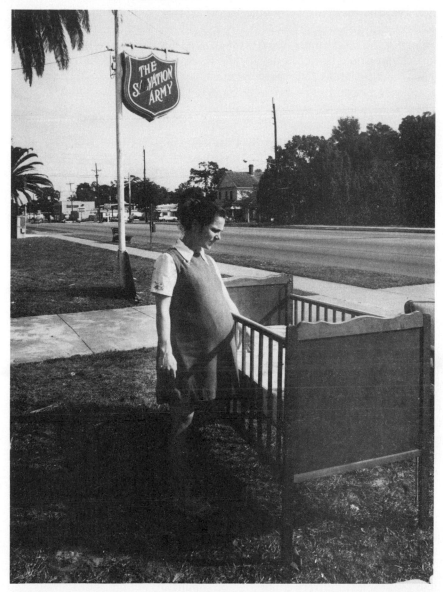

Many teenage pregnancies either are unplanned or are undertaken for the purpose of re-solving some personal problem. The difficulties that can arise from early pregnancy (parental censure, separation from peer group, interruption of work or schooling, financial strain, health complications, conflict between the parents-to-be, etc.) may become crises that threaten to overwhelm the young woman. (*Copyright © 1980 by Anne Campbell.*)

experienced by Ann's parents, crop up again in later generations. Ann's parents, like many other people, used a head-in-the-sand approach for dealing with their pregnancy. As is usually the case, it didn't work. In order for Ann's feelings about herself and her pregnancy to be worked through, it would be necessary for the family to take a look at themselves, a task that the family felt would be an impossible undertaking. The parents again used a head-in-the-sand approach for dealing with Ann's pregnancy. There is no magic or mystery about next-generation repetition of a problem. People learn coping styles from those around them, and Ann copied her parents' method of ignoring the facts, first with her attitude of "it won't happen to me" with regard to the risk of becoming pregnant and later with the pregnancy itself. By the time Ann's parents learned that she was pregnant, she was two months from term—in spite of the fact that Ann was a small, slender young woman who lived at home. The discovery came only after Ann was admitted to a hospital for "intestinal upset and abdominal discomfort."

Not until the child was born and adopted out did the parents seek counseling for their daughter, and then their stated reason was to "be sure we can control her" and so "it doesn't happen again." Ann reluctantly came along for counseling because she wanted to earn her parents' "respect and trust" after the "awful thing" she had done. However, no one was willing to discuss anything beyond the immediate past. Ann refused to consider that having given up the child for adoption might ever present psychological stress in her later life: "I want to shut it out of my mind and never think about it again," she said, quite in conformity to the family's coping style.

While it is advisable to impress individuals with their responsibilities for their own actions, it is necessary for them also to realize the interactional or transactional nature of their behavior. That is, rarely does an individual act as a wholly independent agent uninfluenced by others. This is particularly true of adolescents. Perhaps one of the hardest things for parents to cope with is that their children are in many ways mirrors of the parents themselves. Adults often prefer to see adolescents as entities in and of themselves instead of an integral part of a larger whole.

Adolescents do not have the life experiences or knowledge to act totally independently. Consequently they look about themselves, often not consciously, and try by studying others to learn ways to act, think, and feel. Selecting from a number of significant people, both adults and age-mates, adolescents try out behaviors and experiment with roles until they find some that seem to fit well. More often than not, much of the role acting comes from what teenagers see their own families do over the years. This is often mixed with what other teens are doing and what others' parents have done. In order to see a pattern or find meaning in adolescents' behavior, it is often necessary to look at what the adults around them (family, neighbors, schoolteachers, and community figures) are doing. These people, in addition to peers who are also influenced by adults, are "shapers" of adolescents' minds and behavior. As others' actions and attitudes are absorbed and integrated into the teenagers' overall repertoire of behaviors, the adolescents work toward becoming interdependent with other people, in later years taking responsibility for their own behavior as well as for their influence on others. Many adults find it unpleasant if not impossible to acknowledge their impact and influence on young people. Many operate under the illusion that their lives and actions affect no one but themselves. In real life, nothing is farther from the truth.

While adolescents do not always take direct action based on what parents may say to them or think about them, they hear and absorb more than most parents and other adults are aware of. A frequent complaint among parents is that they don't have any control over what their children do. Generally, what that means is that the adolescent does not agree with or act in a way which corresponds to what an adult thinks ought to be done. It is difficult for the adult to let the growing child experiment with the values, beliefs, and principles that adults come to take for granted. The adolescent's testing is interpreted by many parents as a form of defiance or open rebellion. It probably also serves to open old wounds and dredge up old doubts that the parents thought had ended with their own adolescence.

UNRESOLVED DEVELOPMENTAL CRISES

Defiance and Rebellion

Whether or not adolescents successfully complete the period of testing and experimenting and move on to incorporate adult ways of thinking and acting depends very much on how those around the teenagers treat them during this period of chaotic growth. Adolescents, reaching and searching for their own identity, do not intentionally set out to do harm to parents or parents' ways of living. However, if parents perceive much of an adolescent's behavior as defiance of them, the adolescent will probably stall at this point of development and become more of a rebel and less an integrator of adult norms and beliefs as he or she emerges from the adolescent years.

Often the attention that the testing brings leads to a cyclic repetition of testing. Karl Lanier is a good example.

Karl is the only son of energetic parents. Both parents work and have worked since Karl was a small boy. His grandmother has been primarily responsible for Karl during the day. Until his fourteenth year, Karl was a "model child," quiet, cooperative, orderly, and studious. However, when he was old enough to get a driver's permit and began learning to drive the family car, "the trouble began." Karl began taking the car without permission. These episodes ended with his driving the car off a high embankment and demolishing it. Karl was uninjured.

From the beginning of his trouble over the car, it was evident that Karl wanted to have more time with his father, who was a high-achieving, hard-working, intense businessman. Karl's mother, who had many of the same attributes with the exception that she was able to share her feelings with Karl, assumed the major responsibility for Karl when he was not under the supervision of the grandmother. Karl learned from the car incident that the best way to get his father's attention was to "act out," particularly in a way that brought outside authorities (police, school) into the picture.

Unable to provide Karl with the time he wanted and needed, the father bought him a car, thinking that the responsibility would help him grow up. Karl wrecked that car and two others before his junior year in high school. By the time he was a senior, he was drinking heavily and had engaged in "minor" acts of thievery. Within two years after high school, Karl was heavily involved in drugs. He had fathered a child and married the child's mother somewhat unwillingly but at his own father's insistence. He was involved in major acts of theft. At each bend of the developmental road, Karl did his best and then his worst to get his father to spend more time with him and give more of himself to Karl. Each time, Karl got just enough to keep him reaching. Each time his father either bought Karl's way out of trouble or insisted that Karl needed to "learn the hard way" and left him in jail for a day or two.

While it is clear that Karl's father related inconsistently to him, there is one markedly consistent pattern: No matter what Karl did, his father was unable to provide him any emotional closeness or fatherly recognition. It was not until Karl finally sought psychological help following an unsuccessful suicide attempt that his father began to recognize the important role that he had played, or failed to play, in Karl's life. By Karl's own admission, "All I ever wanted was for him to spend time with me." It was a simple need, but drastically hard for Karl's father to respond to.

Several themes are evident in the above case illustration. The first and probably the most glaring is the adolescent's need for recognition and close contact, particularly with a significant other. The need to be acknowledged and cared about by his father was a driving need that propelled Karl from minor to major acting out.

Second, what begins as testing and experimentation may, if unrecognized, lead to a more serious and consequential set of events. In other words, if the adolescent is unable through appropriate behavior to achieve the recognition and approval of a parent or significant other, then inap-

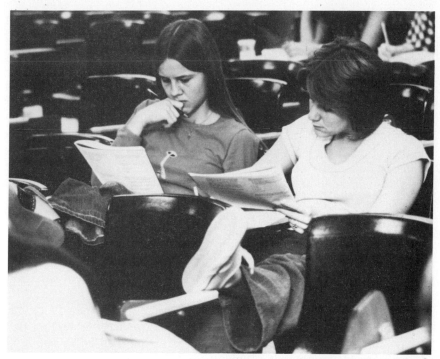

Adults sometimes take an idealized view of being young and forget that going to school, dating, and engaging in other activities of adolescence are far from all fun, opportunity, and lack of responsibility. Competition can be considerable, and pressure to achieve in activities in which one has limited experience and ability may be very intense. Falling school grades are a common early sign of inadequate coping. (*Copyright © 1980 by Patricia Yaros*.)

propriate behaviors will be used. The extent of the deviant behavior is correlated with the depth of need that propels it. Great needs lead to drastic measures to see that they are at least recognized.

The worst behaviors begin as smaller, less offensive actions, but actions that are geared to achieving the adolescent a place in the family arena. Even the most drastic behaviors, such as stealing, drug abuse, or excessive drinking with uncontrolled social behavior, usually begin as less abusive behavior which is annoying but not illegal, such as staying out beyond parental curfew. Major infractions of the law usually arise because minor attempts have failed to achieve for the adolescent the needed attention. Recognition of the smaller acts makes the larger offenses unnecessary and ordinarily is effective in preventing them. Failure to achieve the needed attention or approval is often interpreted by the adolescent as parental rejection.

Suicide

Rejection, imagined or real, is one of the hardest feelings for an adolescent to deal with, and if the feeling is carried too long, suicide may seem the only option. Suicide is a form of communication in a long line of unsuccessful efforts to achieve what is needed for the individual to feel wanted and important to others. Karl's attempts began with borrowing a car without permission and ended up years later with his driving into a bridge abutment, all in order to get his father to make some statement about whether or not his son mattered to him. While Karl's suicide attempt was unsuccessful, it was nonetheless the only act that ever really got the father's total attention. After spending years trying to reach his father, Karl finally came to the conclusion that he must not be worthy of time and attention. For him, suicide was the only response to what he perceived as total rejection by his father and total unworthiness on his part. His failure to gain the love and acceptance of his father was more than he could bear. The need for love and acceptance is an acute need for all humans, but particularly for adolescents, who are not always sure how to love or accept themselves.

The possibility that an adolescent will resort to suicide must be viewed with great seriousness. A suicide attempt or a teenager's feeling that perhaps taking one's life is the only alternative left can be so subtle as to go unnoticed. Automobile accidents and drug overdoses are two methods of suicide attempt frequently used by adolescents. Because each of these methods can be explained away as an accident or the result of poor judgment, the troubled teenager often does not come to the attention of a professional until the second or third attempt.

To consider suicide as an alternative to living, the young person does not necessarily have to come from a broken home, does not necessarily have to have been taking drugs, and does not have to come from what appears on the surface to be a troubled home. An adolescent who considers suicide does, however, generally come from a home or situation where other forms of communication have failed to achieve the love, acceptance, or recognition that the adolescent so sorely needs. Ann, in a previous case illustration, is a case in point. From external appearances her family is a "good" family: socially successful, financially secure, church-oriented, and community-responsible. Karl's family was somewhat similar. What each teenager did not have was a direct link to the parents' understanding or acceptance; there was no flow of emotional investment from parent to child. This is a particularly hard situation to identify until something goes drastically wrong, such as pregnancy, drug abuse, or major crime.

Suicide may be a last-ditch effort by an adolescent to obtain recognition of his or her needs; it may also be a signal that frustration has reached its zenith. The old adage that frustration leads to aggression, particularly aggression directed toward the self, seems related to adolescents' attempts at self-destruction. The period of self-doubt, confusion, and pressure from peers can be for the vulnerable teen a time in life when the scales are tipped and the delicate balance is lost. It must be remembered, however, that most suicide attempts are preceded by some lesser attempt at self-destruction or by some abrupt change in behavior, such as failing grades in the ordinarily successful student. While Ann and Karl are clear examples of the effect of rejection on the adolescent, another case may be illustrative of the principles involved.

> Carol Lewis is a 16-year-old only child of fairly successful parents. Both parents work, the father full-time and the mother part-time. Carol was an average student, but her grades suddenly began slipping and finally she received down slips in five out of her six classes. Her parents placed her on restrictions until such time as she brought her grades up. They did not pursue with her the reasons for the slipping grades, assuming it was a "normal teenage thing." The second week of restrictions, Carol attempted suicide, first by an overdose of pills and, when that was ignored, by cutting her wrists with razors.

Carol Lewis was a vulnerable teen for a number of reasons. She is an only child. She is the child of older parents. She has average intelligence, and her mother is extremely bright. And Carol never learned how to make her needs known through language clearly communicated to the people she lived with.

Because she did not communicate without confusing or threatening her parents, Carol was not always taken seriously. While her parents relied heavily on spoken words to convey information or meaning, Carol instead relied most heavily on symbolic language, particularly physical behavior. When her mother asked her what she wanted to do or what she thought about something, Carol would frequently shrug her shoulders. If pressed for a verbal response, Carol would eventually develop stomach cramps and would find ways to get out of the room. Her parents had difficulty in understanding the importance of Carol's form of communication and expected her to adopt their way of talking about what bothered them. Carol's parents had a great deal of difficulty in letting her grow up. They were older parents, and Carol was not as bright as her mother. She was treated like a child: assigned chores around the house, given a schedule of times for going to bed and getting up, given only a small amount of change for spending money, and told with whom she could associate and when. All in all, Carol was like a prisoner in her own home. Her parents had never been around other children or adolescents and were consequently overprotective and smothering to Carol. This is not unusual in children born to older parents.

Being an only child also put Carol at a disadvantage. There were no other children in the house to divert the parents' time and energy. There were no other children to provide Carol with needed companionship and communication. She was not allowed to do things other young people her age did, because her parents feared that someone would lead her astray. More important, the only child is at risk because it is his or her presence in the home which provides the definition of "family"; without the child's presence and participation the "family" reverts back to "couple." Most social and religious events, therefore, are focused on the child, who in one sense becomes the center of attention with everyone revolving around him or her and who in another sense is like a puppet on strings. One only child described her life as "being the court jester for the family," which meant that she felt terribly responsible for the emotional tone set in the family. This is an overwhelming responsibility for an adolescent.

Carol's suicide attempts were not taken seriously until professional help was sought. Carol recovered from her attempts to end her life but ultimately ran away from home. She did finish high school, got a job, and learned to support herself financially as well as socially. Her parents gained little if any insight into their contribution to Carol's behavior. It will perhaps be years before Carol ever gains the self-respect and sense of self-worth so necessary for personal growth and actualization. Her running away from home was, for her, a healthy attempt at self-preservation. She has not attempted suicide since that time.

Running Away: The Catch-All Solution

There are probably as many reasons for running away as there are adolescents who actually leave home. Inability to meet parental expectations, feelings of rejection, fights with brothers and sisters in which parents take sides against the one who ultimately runs away, drug problems and fear of reprisal for drug use, pregnancy and fear of punishment or abandonment if the parents should find out, and a sense of being different (socially, physically, or religiously) from family members or other adolescents are all reasons given for running away. As in Carol's case, it may be the last alternative in a long chain of ineffective attempts at communication.

An adolescent rarely runs away without giving some prior notice. Glib statements about leaving are the usual indicators. Most people at some time in their lives want to and do actually leave home; often they return without anyone's ever knowing they were gone. These, of course, are less serious runaways than those who are picked up by the police at some distance from their homes, carrying most of their belongings. The recent and more frequent intervention by authorities, particularly the police, has in some ways placed inordinate emphasis on the less serious runaway attempt while at the same time attempting to be of protective service to the more serious attempter, such as the teenager who runs away because she is pregnant or because of a serious beating.

Adolescents want to be listened to and communicated with, and parental attempts to control and dictate to the adolescent are often given as reasons for leaving. Because these adolescents feel they are not being listened to or recognized for their worth, it is sometimes difficult to return them to their homes without outside intervention. Many communities rely on the services of professional counselors as well as juvenile authorities in helping parents and adolescents work out their misunderstandings and communication blocks. In many cases, it is the school nurse working with the juvenile authorities and the family who aids considerably in patching up what may be a simple misunderstanding.

The school or community nurse not only knows about the community in which the family lives but generally knows something about that family in particular. This familiarity with the adolescent's setting makes possible a holistic approach to the problem solving. We believe that the holistic approach is not only desirable but necessary in order both to ameliorate the immediate crisis and to prevent further breakdown such as family dissolution, loss of self-esteem, faulty social involvement, and academic failure.

THERAPEUTIC INTERVENTION: A HOLISTIC APPROACH

The holistic approach to working with adolescents entails working not only with the adolescent but also with families, other professionals, and the community (school, church, neighborhood) in which the family resides. It is one thing to recognize a troubled adolescent; it is quite another to begin to take steps to alter the course of that adolescent's development. It is necessary to be aware that each institution that has some accountability for adolescents is quite protective of the adolescents' rights. This concern grows out of recognition of the adolescent's vulnerability as well as out of the human need to protect the child within each of us and, hence, by identification with others, to protect them. Sometimes these two concerns overlap and fog the issue at hand: to restore healthy functioning and to initiate family understanding.

The first step in working with adolescents, and this seems truer of working with adolescents than with other age groups, is to remember that adolescents do not belong to the professional: They belong to themselves and their families. Although we work with and through the family system, we cannot assume a role of family member. This seems to be a difficult area for most professionals, who easily lose their objectivity when working with adolescents. Lack of control over feelings may lead to a distorted perspective or to taking sides. Once the feeling of taking sides emerges, the ability to work with the family as a unit is diminished. Working with a co-clinician is an important means of keeping enough distance to maintain emotional objectivity. Siding with the adolescent only serves to provide him or her with an advocate *outside* the family, when what most adolescents want and need is to be an integral part of their own family and peer group.

Another component of working with adolescents is to remember their emotional lability and their budding social judgment. Adolescents, troubled or not, often feel like miniature adults and are able to convince others of the myth. By the perpetuation of such a myth, the growing adolescent does not receive the guidance necessary to successfully circumvent developmental and situational barriers to positive growth during these years.

Many adolescents, as well as younger children, are given responsibilities beyond their years, such as care of siblings; unsupervised use of the family car; household chores including preparation of meals, washing, and cleaning; decision making regarding other children; and disciplinary responsibility. Many working parents look to their children to assume a parental role for themselves as well as for siblings. This kind of responsibility gives the adolescent an exaggerated estimate of his or her abilities. A role analysis of the part the adolescent plays in the overall family is helpful in working with the troubled teen. A role analysis entails taking a look at the allotment of family responsibilities and who carries out those functions. Restoration of balance of responsibility is necessary for the adolescent to gain an accurate picture of his or her potentialities.

As background data for work with families, it is helpful to know how the family relates to the community—church, school, legal authorities, and medical and professional services, for example. Use as well as abuse of services provides a social character analysis of the family unit. Much of what adolescents do and think is reflective of the social unit from which they originate. This backdrop gives some indication of the family's ability to change or adapt to the needs of its members; it also shows what behavior may be expected from individual family members.

Nursing intervention requires (1) knowledge of one's own feelings about the adolescent, the family, and the problem itself; (2) a role analysis of the family, including assessment of the adequacy and appropriateness with which these roles are performed; and (3) a social analysis of the family vis-à-vis the community. These are assessment tools for learning about the adolescent and the family, as well as clinical tools for nursing intervention, and they are all preventive as well as therapeutic tools. Equally important for the nurse clinician is a knowledge of the growth and development of adolescents. All adolescents in this society are in a delicate balance; this is a fast-moving, highly technological, perfection-oriented, and somewhat egocentric society. Whether we like it or not, humans are an interactive species, and we must learn to live with the interactions or we will have problems.

Numerous high-risk interactive family situations are known. Children from these settings become adolescents at risk. They include only children; children whose families are outstandingly different from other families in the community; children of families where social status and material gain are of more importance than personal growth of family members; unwanted children, particularly eldest children whose mothers were pregnant at the time of marriage; children of working parents, where the parents delegate adult responsibility to the children and do not provide adequate love and attention; children of families where threat and rejection are used as tools to gain cooperation; children for whom the loss of a significant other is not compensated by acquisition of another source of positive regard and sense of self-worth; children of families where inadequate parenting skills lead to physical and psychological abuse or neglect; and children who for other reasons do not gain a sense of self-importance, self-respect, or the ability to love and be loved in return.

Not any one situation will produce an adolescent with a higher risk factor than others; the interaction of variables and the family's workings both internally and in relation to external systems determine the outcome in any one case. In intervening and working toward long-range solutions with adolescents, each variable must be taken into account: the individual, the family, the community, the church, the school, and the peer group.

Intervention in Acute Situations

It is well to remember that shoplifting and suicide, for example, are levels of severity and not substantially different problems in and of themselves. Adolescents who experiment beyond the point of curiosity and who get into serious difficulty with the law, at school, or in the home are basically adolescents in trouble; the coping mechanisms they use to signal others for help or to act out their problems are marks of how severely they experience the problem as well as what they have seen others around them use as a means of coping. In the case of Carol, who attempted suicide by taking pills and then by cutting her wrists, her father had in earlier years become despondent over a situation at work and had tried to poison himself. His way of handling severe frustration and disappointment influenced the manner of coping that she selected in dealing with similar feelings.

The intent of intervention in acute situations is to convey concern, demonstrate warmth, exhibit respect, and lend support. It is essential that the professional remain aware of adolescents' limited ability to utilize the knowledge and skill which, although the teenager may be experimenting vigorously and seriously with them, have not yet been mastered.

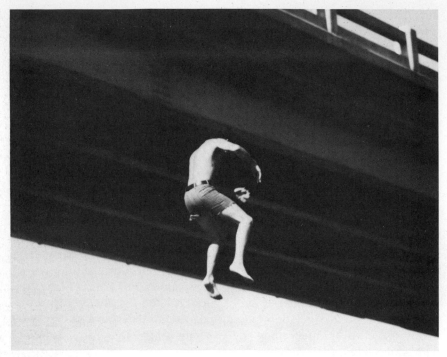

Impetuous acts or extremes of risk-taking may actually be suicide attempts. Suicide is the second-largest killer (after accidents) of older adolescents and college-age young people. It is believed that many incidents that are interpreted as accidents or episodes of poor judgment are in fact unrecognized suicide attempts. (*Copyright © 1980 by Anne Campbell.*)

Caution must be exercised in intervening in acute situations, for management mistakes are made in thinking that the acute situation is in fact the whole problem. In most cases it is the tip of the iceberg. Handling the acute outburst—running away, shoplifting, teenage pregnancy, or suicide attempt—involves handling the situation with an eye to the future as well as to the past.

Adolescents want to be dealt with honestly and warmly but with firmness. Nothing scares a growing person more than being able to push adults or manipulate them into giving in just for the sake of proving a point. One must avoid losing sight of the fact that there is a lot of child in an adolescent, particularly an adolescent who is having an inordinate struggle with growing up. Kind firmness by an adult *who maintains an adult role* is reassuring for the adolescent and provides a role model to emulate in handling future problems.

There are legal reasons, as well as therapeutic ones, why the family must be involved. In fairness to the adolescent who seeks help, this fact should be conveyed early in the contact. The adolescent's particular problem rarely belongs totally to the individual, and those others having impact must be involved in order to take care of the immediate situation as well as to begin working on its resolution for the future. Because it is necessary for the family to be involved, it is important to remember that, while the adolescent has rights, parents legally are ultimately responsible for their children.

It quickly becomes obvious that self-awareness and being in touch with one's own adultness is absolutely necessary in working positively and productively with adolescents, particularly adolescents in trouble. There is some question as to whether a young clinician, young in years or in professional experience, should work with adolescents at risk, particularly without the aid of a more experienced and more mature co-clinician. There is danger to the young clinician as well as to the client. Loss of perspective, overinvestment of feelings, lack of certainty about one's own life or life goals, inability to work with the entire family, and taking sides with the adolescent are all barriers to successfully navigating an adolescent through troubled times.

Interview skills, assessment techniques, and intervention strategies for working with healthy and unhealthy people must be well established within the intellectual grasp and clinical experience of any clinician who desires to work specifically with adolescents. A troubled adolescent—moody, volatile, vulnerable, confused, and fearful—is not a good starting point for a beginning clinician, especially without close supervision and involvement by another clinician. This point cannot be stressed enough: When an inexperienced and inexpert nurse undertakes to intervene with a troubled adolescent, far too much responsibility for performance is placed on the young clinician and far too much uncertainty results for the adolescent.

Intervention Strategies: Basic Dos and Don'ts

Some basic dos and don'ts have been suggested in this chapter and can now be summarized.

Do take what the adolescent does and says as important. *Do not* underestimate an adolescent's seriousness about even what appears to be a transitory or minor problem.

Do listen with extreme care—for feelings, for facts, and for family contribution to the overall problem. *Do not* interpret, analyze, or confront the adolescent with the meaning of his or her behavior.

Do maintain an adult, competent manner, one that conveys warmth but also security for what seems to the adolescent to be an uncontrollable problem. *Do not* take a cold, hard, indifferent attitude in order to appear detached or objective.

Do let the adolescent know that help is available and the problem manageable. *Do not* let him or her convince you that the situation is hopeless.

Do realize how energetic and tense the average adolescent can be— physically, psychologically, sexually. Let the client walk around and feel physically unconfined while with you. *Do not* try to confine or constrain during discussions; adolescents are by nature somewhat fearful of being tied down.

Do involve the parents, and *do* let the individual know that parents are necessary and, in fact, important to the handling of the problem. *Do not* give the impression that you are not going to be of assistance and support for the adolescent as well; make it clear that the client is part of a family unit and that you are not taking sides.

Do include a co-therapist or co-clinician in collecting data as well as in developing a care plan. *Do not* assume that you can do everything for the adolescent; you are as much a part of a larger unit as is the adolescent.

Do treat the adolescent with respect; let the adolescent have a part in working out the problem. *Do not* belittle feelings, ideas, or actions by calling them adolescent. Like many others, adolescents have extreme difficulty in separating in their minds the act from the actor, and they will assume you mean them in particular if you talk about what ''adolescents'' do.

Do realize that no matter how troubled the adolescent is, there are healthy components to the personality. *Do not* assume that once a troublemaker, always a troublemaker. Behavior can be changed and situations made better.

Do be aware of nonverbal language. *Do not* assume that words describe the entire picture.

Do recognize that small acts may grow to larger ones if they go unnoticed. *Do not* assume that any behavior is meaningless or unconnected to other events in the adolescent's life.

Do recognize that the adolescent is reflective, not only about his or her inner feelings but also about what is going on in the family at the moment or has happened in the near past. *Do not* assume that what you see on the surface is the entire picture.

While the dos and don'ts are broad and applicable across all high-risk situations, the guidelines can be made specific with knowledge and sensitivity about the individual situation at hand. Knowledge, empathy, adult demeanor, and family involvement are essential tools for working with every adolescent at risk, but each case must be approached with awareness of its uniqueness and potentialities for growth. No matter what else the troubled adolescent is, he or she is part of a larger whole; to approach the adolescent, the entire system must be included at some point along the therapeutic process, for the majority of adolescents ultimately desire to return to and be an active part of their families. The professional is a bridge that can make the return easier and more lasting, the one who can tip the scales, which exist in delicate balance, in a direction from which all benefit, particularly the adolescent at risk.

CONCLUSION

Being at risk is in some ways a subjectively determined phenomenon. When adolescents believe that they are unwanted, rejected, in trouble, or failures, then for them that situation is real and the feelings are genuine.

The professional facilitates the expression of those feelings, both from the person to the professional and from adolescent to pertinent others. At the same time, the clinician maintains an awareness of self and of emotional investment in order to keep as clear a perspective as possible. It is often helpful to meet regularly with other clinicians to compare assessment data, analyze intervention strategies, and assess personal involvement with clients. This is important for any clinician, but particularly true for clinicians working with adolescents.

An adult attitude; a warm, firm, positive regard for the client; and the ability to work with families and communities are essential to working effectively with adolescents at risk. Scheduling appointments that include significant others (school personnel, family members, community people) helps adolescents to see that their problem is a shared one and that they are not solely responsible for their actions. There is relief in knowing that adolescence is a process between childhood and adulthood and not an end in itself.

BIBLIOGRAPHY

Alvarez, A.: *The Savage God: A Study of Suicide*. New York: Random House, 1972.

Anthony, E. James and Cyrille Koupernik (eds.): *The Child in His Family: Children at Risk*, Vol. 3. New York: John Wiley & Sons, 1974.

Bakker, Cornelis B. and Marianne K. Bakker-Rabdau: *No Trespassing: Explorations in Human Territoriality*. San Francisco: Chandler & Sharp Publishers, 1973.

Bellak, L. and L. Small: *Emergency Psychotherapy and Brief Psychotherapy*. New York: Grune & Stratton, 1965.

Canning, Ray (ed.): *Social Psychiatry: Readings in Mental Health*. San Rafael, Calif.: Leswing Press, 1972.

Coleman, James: "Life Stress and Maladaptive Behavior," *American Journal of Occupational Therapy*, **27**(4):169–179, 1973.

Fagin, Claire (ed.): *Readings in Child and Adolescent Psychiatric Nursing*. St. Louis: C. V. Mosby Co., 1974.

Jourard, S. M.: *Healthy Personality*. New York: Macmillan, 1974.

Lewis, Melvin: *Clinical Aspects of Child Development*. Philadelphia: Lea & Febiger, 1973.

Petrillo, Madeline and Sirgay Sanger: *Emotional Care of Hospitalized Children: An Environmental Approach*. Philadelphia: J. B. Lippincott Co., 1972.

Schwartz, Pepper and Judy Lever: "Fear and Loathing at a College Mixer," *Urban Life*, 4(4):413–431, January 1976.

Sedgwick, Rae: "The Family as a System: A Network of Relationships," *Journal of Psychiatric Nursing and Mental Health Services*, 12(2):17–20, March-April 1974.

Sedgwick, Rae: "Psychological Response to Stress," *Journal of Psychiatric Nursing and Mental Health Services*, 11(6):20–23, September-October 1975.

Chapter 10

Dying and Death

Evangeline C. Gronseth
Dorothy P. Geis
Mary Ann Anglim
Ida M. Martinson

Dying is not usually listed among the developmental tasks of adolescence. But some adolescents, of course, do die, and many more experience the death of someone they know. This chapter addresses itself to death and dying as they particularly pertain to the adolescent stage of development. The chapter will focus upon (1) the dying adolescent's ways of enacting age-typical traits (achieving independence, planning for the future, etc.); (2) the nursing care of the terminally ill adolescent in the home; (3) the effects of the illness, dying, and death upon parents and adolescent siblings; (4) interactions with members of the extended family, peers, and the wider community; and (5) the restoration and reintegration of the family following the death of the adolescent.

THE RESEARCH ON WHICH THE CHAPTER IS BASED

This chapter is based on a study initiated by the School of Nursing of the University of Minnesota, "Home Care for the Child with Cancer."* Of

*The study is funded by the National Cancer Institute, Department of Health, Education and Welfare, Grant CA19490.

the 35 families with terminally ill children who have participated in the study since its inception in 1976, 11 have been families with dying adolescents. There were seven females and four males among the fatally ill adolescents: two each at ages 13, 14, and 15; four who were 16 years of age; and one who was 17. These 11 adolescents had 20 adolescent siblings. Four of the families resided in the Minneapolis–St. Paul metropolitan area and seven in nearby small towns.

The educational preparation of parents was largely limited to secondary school. Three of the fathers were laborers, two were engineers, and the others were an engineering assistant, a store manager, a production manager, and a contractor. Seven of the mothers were housewives. The others worked as telephone operator, restaurant manager, office worker, and waitress. Two mothers were divorced and functioned as single parents.

The adolescents' illnesses were acute lymphoblastic leukemia (four adolescents); Ewing's sarcoma (three); and acute nonlymphoblastic leukemia, malignant astrocytoma, neuroblastoma, and malignant histiocytosis (one each). The duration of their illnesses ranged from 10 to 69 months. The period of care provided by home care personnel ranged from 2 to 95 days. Ten of the adolescents died at home, and one reentered the hospital, where she died the following day.

DEATH AND DYING AS RELATED TO ADOLESCENT DEVELOPMENT

The ill adolescents in our study demonstrated many of the behaviors and attitudes that characterize the teen years. They expressed great concern, especially in the early stages of disease, about body changes and appearance, particularly loss of hair from chemotherapy, emaciation, disfigurement from body lesions and multiple tumors, cushingoid features secondary to drug therapy, and loss of control over body function. Pain may heighten body awareness and thereby affect body image. Some adolescents requested that their bodies be kept covered and used wigs and other means of concealment. As disease processes progressed, even these measures failed.

All the adolescents in the home care study wanted to assist themselves and to maintain independence in their daily care activities. A primary nurse claimed that attempted self-reliance was one of the most striking characteristics of the dying adolescents. One adolescent prepared her own lunch, despite a fractured hip, just hours before her death. Others participated in activities such as bowling, dining in restaurants, attending church with their families, and visiting with friends until shortly before death occurred. One 14-year-old boy insisted upon feeding himself, even though it took him more than a minute to get a glass to his mouth. Other

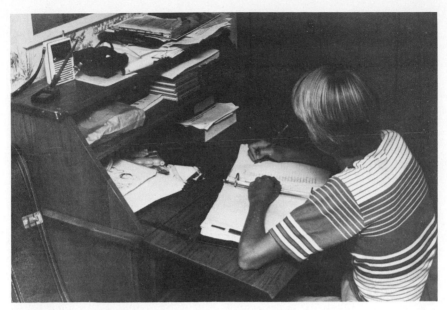

Most adolescents, especially during remissions, continue their regular day-to-day activities, including preparations for the future. (*Copyright* © *1980 by Patricia Yaros*.)

adolescents administered their own medications. During remissions, most of the young people reportedly continued their usual activities at home and in school. They even pursued sports and athletic activities within the limits of their physical capabilities.

Despite the imminence of death, the adolescents expressed interest in future goals. A 14-year-old girl continued to talk about her future, even when she realized that she would not live to experience the things she was describing. The mother of a 17-year-old leukemic boy from a rural community stated:

> He always set goals for himself. He'd plan to get home from the hospital in time for crop plantings. When that didn't happen, he'd be determined to get home for the harvest. He kept up his morale in spite of disappointments. It was only after the last treatment that he didn't mention another goal.

Planning and goal setting were most prominent during remissions, at which times both parents and patients expressed hope for their future. Other people sometimes abruptly reminded them of their limited future, however. A 15-year-old girl was greeted on her return to school after a period of rehospitalization, "We're glad you didn't do you-know-what" (die).

Plans and goals often included the hope of completing certain activities or participating in certain events before death occurred. A 15-year-old hoped to "put off death" until a cousin arrived from another part of the country. Some included death itself or the afterlife among their stated goals. Several were comforted by the prospect that their pain would "go away" when they died. An aspiring baseball player looked forward to the possibility of meeting the baseball star Lou Gehrig in a future life.

Other adolescents expressed regret over goals that would never be attained. A 16-year-old girl rued the fact that she would not marry and have a family; a 15-year-old boy was disappointed that he would never possess a driver's license.

Adolescents' Awareness and Responses Concerning Death

It is during the adolescent years that the growing child first becomes cognitively mature enough to understand the phenomenon of death as adults do. Preschool children consider death as sleep, a kind of separation, and as a temporary, reversible condition. School-age youngsters develop the concept that death is permanent and believe that everyone will die, but they inject magical and fanciful ideas (e.g., animated skeletons, bogey men who come after those whose time to die is at hand) into their concept of death. Both preschoolers and school-age children are likely to believe that death can result from their wishing someone dead, or that death is a punishment for misbehavior. During the cognitive stage of formal operations, which extends approximately between the ages of 11 and 15 years,[1] youngsters develop an adultlike understanding of death. They may, of course, still be naive and mistaken about, for example, what illnesses do and do not lead to death or what physiological events accompany dying. But, by the middle of the teen years, adolescents know that they, like everyone else, are mortal. It hardly need be said that the cognitive understanding that everyone will eventually die is often *not* accompanied by the emotional acceptance that that generality applies to oneself or to persons one knows well and cares about.

Most of the dying adolescents in our study spoke realistically and openly of their own deaths. They also discussed the deaths of acquaintances and persons who had become friends during periods of hospitalization.

Some children spoke of preparations for their own funerals. The mother of a former member of a baseball team had placed his baseball uniform in a box beneath his bed, so that it would be ready for his funeral. He periodically checked to ensure that it remained there. An adolescent who had struggled for 5 years with metastatic neuroblastoma gave her minister permission to share the tape-recorded story of her illness, progress, and prognosis with members of the congregation to which she and her family belonged. Later, she played the tape to friends. She also wrote a letter, addressed "to my friends," concerning the nature of her illness.

> To my friends:
> I'm writing this summary to bring you up to date on my medical problem.
> I first became sick in May of 1972 and was diagnosed on my 10th birthday, June 14, as having neuroblastoma, a type of childhood cancer.
> Since then, I have gone through two surgeries and various courses of chemotherapy, some at the hospital, and some at home. I have also had many areas treated with [radiation] therapy. Along with many check-ups and lots of trips to the hospital, I have faced many ups and downs over the past four and one half years.
> Last fall I spent 32 days in the hospital at which time I was given a four-drug hard chemotherapy course. I was fine for two weeks before being stricken with more pain. I had more [radiation] therapy along with pain pills, and managed to have a nice Christmas.
> By December 28, 1976, I was back in the hospital because of so much pain. During my check-up tests and evaluation, they tried different combinations of pain medication for me. Then I received a new drug, VM 26, once a week for three weeks in January. The tests showed no improvement in my condition.
> They have other drugs that could be tried, but with about the same percentage of success. So I have made my decision—no more drugs. It gets very discouraging when there aren't any more veins left to start IVs in. I want to spend my time at home with my family and new black cat named Lucky.

Some adolescents, while aware of the critical nature of their illnesses, avoided talking about their impending deaths in order to prevent the hurt and distress that their remarks would be likely to impose upon parents. For example, a 14-year-old girl never spoke of death in the presence of her mother. She did, however, talk about her death with her minister. A 17-year-old boy demonstrated the protectiveness some of the adolescents showed for others when the inevitability of death was discussed:

> When curative procedures had ceased, the doctor said, "You've always wanted to know the truth. You've said you wanted to know when there wasn't anything else that we could do for you . . . we've come to that now." There was no reply; the boy just looked at his mother. Finally, the doctor said, "Well, what do you think? What do you want to say?" The dying boy said simply, "I feel sorry for you. You're the one who had to tell me."

NURSING CARE

Whether the dying adolescent is cared for in the hospital or at home, as in our study, certain aspects of physical care are similar. While the ther-

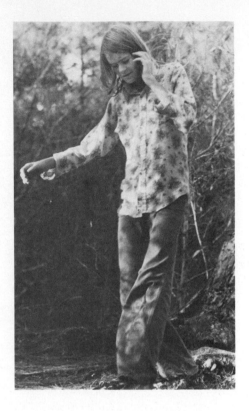

Disbelief that time is limited and sorrow over impending separation are parts of the grief response experienced by the ill adolescent, peers, family, and others, including health professionals. (*Copyright © 1980 by Patricia Yaros.*)

apeutic regime depends to some extent upon the disease processes involved, the aim when curative procedures have been discontinued is to maintain comfort and as much physical, emotional, and social integrity as possible. When heroic measures are largely abandoned, as in the care of the dying adolescent in the home, the efforts of the nurse center around relieving pain and discomfort, assisting family members in the observation and management of signs and symptoms, and administering some aspects of care. Although the primary nurse assigned to the care of the patient in the home care program is available on short notice and is on call 24 hours a day, family members usually perform the direct care, including drug administration, bathing, changing of position, and assisting with ambulation and the use of ambulatory devices.

The study has shown that pain can be successfully controlled at home with available medications. Methadone, administered orally at regular intervals, has been found to be particularly effective. In a few instances, morphine sulphate has been used together with chloral hydrate, and Demerol has been given with Vistaril and Tylenol. The drugs have usually been effective for periods of 4 to 8 hours and have been administered at regular intervals rather than "as necessary." One reason for giving pain medicine at regularly scheduled times rather than on request has been the adolescents' manifest reluctance to seek medication for fear of "being drugged." They have resisted anything which would result in the loss of control. The importance to them of being "in command of the situation" has been expressed in several ways. One adolescent refused pain medications because she was afraid she would be denied permission to attend school if it appeared that she had to have them. Some adolescents associated drugs with untoward effects which had been stressed in school drug education programs; some were afraid of building tolerances to them prior to anticipated periods of increased need.

In other aspects of care, as well as in the administration of drugs, adolescents may present more care problems than either the adult or the younger child. Cooperation with the care plan is one such area. Often parents have hesitated to discipline terminally ill adolescents when the adolescents have actually been seeking behavioral limits. The plan of care has usually been more effective when the adolescents have participated in planning and carrying out their care and have been made to feel that they could do so successfully and were expected to do so.

One of the home nurse's functions is to prepare the family for all possible symptoms likely to be experienced by their child prior to death, particularly changes in respiration, difficulty with breathing, seizures, hemorrhage, and symptoms of infection. These symptoms can be frightening to the adolescent as well as to family members, and the adolescent also should be prepared for them, whether death is expected to occur at home or in the hospital.

Advantages of Home Care

A major advantage of home care for the dying adolescent is that the entire family participates in the care process. Siblings, as well as parents, other relatives, and friends of the adolescents included in our research program have taken part in various aspects of care. The mere presence of these persons is an important supportive measure when the adolescent desires to have them present. The interpersonal richness of being in the home stands in contrast to the isolation sometimes experienced by dying patients in the hospital. The participation of the family in the care of the hospitalized patient may be minimal, and there is less opportunity for family and friends together to discuss feelings related to dying and death.

Home care keeps the family together rather than, as commonly happens when a dying child is hospitalized, separating the patient and a parent or other family member or two from the rest of the family. The mother of a 14-year-old with four teenage siblings stated that home care had enabled her to "keep track of" the other children. When she was with the dying child during periods of hospitalization, the other teenagers just "went off" and she didn't know where they were. There was also more regularity of schedule in the home, including that of meal hours. Older siblings frequently remained at home to help with patient care and thus provided intermittent relief for their parents. One 14-year-old prepared sandwiches, brought drinks, and helped to move his dying brother. Well siblings also played games with ill adolescents. When one adolescent became too ill to play, his sister informed him that she would "play for both of us." Often the ill adolescents included in the home care study spent much of their time in the living room, in the center of activity, rather than in comparative isolation in the bedroom. Families thus congregated around them and, as one mother maintained, the dying adolescents could feel as if they were "participating in the family structure without inconveniencing the family members." A large percentage of adolescents cared for at home have died while in the living room.

Because it tends to keep the family members in continuous interaction with one another, home care allows opportunities that could otherwise be missed to redefine and revise their relationships. In many instances, it has appeared that the family's provision of care and comfort measures has helped both the ill adolescent and the other family members to an enhanced appreciation of one another and a resolution of old conflicts.

> Had J. died 2 years ago, I would have had the feeling that my son was a troublesome teenager, and he would have felt that I was a meddlesome mother. We grew with J. through the months. Near the end he said, "You know, Mom and Dad, I never really liked you very much, but now I love you both so much."

EFFECTS OF THE TERMINAL ILLNESS ON PARENTS AND SIBLINGS

Parents

A physician oncologist involved in our study has identified three phases parents go through following the diagnosis of their child's fatal illness:

1 In the initial phase, they want to know about the future. They press for answers. The physician is truthful with them in this phase, emphasizing that there will be no miracles. The possibility of remission is discussed.

2 In the second phase, and particularly if the initial treatment is successful, parents are more hopeful. There is less talk of dying, and some denial is usually evident.

3 In the third phase, remissions become shorter. The family is faced with death. Siblings are informed of the impending death, if they have not

realized it before. The imminence of death is again clarified for the parents, to whom the inevitability of death may not yet have become a reality.

In the first phase, parents typically express disbelief and anger over the diagnosis. "Why did it have to be us? Why should we have to go through this?" repeated the father of an adolescent with Ewing's sarcoma. The mother of an adolescent with a diagnosis of metastatic neuroblastoma stated, "You get married and have a baby and you expect the child to grow up. You never dream that something like this could ever happen to you." Sometimes the disbelief has led parents to search for several medical opinions. When radical therapeutic measures have been suggested to halt the progression of the disease and to facilitate remission, some parents have delayed the treatment by instituting folk measures and "cures" suggested by friends and relatives.

Anger has frequently been directed toward medical personnel and hospitals. Some families have severed contact with the physicians who made the initial diagnosis. One family spoke bitterly of the staff of the small hospital where their adolescent son was initially hospitalized. They had been told bluntly that their child had cancer and that he would die. They had not been encouraged to seek further treatment, but rather to "just let the child stay in the hospital until he dies."

Remission brings a sense of relief and, as has been previously mentioned, encouragement. With repeated remissions, however, parents manifest both hope and despair. The remissions become almost as painful and difficult for some families as the critical phases of the illness because of the contradictory expectations and the false hopes which are engendered. One mother described remission as the period of "ups and downs. Is he going to live, or is he going to die?" A primary nurse related the experience of an adolescent boy: "Apparently there has been a lot of hope for a long time. It has been recently discussed that it is all right for him to give up hope. He has been pushed to hope and hope and hope." After several remissions, one adolescent explained that he was tired of being "revived" and just wanted to go home to die. He expressed regrets, however, over the effect this would have on others, particularly his mother.

Disbelief expressed by parents in the initial phase often reappeared during the periods of remission. The mother of an adolescent whose illness had extended over a period of 5 years was reluctant to use the word "cancer," which she referred to as "that six-letter word." The mother avoided the topic of death, despite her knowledge that the dying daughter wished to discuss that eventuality with her. The primary nurse reported:

At no time was dying discussed with J. by the mother. The child never said anything, never brought it up. The doctor wanted to discuss dying with the child, but he couldn't talk with J. by himself. The mother wondered if he had approached the subject. She stated the children in school would associate leukemia with dying, and she wondered how J. would respond to that. If J. was aware of their thoughts, she didn't show it. Despite the fact the mother didn't want the child to know the diagnosis, she stated she would have told her if she had asked.

It is in the third phase, when hopes for further remissions have been abandoned, that the home care program has had most contact with adolescents and their families. Several mothers of the dying adolescents stated that they felt much closer to the child during this time. Death was often discussed openly, and questions concerning the final stages of illness and death were answered when the child was ready to or wanted to discuss them. Most of the mothers had developed some technical expertise in the care of the children by this phase, including the administration of medications. In some instances, the care became exhausting and family members and nurses on call helped to relieve the mothers. In our study, the role of the primary nurse included the care of families at the time of death, and, in four instances, the nurse was with the adolescent and family when death occurred.

Several of the mothers in the home care study were employed outside the home and continued with at least part-time employment until the deaths of their children. Other family members, including siblings, cared for ill children during the mother's absence. One mother preferred to be employed at home in the day care of young children, and her terminally ill daughter assisted with the baby-sitting activities until shortly before her death.

Funeral preparations were discussed openly with parents by home care personnel prior to the death of the child. The topic was introduced to help parents focus on reality and plan in advance for whatever assistance might be needed. Parents reacted in different ways to this task. While most of the mothers in the study were able to discuss such preparations, many of the fathers could not.

The tendency for the fathers of terminally ill children to absent themselves from the home situation to the extent that they would be unable to participate in the care of their children is documented elsewhere in the literature.[2] There were several examples of this tendency among the fathers of adolescents included in the present study. In one instance, the mother of a dying child informed the child's father that he would have to accept the child's illness and help the family, or he would be told to "leave the premises." The father claimed he would not attend the child's funeral, and he refused to discuss the matter with the well adolescent family members who had questioned him about it.

Another father who reportedly "kept everything in" withdrew and would not share his feelings after he was told of his child's diagnosis. He was frightened of the disease and the fact that his son would die. But when the child arrived home from the hospital, the nurses noticed he not only verbalized how he felt, but also actively supported his wife and his two other children.

When there appeared to be a particularly close relationship between the fathers and the dying adolescents, the fathers were sometimes unrealistic in their expectations for both the dying adolescents and their well siblings. When the well children requested to participate in certain activities, they were frequently told that they could not do so until the ill child could take part also. This occurred when the participation of the dying child was an impossibility.

In the instance of the two divorced mothers included in the study, the fathers did participate to some extent. Absent fathers assisted with financial support, including insurance, and by visiting the adolescents.

Siblings

There were many similarities in the reactions to death and dying evinced by the 20 adolescent siblings in families included in the home care program. They reported shock and disbelief at the diagnosis and prognosis. The siblings, especially those who had been told by the dying siblings themselves, stated it was "such a shock," but they said they had been temporarily comforted by the thought that perhaps the ill adolescent would eventually get well. Later, the realization that death would actually occur was reinforced by movies such as "Brian's Song," in which death from leukemia occurs, and by articles in popular magazines.

While the adolescents expressed sorrow over the impending loss of their ill siblings, there were also feelings that they were being comparatively neglected. The loss of the attention of the mother was particularly emphasized. In one family, after a mother had been with her hospitalized child for some time, the well adolescent sibling called to inquire, "What do you look like now, Mom?" Similar feelings were expressed by four adolescent siblings ranging in age from 14 to 19 in an excerpt from a scheduled interview:

> "How did the illness of your sister change your lives?" J. spoke up immediately, saying, "Mother was more crabby," and T. shot back, "J. was more crabby." D. added, "Everyone got bolder in what they said. Everyone has his own makeup, but in a crisis you have to build yourself up, mostly by cutting someone else down. We argued a lot; there were lots of arguments between mother and children." T. continued, "Mother wasn't around very much and some people got used to that, so they yelled when she *was* at home. That wasn't very often, but it seemed like all the time."
> They added that sometimes, when the dying sibling was limping around

the house, they reproached her. They accused her of trying to get attention, when actually she had broken her hip. "It was a sort of jealousy of her, because she was getting all Mother's attention," they explained. They felt she should be "treated as always" and should not be "spoiled," for "you [the well siblings] have to adjust your lives, too. You don't get to do as many things as you would like to."

Siblings sometimes expressed guilt because of their own good health. The 15-year-old sister of a dying adolescent subsequently began to "act out" some of her feelings. She was truant from school for a few days and was caught drinking with friends. She complained that it was unfair that her brother was dying while she was going to live on. The family subsequently discussed the matter with her with some success, and she changed her behavior.

Several of the adolescent siblings reported physical symptoms such as fatigue and vomiting, and some feared that they would also succumb to the terminal illness of the dying sibling. Some reported problems related to school attendance and performance. They found it difficult to concentrate, and several siblings reported that they had received lower grades.

They had also missed a number of school days to enable them to be with the dying adolescents. Adolescent siblings were frequently absent from school during the final stages of their siblings' illness so they could participate in the care of the dying adolescents. They conversed with and entertained them and slept beside them at night. In one instance, a brother administered medications. Others relieved their mothers of various tasks. While most well adolescents were able to assist with care activities, others withdrew from them.

For most adolescents included in the study, the death of a sibling constituted the initial experience with dying and death, and there were mixed reactions to the actual moment of death. The fear of dying was expressed, but there was also satisfaction in being with the dying sibling at that time. Several teenagers commented upon how peacefully their brother or sister had died. While some teenagers were positive about their own experience at the time of death, they felt that such experience would have been too difficult for younger siblings.

Finally, the well adolescents expressed some of their feelings concerning the general phenomena of death and dying. "Death is a part of our lives. We should brace ourselves for it every day," a 19-year-old stated. His 16-year-old brother agreed, saying, "But we shouldn't mope for nine years after it. It's okay to be sorrowful for a couple of weeks, or three, or four, but you have to go on living." There was unanimity of opinion that an adolescent should be informed if he or she develops a terminal illness. The adolescent siblings of a dying 15-year-old girl were very angry that their sister had not been told. "Perhaps she knew already,

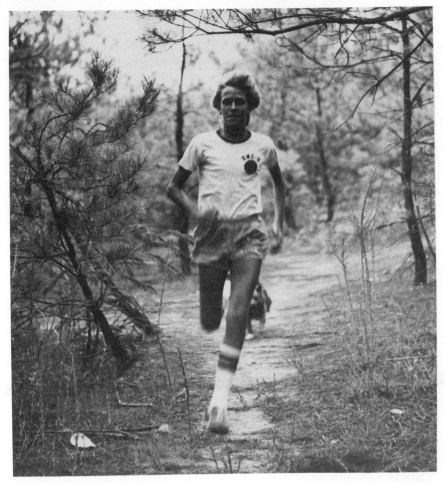

The abundant health and vitality of siblings of a dying (or handicapped) adolescent can engender resentment in the ill person and parents and can lead the healthy youngsters to feel guilty. (*Copyright © 1980 by Patricia Yaros.*)

but she should have been told." Some adolescents believed that religion could help one to accept a sibling's death, while others either had no opinion concerning religious belief or felt that it would not be of any particular benefit.

The well adolescents also felt that they personally needed someone with whom to discuss their feelings. The mother of a 15-year-old adolescent was described in this context as "both a friend and a mother to me. I can talk things over with her." Others preferred friends to parents. A 19-year-old boy maintained, "It would have to be a very close, a very tight friend. Someone who could understand you. Someone you'd trust."

The teenagers offered several suggestions for families with dying children. For instance, "They should sit down and talk together. Not all the time, but sometimes." This recommendation resulted from a situation in which the divorced father of a dying daughter wanted the other children to tell him what was happening to her; but the mother did not communicate with the children, and they, therefore, could not inform the father of the dying child's condition. This disturbed both the father and the children. The teenage children felt that all family members should be informed of "almost everything," including various aspects of treatment. They believed that it was best to "get close to" the ill child. If the child survived, there would be a closer relationship. If death occurred, everything would have been done.

The prolongation of life and, together with it, prolonged suffering were also discussed by the well adolescents. They placed particular emphasis upon the debilitating effects of pain, and some observed that when animals were in such great pain they were "put to sleep." The adolescents not only associated pain with death, but several of them suggested that, while death was an unpleasant event even to contemplate, life should not be sustained in the presence of intense pain.

EFFECTS OF THE TERMINAL ILLNESS
ON EXTENDED FAMILY, PEER GROUP, AND COMMUNITY

Some members of the extended families of adolescents included in the home care program have been actively involved with the care of the dying adolescent, and some have absented themselves from such care. Grandparents sometimes provided household help, transportation, physical care for the ill adolescents, or financial assistance. The aunts of one adolescent not only provided entertainment for the child, but also assisted the family in numerous other ways.

The importance of the peer group to the adolescent has been emphasized in the child development literature. While the family constituted the primary source of comfort in the home care of adolescents in their final days, peers entertained and assisted the ill teenagers and members of their families during remissions and periods of illness when the adolescents were able to respond. One mother was especially appreciative of her son's friends: "We can really learn from them; they are both faithful and devoted." One such friend drove some distance to visit the dying adolescent during his hospitalization. When the patient returned home, the friend stayed in the home and slept on the floor with the boy's brother during the dying adolescent's last night. When the friend was awakened and informed that death had occurred, he stated, "That's why I didn't want to leave. I knew if I left, I would not see him again." Some friends called daily, and it was very important to the dying adolescents to know that their friends had called. This was particularly evident in an instance in which a patient's family moved shortly before her death and she became separated from her close friends.

While most adolescents welcomed the attention and the interest of friends, some objected to the noise and activity and requested that friends be kept away. They preferred to limit social contacts to the immediate family and to adult relatives. Sometimes the assistance of family members and friends was considered "too much of a good thing" by both the adolescents and their parents. Some mothers complained of "weekend advice" from relatives and friends.

The response of the communities in which the dying adolescents resided depended in part upon the length of time the family had been in the community and upon the size of the community. In the small towns, a considerable amount of support was provided to the families. Neighbors helped with household tasks and provided food. Community fund-raising events, such as dances, were held. In an urban neighborhood, tears were shed when an adolescent who had been active in baseball events was wheeled around the baseball field for the last time. Members of the neighborhood not only cooperated to assist the family financially, but stated that they had been brought closer together as a neighborhood because of the child's illness. "There is more emphasis upon what is real now" was the comment of one neighbor.

A community institution of particular importance to some families was the church. Support from religious institutions depended upon personal relationships with the clergy and upon individual participation in the respective congregations. While some ministers were castigated for failing to "personalize religious support," others were considered the most important sources of emotional support. Some adolescents could discuss death and dying with ministers when that possibility did not exist with family members.

THE AFTERMATH: FAMILY RESTORATION AND REINTEGRATION

The nursing care of the family continues after the adolescent dies. A death in the family leaves a void, and reestablishing individual and family function takes time. The continuing contact, concern, and counsel of the nurse with whom the dying and death were shared can be quite helpful to the families as they recover. Singher states that professional responsibility "does not end with the death of a child. . . . Inviting families to return for a talk, after an appropriate interval, is often of vital meaning."[3] In our home care program, families are seen at intervals of 1 month, 6 months, and 1 year following the death of a child. Our data are yet incomplete.

Findings to date from the 1-month visit have included occasional parental expressions of anger about the sympathy which people have extended to them. Some parents have complained that others say they understand when they "can't possibly know what we have gone through." Some parents have described a feeling of relief following the death of the adolescent. Loneliness and emptiness have also been reported by parents, particularly at the 6-month interval. A primary nurse's interview excerpt depicts these feelings:

> The hardest part for Mrs. R. since D.'s death has been the loneliness, the emptiness. The neighbors are still sympathetic, still interested, but not quite so present as they were. One day a brother-in-law said to her, "You've got to put that picture away. You won't be able to stand that. It will be a constant reminder." Her reply was, "You can't take the memories out of this house. That's where D. used to sit when he ate his breakfast; that's the couch where he always watched TV; and that's the cupboard where I kept his medicines. You'd have to burn the house to get rid of the memories. Besides, I don't want to forget. The memories are all I have."

Parents sometimes reflect with regret upon past actions and events. One mother who had continued her employment throughout her son's illness evinced some regret concerning this endeavor, stating, "If I had known J. would die, I wonder if I would have done things differently." The primary nurse assigned to her son thought this was astonishing, since the mother had seemed during the illness to accept her son's impending death. Intellectually she knew he was dying, and she had spoken openly of what would happen and how she would cope with future events.

Some parents commented upon the difficulty they had with restoration of the household operation and the pursuit of their former activities. In many instances, the family could not face the room of the deceased and left it as it was for some time. Going through belongings was painful. Often notes and other materials of which the family had not previously been aware were discovered. One mother expressed regret about discovering that there was so much of her daughter that she had not known and now would never know. Families often had lost social contacts during the period of illness. Some parents not only were concerned about the low ebb of their social lives, but also described their worry about losing their ability to work. Siblings who had missed school for long periods had to reorganize their peer relationships. For some other children there were no marked changes in life-style; they kept up with their activities, such as hockey and dancing lessons.

A number of parents in the study were young, in the 30- to 39-year-old group. The death of a child may be particularly devastating to parents at that stage of life. Not only did most have limited experience with death,

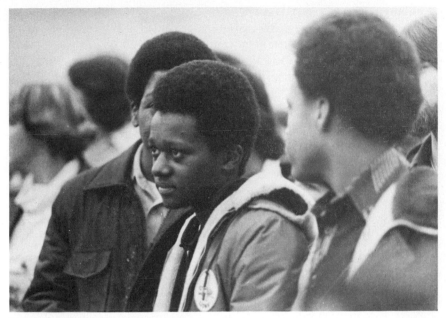

A teenager whose sibling is dying may decrease involvement in usual activities or may find it difficult to resume them after the sibling dies. Peers sometimes are highly supportive to the dying adolescent and other family members. (*Copyright © 1980 by Patricia Yaros.*)

but also they had not accrued financial resources to cope with hospital expenses and other financial burdens at a time when they were preparing their young families for the future.

Sometimes young friends of the dead child facilitated the family's healing process. Those who had visited dying adolescents sometimes continued to visit the family. One boy came to the home of his deceased friend every Sunday. He would announce that he was there "to fill the empty chair." His visits meant a great deal to the family. The mother contrasted his behavior with that of other friends who seemed to "pull away when it was all over."

Despite the extreme difficulties families experience in the loss of a child, we have been impressed by the strengths that many of the study families have seemed to derive from their involvement in their adolescent's dying. Some husbands and wives maintain that the experience has brought them closer to each other. One couple specifically mentioned that they had found the greatest strength in one another. They had been told that the experience would make them either "bitter or better" and they concluded that it had made them "better." Improved relationships between parents and their surviving children have been reported. It has been suggested that impressions and attitudes the well siblings have acquired from their experience may positively affect their future parenting behavior. Fathers, who have been described in the literature as withdrawing from their dying children and even from their families, and who have also been largely excluded from the caring process in many cross-cultural settings, have actively participated in a number of the home care situations. Parents and adolescents have attributed much of their cohesiveness to having cared for the dying adolescent in their home, which had led them to understand not only death but also one another in a way they felt would not have been possible in the hospital. They have made statements such as "We know now what can happen, so the whole family is much nicer to one another" and "We all appreciate one another more now." Finally, there has been the possibility for self-actualization on the part of the dying adolescent, whose time for fulfillment in any sense was drastically curtailed.

REFERENCES

1 John L. Phillips, *The Origins of Intellect: Piaget's Theory*. San Francisco: W. H. Freeman and Co., 1964, p. 64.
2 Lawrence J. Singher, "The Slowly Dying Child," *Clinical Pediatrics*, **13**(10):863, October 1974.
3 Singher, op. cit., p. 866.

BIBLIOGRAPHY

Erikson, E. H.: "Identity and the Life Cycle," *Psychological Issues*, Monograph 1, 1959.
Erikson, E. H.: *Identity: Youth and Crisis*. New York: W. W. Norton, 1968.
Gyulay, Jo-Eileen: *The Dying Child*. New York: McGraw-Hill Book Co., 1978.
Havighurst, R. J.: *Developmental Tasks and Education*, 2d ed. New York: McKay, 1952.
Inhelder, B. and J. Piaget: *The Growth of Logical Thinking*. New York: Basic Books, 1948.
Lacasse, Christine M.: "A Dying Adolescent," *American Journal of Nursing* **75**(3):433–434, March 1975.
Leininger, Madeline: "Caring: The Essence and Central Focus of Nursing," *American Nurses' Foundation Nursing Research Report*, **12**:1, February 1977.
Phillips, John L.: *The Origins of Intellect: Piaget's Theory*. San Francisco: W. H. Freeman and Co., 1969.
Schowalter, John E.: "The Adolescent Patient's Decision to Die," *Pediatrics*, **51**(1):97–103, January 1973.
Singher, Lawrence J.: "The Slowly Dying Child," *Clinical Pediatrics*, **13**(10):861–867, October 1974.

Chapter 11

Health Counseling
and Teaching

Judith B. Igoe

Health is more than well-regulated physiological functioning. For adolescents, personal-social issues frequently constitute the harshest form of health disturbance. Problems of this kind in all likelihood originate from the adolescent's struggle to master the particular developmental tasks for this age period. Sexual identity concerns, continuous emotional fluctuations, and ever-changing relationships with peers, family, and school associates are but a few examples of the arduous developmental crises with which an adolescent must contend. Tension, anxiety, apprehension, and stress are not uncommon during adolescence. If these stressors are sustained for long periods of time at heightened levels, serious consequences can be anticipated. Specifically, susceptibility to mental and physical illness may develop, thereby jeopardizing the adolescent's total well-being.[1]

Social and emotional problems during adolescence are not unique to certain income groups, areas of the country, or particular cultural backgrounds. Numerous surveys of adolescents' health needs in ghetto street clinics, private physicians' offices, and rural health facilities document the fact that personal-social problems remain essentially the same in every environment and among diverse populations. For example, Garell's survey of health professionals in hospital adolescent clinics throughout the country reported that the following disturbances had nationwide distribution and occurred commonly:

- Adjustment reaction to adolescence
- Behavior problems
- Scholastic failure
- Personality pattern and trait disturbance
- School phobia
- Psychoneurotic reaction
- Psychosomatic complaints
- Enuresis
- Delinquency[2]

Further studies, which have included the viewpoints of adolescents themselves, have also shown that practices such as alcohol intoxication, drug abuse, and cigarette smoking are prevailing habits among this age group. This is in spite of the fact that adolecents acknowledge the health strain inherent in dependency practices of this kind and worry about the consequences.

Although social and emotional problems are found among all teenagers, the incidence is reported to be higher among impoverished minority youth than other adolescents. The Hofmann and Gaman study exemplifies this point.[3] According to the findings of these investigators, the maturation and life functioning of one in four adolescents living in poverty had been seriously impeded by home and school difficulties; acting out behaviors; or pregnancy, drug abuse, and emotional disturbance. Brunswick and Josephson also found a higher percentage of personal-social problems among minority adolescents who are poor, as evidenced by the occurrence of nervous and emotional disorders among Harlem youth at rates of 11 percent in girls and 6 percent in boys.[4]

Unfortunately, in the minds of many adults, the social and emotional problems facing adolescents signify no more than the normal hallmarks for these years. ''Leave them alone—they'll soon grow up'' is an often-stated adult response in discussions about these types of problems. However, the reality of the matter is that, left alone, many adolescents experiencing the difficulties of depression, peer pressures, drug abuse, etc., may not have the opportunity to grow up: Emotional-social problems do not always resolve spontaneously and, in fact, may intensify if not recognized and treated early. Suicide, the third leading cause of adolescent death, serves as alarming evidence of the need to pay special attention to the personal-social problems of teenagers.[5]

Nurses have an important role to play in helping adolescents to recognize and resolve many of their personal-social health problems before serious difficulties arise. In most instances, the skills and knowledge needed in assisting with uncomplicated emotional-social disturbances may be found in the areas of health counseling and teaching.

THE HEALTH COUNSELING AND TEACHING PROCESSES

Counseling is "a broad name for a variety of procedures for helping individuals achieve adjustment such as the giving of advice and guidance, therapeutic discussion, administration and interpretation of tests and vocational assistance."[6] *Teaching* is defined as "activities by which the teacher helps the student to learn" and "any interpersonal influence aimed at changing the way in which other persons can and will behave. Activities are used in which the learning of one or more persons is being deliberately controlled by others and there is the controlled introduction of discontinuities in the form of new or novel objects, events or information into the learner's environment."[7]

Often the terms *counseling, teaching*, and *interviewing* are used interchangeably, and the nurse is confused as to the nature of the relationship among these three types of nursing activities. Actually, teaching, counseling, and interviewing are three separate and distinct functions, all of which are necessary in helping the adolescent.

Interviewing as a Precursor to Health Counseling and Teaching

Interviewing, which is a process of data collection through questioning, always precedes any attempts at counseling and teaching. The focus of the interview should be the discovery of the adolescent's self-perception, method of communication, previous knowledge and experiences, problems, expectations of the counselor, and learning style. Without the benefit of preliminary interviewing sessions during which a specific and comprehensive data base is established, teaching about health and giving advice or recommendations to adolescents are meaningless. Adolescents have a prominent need to be closely involved in the identification, as well as the resolution, of their own problems. Because this period of life is a time of self-concern and self-identification, adolescents experience a strong sense of uniqueness about their own particular worries, viewpoints, and philosophy. Whether or not others share the same feelings, problems, or anxieties is not as important to teenagers as the others' recognition that the young person's particular circumstances require his or her personal interpretation. When health professionals disregard this normal devel-

opmental characteristic of adolescence and bypass the interview in favor
of their own preconceived assumptions, the counseling or teaching that
results is inevitably too general, authoritarian, rigid, impersonal, and inappropriate to be of any value to the adolescents. Successful interviewing
requires the implementation of a number of communication techniques.
Vander Zanden and Vander Zanden[8] provide some useful guidelines in
this respect.

1 Allow adolescents to describe themselves and the situation in
their own words. The nurse may wish to take notes during this phase of
the interview. If such is the case, an explanation about the reason for
recording and what happens to the information will be of interest to most
adolescents.

2 Explain the purposes for asking questions. For example, asking
adolescents if they've experimented with sex, drugs, or alcohol may generate unnecessary confusion, anxiety, and suspicion unless they understand the reason for the nurse's interest in these experiences.

3 Do not hurry an interview by either verbally or nonverbally
demanding instantaneous replies to questions. This is especially important
with younger adolescents who, because of their acute awareness of the
physiological changes occurring within their bodies, often have difficulty
in clearly articulating their views and opinions in a conversation with
adults.

4 Consider the adolescent's past experience in interviewing situations. What does the process of questioning mean to the interviewee?
Has she or he experienced unpleasant consequences as the result of having
to provide answers? Certainly this is true for those adolescents who have
previously come to the attention of law enforcement agencies. In these
instances, continual reassurance of the ways in which the information is
to be used will be necessary.

5 Delay extremely personal questions that may provoke anxiety
and embarrassment until a relationship has been established with the
adolescent.

6 Even in very positive relationships with health professionals,
adolescents may be extremely hesitant to verbalize information about
themselves with regard to such issues as masturbation, homosexuality,
or venereal disease; therefore, many experienced nurses dealing with
adolescents elicit this information initially in a depersonalized way by
asking that a preprinted questionnaire be completed by the teenager.

7 Keep in mind the overconcern with bodily functions which normally accompanies adolescence. In terms of the interview, this means the
nurse must continually reassure the adolescent that he or she is not plagued
with all the conditions about which inquiries are made. For example, if
the nurse has found it useful to establish the prevalence of such complaints
as headache, nausea, or dizziness in stressful situations among all adolescents and regularly poses these questions in interviews with teenagers,

the adolescent must be promptly assured that the questions are a matter of routine and not the direct result of evidence that indicates the interviewee may be ill.

8 Using a carefully formulated set of questions for adolescents helps ensure that the nurse will communicate effectively and obtain useful baseline data. Table 11-1 provides a synopsis of material that is traditionally included in an adolescent interview for health counseling purposes. The actual development of interview questions in terms of wording and syntax is best handled by the individual nurse and adapted as necessary for particular interviews.

9 Limit questions to one single idea and avoid complicated wording.

10 Use language that is understandable to the adolescent. This does not mean, however, that nurses must adopt adolescent jargon and expressions unless these particular mannerisms are their customary form of communication.

11 Ask adolescents to describe specific recent events instead of what they "usually do" in a certain situation. Research has shown that people tend to distort information when asked to generalize about their "usual" behavior in a given situation.

12 The adolescent's need to develop self-esteem can be positively or negatively influenced in an interview situation. Therefore, it is especially important to avoid asking adolescents a lot of questions that call for answers they do not have. Nothing can be more deflating to one's sense of identity and self-confidence than the experience of repeatedly having to respond "I don't know."

Differences between Teaching and Counseling

Having collected a sufficient amount of information about the adolescent during the interview, the nurse is now in a position to develop a plan for health counseling or teaching. While both these nursing interventions involve an exchange of information between the nurse and the adolescent out of which some positive behavior change is expected, counseling and teaching methods are not exactly alike. Differentiating health teaching from counseling was less complicated in years past than it is today. This is largely because of the changes in educational philosophy in more recent years which have tended toward the incorporation of a number of counseling principles into teaching situations. Previously, health *teaching* has been viewed as a process in which the student assumed a role of dependence and passivity, while the individual assigned the role of teacher was expected to assume an elevated position of authority from which knowledge was dispersed downward to the learner. The quality of the relationship between teacher and student, an exchange of questioning and challenge between student and teacher, and actual student involvement

Table 11-1   Diagnostic Evaluation of an Adolescent in Preparation for Counseling

1   Mental status
   a Orientation: knows full name, age, today's date, home address, school name
   b Memory: digit span, sentence recall, list of words recalled 5 minutes later
   c Planning and organization: puzzles
   d Reasoning and judgment: analogies, resolution of simple and complex problems
   e Concentration and attention span: memory tasks, counting, calculation
   f Intelligence: Slosson test, Peabody Picture Vocabulary test
   g Coordination skills: balance, hopping, ocular pursuit, copying, catching, throwing
   h Comprehension: story recall, ability to follow commands
   i Personality
      (1) Activities/hobbies
      (2) Questions about self:
          Three wishes
          Likes and dislikes at home and school
          Describe self
          Questions specific to symptoms and presenting problem
      (3) Questions about relationship of self to others (peers, parents, siblings):
          "Why was your name picked for you?"
          Describe mother and father
          Describe ways in which parents give praise and discipline
          "How would your best friend describe you?"
2   Symptom inventory and recent behavior
   a School adjustment: behavior, achievement, truancy
   b Aggressive and antisocial behavior: fighting, stealing, alcohol or other drug use
   c Affective state: depressed, elated, sleeping and eating habits, suicidal thinking or behavior
   d Neurotic symptoms: fears, phobias, excessive worry, unusual rituals or habits, obsessive thought
   e Psychotic symptoms: hallucinations, delusions, suspicions, control of mind, consistently held strange beliefs
   f Sexual behavior: interest in opposite sex and how shown, sexual development
   g Neurologic symptoms: headaches, memory loss, convulsions, fainting
   h Peer relations: close friends, group membership, making and keeping friends
   i Relationships with adults: quality of associations with parents, relatives, neighbors, teachers; attachment
3   Personality and temperament: What was the adolescent like before and after onset of the problem?
   a Meeting strangers: friendly or withdrawn?
   b Dealing with new situations: how adaptive?
   c Emotional expression: how does adolescent express feelings when angry and when happy?
   d Affections and relationships: expressive or reserved?
   e Regularity of bodily functions: sleeping, eating, bowel
   f Sensitivity: how does adolescent react when he or she has done something wrong, seen something or someone hurt?
4   Developmental history
   a Prenatal and perinatal history: mother's health during pregnancy, complications at delivery, premature or postmature

    b Neonatal and infancy: feeding, sleeping, colic, active or passive baby
    c Milestones: walked, talked, sentences, bowel control
    d Medical history
    e Early experiences: losses, separations
5 Family history
    a Family structure and home circumstances: living situation, others in home, employment
    b Family history of illness
    c Family interactions and relationships: observe positive or negative interactions, what is said and how it is said, value system, rules and regulations, discipline, how parents get the adolescent to do something

---

in learning were thought to be of no particular consequence. Teachers were responsible for dispatching information to students but not necessarily held accountable for learning.

Counseling, on the other hand, has generally been viewed as an activity that couldn't succeed without the foundation and maintenance of a positive, trusting relationship between counselor and counselee. Unlike the superior-inferior position of teacher to student, the counselor and counselee have generally tended to share a more reciprocal relationship with respect to the issues of authority and accountability. There is a mutual bond of closeness and shared decision making between those involved in counseling—a joint desire and motivation for behavior change. That is, effective counseling depends on client feedback and involvement.

One of the main goals of counseling with adolescents is to facilitate the formation of ego identity. Helping the teenager discover "Who am I and how do I cope independently in an adult world?" is the issue at hand. As change occurs through counseling, the nurse provides support by encouragement and by acceptance of failures as they occur. Counseling, therefore, provides an opportunity for adolescents to discuss their new sense of awareness and to work with the nurse counselor in resolving the developmental difficulties of identity formation.

At present, the noticeable difference between health counseling and health teaching has to do with the methods employed to facilitate behavior change. Generally, counseling sessions are periods of time in which the counselor and adolescent explore the ways a situation might be handled. Existent coping methods are explored for current usefulness, and the adequacies of the teenager's problem-solving abilities are investigated. The goal frequently involves searching for alternative approaches for handling and integrating new experiences, impulses, and social rules. Moreover, counseling is a process whereby feelings are put together with ideas and reflected back and forth between counselor and teenager. In this way, the adolescent gains insight into his or her own problems; develops an understanding for the intensified drive toward maturation which is typical of this period; and acquires a sense of control over his or her own life.

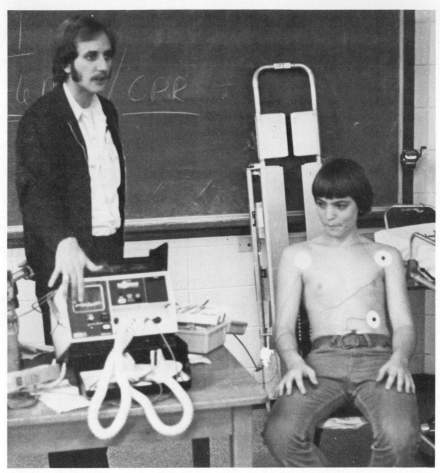

Health teaching programs must prepare young people to become skilled and knowledgeable as consumers of health care services. Information about the work roles and training of various members of the health team may be useful to students not only as health care consumers but also as persons who are in the process of selecting a career. (*Copyright © 1980 by Anne Campbell.*)

While some counseling sessions may incorporate technical instruction in some area of health which is unknown to the adolescent (e.g., hormonal changes), learning factual knowledge is not the primary purpose of the counseling session but, rather, a secondary means of assisting the adolescent with personality growth. Health teaching, on the other hand, is directed at changing the adolescent's behavior through a formal process of instruction in which the emphasis is generally on the dissemination and integration of new knowledge and skills. Obviously, most teachers are aware that there is an affective component to learning. Consequently, counseling can and does take place during teaching sessions but is generally of secondary importance in relation to the factual material to be learned.

THE IMPACT OF COMMUNICATION PATTERNS, MOTIVATION, AND LEARNING STYLES

The nurse who provides health counseling and teaching services for adolescents needs a well-developed understanding of various communication patterns, an awareness of the factors that motivate adolescents toward behavior change, and some knowledge of the differences in learning styles. Early recognition of the adolescent's manner of communication, motivational attributes, and learning style will enable the nurse to effectively personalize the counseling or teaching sessions. Individualizing in this way positively influences the sessions toward an effective outcome.

Communication Styles

Paul Mok, a psychologist who has been interested in Carl Jung's work in the area of personality development, has identified four main styles of communication.[9] Mok believes these styles represent the various ways in which people interact with one another. He has further theorized that, although one individual may use all of these styles interchangeably, the tendency for most people is to select one primary style over the others during childhood and, subsequently, to use this style most frequently in their communications. The four communication styles identified by Mok can be recognized as follows:

The Intuitor This adolescent communicator is particularly intent on discovering why something is as it is. Accepting something because the nurse counselor says it's so is not enough.

> John, age 16, has developed a chronic morning cough, and his family is insistent that he stop smoking. Everyone has spoken to John about the statistics relating smoking to cancer and heart and respiratory disease, but John still smokes. "He won't face facts," complains his father. The school nurse, however, takes a different approach with John, encouraging him to examine the physiologic and anatomic effects of cigarette smoking on a lung in biology. John is also given free access to a variety of anatomy and physiology books in the school clinic. When the school physician is in John's school, he invites John to view some x-rays of individuals experiencing lung problems. In every instance, John is really told very little about smoking, lungs, etc., and allowed to think through the situation on his own. When he

seeks out the nurse and others for answers to his questions, they willingly provide the information requested but stop short of providing unsolicited advice. The health professionals do, however, frequently ask John what he thinks about the basic reasoning behind the public health campaign to ban smoking because it is a detriment to health. Shortly thereafter, John stops smoking.

Teenagers whose primary communication style is that of the intuitor can be identified by their desire to think things through verbally as well as nonverbally and to draw their own conclusions. Closely listening to the adolescent's conversation over time will enable the nurse to make a determination as to the preferred communication style.

The Thinker   This adolescent is most concerned with being right (correct, accurate). He or she is interested in gathering facts and figures as a means for deciding what to do. Generally, the information collected is taken pretty much at face value with no particular interest in subjective interpretation.

Maureen, age 15, is interested in birth control measures for herself. She therefore seeks out the advice of counselors at the Planned Parenthood clinic. She meticulously reads numerous articles and reports in an attempt to determine the most effective means of contraception. Maureen selects the most effective method with little concern for the issues that would be of interest to an intuitor-type communicator (e.g., ''Should I engage in sexual relations with this person?''). The nurse who attempts to establish effective communication with the thinker must begin with facts and figures as a basis for understanding.

The Feeler   This adolescent responds to his or her own and others' emotions, because learning occurs through ''gut level'' responses. Meaningful memories of personal experiences (rather than facts or self-discovery of the essence of something) are the crucial determinant of the way in which this adolescent will respond to new and different situations. This teenager has an almost uncanny ability to interpret nonverbal as well as verbal subtleties in conversation.

Mike, age 14, has had trouble sleeping for the past 2 weeks, following a termination of his relationship with his girlfriend. He is increasingly depressed and spending most of his time alone. Generally, he's become noncommunicative with his friends and family. His counselor at school has tried unsuccessfully to work with Mike in a reflective manner, trying to have this teenager analyze the situation in terms of the circumstances surrounding the termination. A friend has given Mike several articles on cures for insomnia, but Mike has had no interest in reading them. During a visit to the school nurse one afternoon, however, Mike begins to pour out his feelings of despair, sadness, and fear over the loss of his girlfriend. The precipitating circumstance that resulted in this behavior was the nurse's inquiry as to *how Mike had felt in the past* when confronted with a loss. The nurse decided on this approach while interviewing Mike and listening closely to his conversation, which included telling the nurse what others had tried to do to help him.

The Sensor   This adolescent is a doer. He or she learns primarily through action and not by thinking, imagining, or feeling. His or her conversation reflects this style.

Ann, age 13, has trouble meeting new friends. She finds these situations terribly uncomfortable and usually "clams up" in interactions with people she doesn't know. Although she's thought about the reasons behind this behavior in sessions with the nurse counselor and imagined how she would like to act in new situations, her behavior hasn't changed. She's read numerous books on making friends and asked close friends to tell her what they do in new surroundings, but her problem still persists. Finally, the nurse suggests to Ann that they role play a situation involving meeting new friends. These role playing sessions continue for several months on a weekly basis. Soon Ann begins to experience greater comfort in actual interactions with other adolescents whom she doesn't know. Eventually, Ann is able to carry on a conversation easily in situations which previously left her speechless.

As stated earlier, all adolescents are reflective, interested in specific data, emotional, and action-oriented because of the developmental tasks for this age period. Consequently, they may frequently interchange one style of communication with another. The nurse's ability to assess which style is primary during a particular counseling or teaching session and to adapt his or her own style to harmonize with that of the adolescent's will significantly influence the nurse's effectiveness. Only through repeated experiences and concentrated listening does a nurse achieve the necessary skill to identify communication styles.

Motivation

Motivation is defined as "an intervening variable which is used to account for factors within an individual which arouse, maintain and channel behavior toward a goal."[10] Motivation is an important determinant in any counseling or health teaching situation. A number of elements have been identified as contributing toward motivation. Nurses need to be aware of and implement some of these factors if they wish to encourage motivation and subsequent behavioral change. In interactions with adolescents, the following ingredients are believed to enhance motivation:

- Two-way communication
- Involvement in decision making
- Commitment to the goal
- Training as a means to increased understanding and interest
- Meaningful participation in problem solving[11]

Learning Styles

Individual learning styles are the personal ways in which the learner acquires and organizes information. Some adolescents, for example, may learn best by listening to a lecture or a cassette tape recorder, whereas other teens prefer reading a text, working with programmed instruction, or seeing slides.

A *learning style* refers to sensory modality preference and cognitive patterns.[12] There are three sensory modalities that are closely related to learning. These modalities are auditory, visual, and tactile, or kinesthetic. The auditory (verbal) learner prefers to acquire knowledge by listening rather than reading or observing. The visual learner, on the other hand, prefers to learn by reading or observing. A kinesthetic individual needs to get a "feel" for the task to be learned and, consequently, learns by doing or physically manipulating objects in his or her environment.

Cognitive style has been described as "those habits in acquiring information that are the learner's typical mode of perceiving, problem-solving, thinking and remembering."[13] An evaluation of the adolescent's cognitive style, therefore, entails observation and tests to determine, for example, whether the adolescent analyzes situations in terms of the various aspects that make up the total environment or, instead, views new information as a total entity and has little interest in the component parts which make up the whole.[14] Does he or she reflect on new knowledge, thereby slowing down the process of learning, or act impulsively and quickly integrate new information with more emphasis on speed than accuracy?[15] There are seven other areas of cognitive style that are assumed to influence learning. These areas are scanning, breadth of categorizing, conceptualizing style, cognitive complexity versus simplicity, level versus sharpening, constricted versus flexible control, and tolerance for incongruous or unrealistic experiences.[16]

Individualized educational plans are becoming increasingly important to nurses teaching adolescents. The ability to personalize health teaching to suit the particular learning style of individual adolescents enhances the likelihood that learning will actually occur.

THE COUNSELING PROCESS

Counseling as a means of nursing intervention for use with adolescents may be initiated in several ways: (1) the teenager may purposely seek out the nurse for advice and counsel; (2) the nurse may, in the process of evaluating the physical health of an adolescent, become aware of the need for guidance with regard to personal or social health; (3) a parent or teacher may confide in the nurse that a particular teenager needs help; or (4) peers may express concern for their friends and make indirect and informal referrals. When the need for health counseling arises, a series of preparatory events must take place before the actual guidance sessions begin.

    1 A functional relationship will have to be established with the adolescent.
    2 An agreement between nurse and adolescent must be reached as to the need and desire for counseling.
    3 A contract needs to be developed which makes clear the conditions under which the counseling will take place and the outcomes anticipated.
    4 A counseling program must be selected.
    5 A plan must be devised for measuring the effectiveness of the counseling.

Throughout the entire process, interviewing as a means for data collection serves a most important function in the development of relevant counseling sessions.

Developing a Relationship

Developing a relationship with an adolescent is a rewarding and challenging experience for some nurses. For others, however, the task is not always achieved easily. Unresolved and difficult experiences related to one's own adolescence may inhibit the nurse. Consequently, the extent to which nurses have mastered their own developmental tasks of adolescence significantly influences their ability to be supportive, honest, objective, and spontaneous enough to create an environment of trust in which a functional nurse-adolescent relationship can emerge. Therefore, the nurse's first step toward developing productive relationships with adolescents is a process of self-reflection, For this purpose, the following tool for self-evaluation has been prepared to enable nurses in the University of Colorado School Nurse Practitioner Program to scrutinize their own progress in accomplishing the tasks of development associated with adolescence. This questionnaire is also useful in reviewing developmental characteristics of this age period.

Adolescent Developmental Task Inventory

1 What is your opinion of the size, shape, function, and potential of your body? (Developmental task: accepting one's changing body and learning to use it effectively.)

2 Look at yourself in the mirror. What's your evaluation of the way in which you're maintaining your personal appearance? (Developmental task: accepting one's body.)

3 Think of all of the situations in your life requiring physical skills. How well do you handle yourself and your body in these situations? (Developmental task: accepting one's body.)

4 What are your feelings about being a woman (man)? Is your sexual identity pleasing or nonpleasing to you? (Developmental task: achieving a satisfying and socially accepted masculine or feminine role.)

5 Do you have friends? Do you date? Are you married? Are your friends from a variety of different settings (e.g., your neighborhood, work settings, community organizations, church, etc.)? How do you feel about these relationships? Are these relationships truly satisfying for you? (Developmental task: finding oneself as a member of one's own generation in more mature relations with one's age-mates.)

6 When you have a conflict with a peer, how do you handle it? (Developmental task: finding oneself.)

7 When you approach decision-making situations, are you generally pleased that you have a decision to make or is decision making difficult for you? (Developmental task: finding oneself.)

8 When it's time for you to make decisions, solve a problem, or deal with a crisis, how important is it to you that someone else assist you with these activities? (Developmental task: achieving emotional independence.)

9 Are you well suited to and satisfied with your career as a nurse? (Developmental task: selecting and preparing for an occupation and economic independence.)

10 Do you have a mutually satisfying love relationship with someone? (Developmental task: preparing for marriage and family life.)

11 Do you maintain your own home or have plans to do so? (Developmental task: living independently, preparing for marriage.)

12 Do you vote regularly in elections? Have you a membership in any community or professional organizations? Do others turn to you for help? How do you feel about others turning to you for help? (Developmental task: developing intellectual skills and social sensitivities necessary for civic competence.)

13 Have you a philosophy about life which has been meaningful and usable for you in today's world? (Developmental task: developing a workable philosophy of life that makes sense in today's world.)

Source: School Nurse Practitioner Program, University of Colorado. Based on Evelyn Duvall, *Family Development*, 3d ed., J. B. Lippincott Co., Philadelphia, 1967, pp. 294–297.

Nurses who discover they have not mastered all these tasks should not automatically disqualify themselves from relationships and counseling activities with adolescents. However, they will need to be fully aware of the areas of adolescent development in which they themselves are continuing to mature in order that they not let their own maturational needs and feelings seriously interfere with their counseling endeavors.

Successful relationships with adolescents require an environment in which the young people (1) feel comfortable admitting their dependency needs, (2) find a satisfactory ego ideal for themselves, (3) discover ac-

Table 11-2   The General Process of Nurse-Patient Relationships

Nurse should:

A *Initiate* the relationship by
1   Introducing self
2   Stating purpose of relationship
3   Stating limitations of relationship including:
   a   Frequency of interaction
   b   Duration of relationship
   c   Nature of relationship
B *Continue* or *maintain* the relationship by
1   Establishing rapport and practicing interviewing and counseling techniques
2   Respecting the adolescent and not being judgmental
3   Keeping within the contract established at the outset
C *Terminate* the relationship by
1   Preparing adolescent for termination well in advance of termination date
2   Summarizing the relationship with the adolescent
3   Encouraging the adolescent to verbalize feelings and/or thoughts about the relationship and termination
4   Expressing own thoughts and feelings about the relationship and about termination

Source: *Family Study and Interviewing Guide—Health Professionals, Health Issues, and Family Study*, mimeographed, University of Colorado Medical Center, Fall 1977, p. 20.

ceptance and support for experimenting with new desires for independence, and (4) feel confident that direction will be available to help them identify achievable and acceptable goals for living. A relationship of this kind begins with the establishment of trust. To facilitate trust, it is important that the nurse both allow the adolescent to get to know the nurse as a person and carefully explain the process of counseling. A humanistic approach is essential. Moreover, relationships develop sooner if the nurse is easily accessible to the adolescent, especially in the event of a crisis. School clinics, for this reason, are ideal settings for adolescent counseling. Table 11-2 describes the general process of nurse-patient relationships.[17]

Contract Development

A contract is an agreement between the nurse and adolescent about the nature and duration of the counseling sessions. Once the diagnostic process of interviewing is completed, it is important to clearly state the purpose of the counseling sessions, enumerate the conditions under which the counseling sessions are to take place, and identify the specific goals to be achieved as a result of counseling. Establishing the contract should be a joint venture between adolescent and nurse, with each person stating his or her particular expectations of the other. While the idea of a written contract for counseling may seem superfluous to some nurses, there is no question that this approach lends an added sense of credibility and seriousness to the sessions and helps to ensure the commitment of both counselor and adolescent to the task at hand. The likelihood of behavior change is far greater under these circumstances than in more informal interactions.

Evaluation

In nursing in general, there has not been a great deal of interest in documenting the effectiveness of nursing intervention. However, if nurses wish to be viewed as legitimate health counselors, it is imperative that they continually evaluate the outcomes of their counseling endeavors. Contracts help with evaluation because the purpose and goals of the counseling session are clearly stated, frequently in behavioral terms. For evaluation to occur, a written record of each counseling session must be maintained. Moreover, the nurse should make ongoing evaluations rather than delay this activity to the end of the sessions. Nurses in clinical settings may wish to seek consultation from their colleagues in schools of nursing for additional help in delineating and refining their plans for evaluation.

Termination

If the counseling sessions have been effective, the adolescent has experienced a satisfactory relationship with an adult, learned new coping mechanisms, and gained a greater sense of self-identity. As the time for termination of the sessions approaches (as specified in the contract), the nurse should bring to the adolescent's attention the fact that they are nearing the end of their work together. Often the adolescent is apprehensive about his or her ability to function well without the support of the counseling. In such a situation, the nurse may suggest that their sessions gradually taper off rather than abruptly end. An important additional point to be made about termination is that the adolescent needs to realize that his or her ability to establish a mutually satisfying relationship with the nurse counselor is indicative of readiness to develop equally significant relationships with other peers and adults. With proper support and encouragement, most adolescents are soon willing to end the counseling relationship.

Counseling Programs

Throughout the diagnostic phase of the counseling process, the nurse, by interview, attempts to determine what developmental issues are of particular concern to the adolescent. The following inventory of concerns common to different periods of adolescence should prove helpful to nurses in these attempts:

   • Early adolescent (puberty to about age 14): Worries about appearance (size, proportions, features, etc.). Worries about health, so-

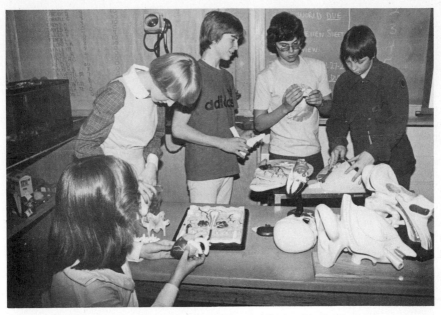

Health teaching deals with information, attitudes, and skills; its objective is to induce students to change their behavior in ways that promote their health. (*Copyright © 1980 by Anne Campbell.*)

matizes. Is critical of adults and younger siblings, admires older siblings. Is easily embarrassed.

• Middle adolescent (approximately 14 through 17 years): Worries about peer acceptance, schoolwork, health, and interactions with opposite sex. Struggles for emancipation from parents.

• Late adolescence (approximately 18 through 22 years): Is concerned about and involved with love relationships, career choice and preparation, and selection and attainment of own life-style.

A variety of counseling approaches are available for the nurse's use. Descriptions of several counseling programs are included here to further clarify the counseling process.

Behavior Management   This form of counseling originates from learning theory. The basic premise is that all behavior is learned and that both appropriate and inappropriate behaviors recur only if they are rewarded. Behaviors are defined as only those actions which can be objectively evaluated. Hence, for example, *joy* is considered a subjective observation and does not describe a behavior, whereas *smiling* or *laughing* does.[18]

A behavior management program includes very specific behavioral goals worked out between the adolescent and the nurse and stated in the contract. These goals (e.g., reduce crying spells) determine the system of giving or withholding rewards. The success of behavior management is absolutely dependent upon the consistency with which the procedure of giving or withholding rewards is applied. Generally, this is a very popular program of counseling because it takes so little time to see results.

Crisis Intervention Adolescence is typically a period of crises because of the imbalance of internal needs and external demands. Consequently, crisis intervention counseling, which involves providing support to an individual learning how to cope in new situations, is particularly well suited to the needs of the adolescent. The nurse's role is to reflect the adolescent's ideas and encourage dependence and independence as indicated. Walkup identifies more specific nursing actions in a crisis intervention program:

1 Identify the change that has precipitated the crisis, focusing on the immediate problem.
2 Define the problem.
3 Solve the problem by modifying external or internal factors, redefining the problem, or giving up.
4 Assess coping mechanisms, explore alternative courses of action, and seek out situational support.
5 Assess self-destructive potential.
6 Do anticipatory planning to prevent future crises.[19]

Values Clarification Based on Louis Raths' model of the valuing process, values clarification utilizes strategies designed to give adolescents in groups opportunities to experience the steps in the valuing process. Raths and his colleagues define the valuing process as follows:

Choosing
1 Freely
2 From alternatives
3 After thoughtful consideration of the consequences of each alternative

Prizing
4 Cherishing, being happy
5 [Being] willing to affirm the choice publicly

Acting
6 Doing something with the choice
7 Repeatedly, in some pattern of life

Formalized value-clarifying strategies are available for use in counseling groups of adolescents.[21]

Problem Resolution   The School Nurse Practitioner Program at the University of Colorado offers instruction in another form of counseling, in which the adolescent is consciously made aware of the steps involved in problem solving and helped to identify his or her strengths and weaknesses in performing at each of the steps. As areas of need are identified (e.g., defining the problem), various techniques based on the adolescent's communication pattern and learning style are used to reduce the deficiency. During this process, the nurse counselor helps the adolescent evaluate the way in which this step of the problem-solving process was handled in the past and to identify new methods that are more appropriate. The basis of this type of counseling is the young person's awareness of the actual steps in problem solving. This counseling approach has been well received by the adolescents who have been involved.

A number of structured counseling programs have been designed to assist with counseling related to drugs, alcoholism, sex, social development, etc. Nurses interested in these programs should make inquiries to local mental health centers and adolescent clinics to determine the availability of materials as well as training sessions for professionals interested in these types of counseling.

Counseling Techniques

This chapter has presented numerous techniques associated with interviewing, communication patterns, motivational factors, and learning styles—techniques that have been found to enhance the process of health counseling by the nurse. The following interpersonal techniques are additional suggestions for improvement of the nurse's counseling skills with adolescents.

  1   Use silence to allow the adolescent to stop and consider what has been said.

  2   Make sure the adolescent's language is understood. Ask for clarification whenever necessary. Example: Adolescent—"I'm completely bagged." Nurse—"Are you telling me you're tired?"

  3   Give recognition. Example: "Mary, I notice you've changed your hair style."

  4   Accept what is said. Avoid cutting the adolescent off or abruptly changing the subject. Examples:

    a   *Helpful techniques*: "Yes." "I understand what you're saying." Interested nod of the head.
    b   *Nonhelpful techniques*: Cutting the adolescent off. Adolescent—"I think I might die." Nurse—"That's crazy. You're fine." Changing the subject: Adolescent—"I really had a fantastic time going out with Tim." Nurse—"You were telling me earlier that sometimes you feel very sad."

   5   Offer yourself. Example: "I'm interested in you."

   6   Give broad openings. Example: "How shall we begin?" or "What happened this week?"

   7   Make behavioral observations. Example: "I notice your hands are trembling." Avoid judgmental statements like "I notice you're angry" (an assumption) in favor of "You slammed that door, yelled at me, and just pounded your fists together. What kind of feelings do you have right now?"

   8   Encourage comparison. Example: "Is this feeling of fear one you've had before in your life?"

   9   Avoid voicing doubt. Example: "I can't imagine that would happen."

   10   Examine the meaning of what is said by both parties.

   11   Be consciously aware of your own behavior and verbal interactions.

   12   Avoid value judgments.[22]

One of the common problems facing nurses who counsel adolescents is the situation in which an adolescent attempts to manipulate the nurse by saying, "I'm going to tell you something serious, but first I want you to promise not to tell anyone." It is a serious mistake to make or insinuate such a promise. If the teenager then reveals some information that the counselor must share with others to protect the adolescent's (or another's) safety, the nurse's failure to keep this promise will, in most cases, signify to the adolescent that the nurse can no longer be trusted. Obviously, when trust is lost, the quality of the relationship is seriously jeopardized and the effectiveness of counseling is lost. A truthful and more realistic response to the request will avoid compromising the counselor's trustworthiness. The nurse may say, for example: "Tom, I can't make that kind of promise. You and I both know that it will be necessary for me to get help if your information indicates that you or someone else is in serious difficulty."

With adolescents in particular, it is important that the nurse role-model responsible, adult behavior. The nurse in the above situation may continue the conversation by saying something like the following: "I'm interested in you, Tom, and it sounds as if you really need to tell someone what's happening. Perhaps our talking about the situation will help you find a solution to the problem." By this approach, the nurse places the decision for discussing the particular problem back on the adolescent, which is where it belongs, and both preserves the integrity of their relationship and supports the adolescent's ability to make decisions.

There are three other things the nurse counselor must keep in mind. First, there is always more than one way to say something. Second, the intonation of one's voice is important because it can communicate a wide range of feelings (e.g., disinterest, happiness, etc.). Third, sincerity is the key to effective counseling, as it will complement whatever words are used.[23]

THE HEALTH TEACHING PROCESS

Much of the counseling material presented earlier is equally applicable to health teaching. It is important that the teacher communicate with students, understand their learning styles, and apply the necessary techniques to motivate learning. While the nurse may interview the adolescents to determine their level of health knowledge and skill, it is doubtful that the extensive interviewing associated with counseling is necessary in health teaching situations.

Curriculum Planning

Increasingly, adolescents are becoming directly involved in the planning for their own learning experiences, and with successful results.[24] Realizing one of the strongest needs of adolescents is to feel they can make a difference in the world around them, many nurses who teach health view this type of participation as important not only to learning but to overall development. Motivation is greater and improved learning occurs. Furthermore, the curriculum developed is far more relevant than curricula produced by the single-handed efforts of one or more adults.

Teaching, like counseling, must be evaluated. Any plans for development of a curriculum for health teaching should include a statement of the desired outcomes to be achieved (e.g., class will learn to take blood pressures). In addition, a series of objectives must be formulated which specify the means whereby the outcome will be realized (e.g., a lecture on blood pressure, practice, and return demonstrations of blood pressure measurements, etc.). Finally, a means for evaluating how much the students learned as a result of the teaching must be developed (e.g., pretest, posttest, return demonstration of a skill, etc.).

Three types of learning should be taken into consideration at the time of curriculum planning, because all three are necessary parts of almost every learning situation.[25] For *cognitive learning* to occur, it is necessary to establish a teaching method that bridges the gap between old and new understandings. For *attitude learning* to occur, the lesson plan must provide opportunity for imitation of a model so that the student adopts the model's attitude (e.g., Weight Watchers, Inc.). Another approach to attitude learning is to offer students such a positive experience in conjunction with a learning situation that the emergent attitudes also are positive. The third class of learning, motor skills learning, requires practice and feedback. In the actual classroom, therefore, it is important that the nurse interested in teaching the adolescent the skill of blood pressure measurement, for example, has considered these three types of learning and planned the method of teaching accordingly. If this has been done, the lesson plan will include the following:

1   A plan to relate what the adolescents already know about the circulatory system to the new knowledge to be taught about blood pressure (cognitive learning).
2   A plan to provide a satisfying experience in conjunction with learning how to measure blood pressures (attitude learning). Such experiences will positively influence the adolescents' attitude toward having their blood pressure taken in the future.
3   A plan of instruction that will allow the adolescent students to take blood pressures under the instructor's supervision and to learn immediately how well they did (motor skills learning).

Two developmental characteristics of adolescence—anxiety and orientation to the present—tend to impede learning. Anxiety frequently scrambles the messages teenagers perceive and makes learning impossible. Consequently, the nurse needs to watch the students for signs of high anxiety such as inattention, hyperactivity, thought disorders, and inability to convey a message without jumping from one subject to another. From the standpoint of learning, it is pointless to keep a student with a severe anxiety reaction to adolescence in a class unless supplementary counseling is provided to help reduce the stress. The adolescent's age-typical focus upon the present leaves him or her for the most part uninterested in the future and unable to conceptualize it. Preventive health education for adolescents hence is difficult, since teenagers are often unable or unwilling to deal well with information about present health hazards whose ill effects may not appear for several years.

Adolescent Health Interests

Learning readiness is an important determinant of whether or not new health knowledge will be gained and skills acquired. The nurse providing health instruction must be capable of assessing the adolescent's readiness to learn. Factors that influence readiness include motivation to learn the material, ability to learn it, and background experiences, attitudes, and skills.[26] In view of the relationships between motivation and readiness to learn, it is important that the nurse be particularly aware of the individual health interests of adolescents. Certainly one is more motivated to learn when the subject matter is interesting and personally meaningful.

To discover the health interests of adolescents in grades 7 through 12, Byler and her associates[27] posed the following questions to adolescents during an East Coast study conducted in 1969: What is good health? How do you know if you have it? What topics do you think should be included in a health curriculum for today's young people? The areas of concern identified by Byler and colleagues appear in Table 11-3. For a more complete description of adolescent health interests, the text *Teach Us What We Want to Know* is an excellent report of the study.

School health services for adolescents are described in Chapter 15, which includes a description of a participatory health education course with which the author has been involved. Readers are referred to that chapter for further discussion of health education programs.

SUMMARY

Adolescent counseling and health teaching have been discussed from the standpoint of need and process, and examples of certain health counseling and education programs have been provided. Specific techniques for interviewing and counseling have also been presented. The ways whereby

Table 11-3 Common Health Interests and Concerns of Adolescents

Grade level	Areas of health interests and concerns	General comments
7	*Body*	Interested in many
	Physical health	things, most of which stem
	Posture	from the advent of puberty. A
	The senses	strong desire to be attractive
	Food, nutrition, diet	to the opposite sex and to
	Rest	understand them is evident.
	Personal hygiene	Sex is a matter of growing
	Grooming	interest. Home problems
	Mental health	continue to threaten
	Emotional control	emotional health, and social
	Results of fright	problems loom larger to these
	Symptoms of mental illness	adolescents than to sixth-
	Work of psychiatrists	graders.
	Social-emotional development	
	Social skills	
	Physical appearance	
	Personality	
	Sex education	
	Other areas	
	Diseases	
	Accidents	
	Alcohol, drugs, smoking	
	Pollution	
	Special groups (hippies, runaways, Hell's Angels, Ku Klux Klan)	
	Events: riots and war	

Table 11-3   Common Health Interests and Concerns of Adolescents (Continued)

Grade level	Areas of health interests and concerns	General comments
8	*Body* Change in adolescence Physical health and appearance Health habits Grooming First aid Self-defense *Mental health* Maturity in attitudes and behavior Results of fright Mental illness Teenage pressures *Social-emotional development* Emotional health Social skills Boy-girl relations Relations with parents Sex and family life education Handicapped people Preparation for marriage Child development *Other areas* Diseases Heart Cancer Venereal disease Alcohol, drugs, smoking Pollution Consumer education	The primary interest is how they think they appear to other boys and girls, whether they feel they are gaining understanding of the opposite sex. Emotional health is threatened if the teen cannot resolve the conflict between fear of losing parents' love and the need to establish themselves with peers.
9	More about life than we already know. How to get along with the other sex. How to plan efficiently in terms of school and daily health habits. What products on the market are irritating or harmful to the body. Some of the terms the medical doctor uses. Half the time we don't know what was said when we get home from the doctor's office.	High point of concern: peer relations, parent relations, sex education. A health curriculum is important as it relates to the teens' need to become independent of parent control. Measure their own growth and development by keeping themselves well groomed. They have a positive view of self if they are poised and have a sense of sureness about themselves.

Table 11-3   Common Health Interests and Concerns of Adolescents (*Continued*)

Grade level	Areas of health interests and concerns	General comments
9		Getting along with others is important. Concerns with disease, alcohol, drugs, and cigarettes are increasing and they want a firm foundation of knowledge about these problems.
10	Personal health habits Sex education Smoking Alcohol Drugs Food, nutrition, diet Grooming First aid and safety Mental illness Abortion Marriage preparation Venereal disease Sanitation Emotional control Relations to parents The body Exercise and physical education Diseases Mental health Dental health Family problems Slums Understanding self Child psychology Pollution Public health Birth control	Major concerns: understanding self, relating to parents, and sex education. Physical changes still of concern and the resulting unpredictability of personal behavior causes young people to question themselves. Beginning search for values—"Who am I?" Peer life more time-consuming. Less tolerance for parents. Want proof as to how drugs, alcohol, and cigarettes are harmful.
11	Sex education Alcohol Drugs Smoking Mental health Birth control Body systems Body functions Mental illness	Major concerns: mental health, responsibilities of parents, sex education. Psychology and values clarification of great interest for self-understanding rather than to help them in dealing with parents (response of ninth graders).

Table 11-3 Common Health Interests and Concerns of Adolescents
(Continued)

Grade level	Areas of health interests and concerns	General comments
11	Personal hygiene Food, nutrition, diet Physical fitness Pollution Diseases Psychology Sociology Social relations Morality	Mellowing desire to understand parents and for harmony. Angry that parents have not taught them about sex. Want to take advantage of talking things over with an older person, definitely interested in self-help measures to defeat colds, sore throats, other conditions impeding their daily obligations. A general sense of approval for the use of alcohol.
12	Physical health Physical fitness Personal hygiene Food, nutrition, diet Mental health Study habits Diseases Venereal diseases Vaccinations Identification of physical and mental illness Defects: sight, hearing Sex education Birth control Abortion Alcohol Smoking Drugs Morals Living conditions	Want a well-organized K-12 health education program. See the school as responsible for physical education and home as responsible for health and sex education. Mental health education is a must.

Source: R. Byler, G. Lewis, and R. Totman, *Teach Us What We Want to Know*. New York: Mental Health Materials Center, Inc., 1969, pp. 50–60. ⓒ Connecticut State Board of Education.

communication patterns, motivation, and learning styles influence the outcome of health counseling and teaching efforts have been explored. A detailed description of the health interests and concerns of adolescents as well as information about their developmental characteristics rounds out the chapter.

REFERENCES

1 H. Benson, *The Relaxation Response*. New York: Avon Books, William Morrow and Co., 1975, pp. 18–22.
2 A. D. Hofmann and M. Gaman, "The Adolescent Outpatient," *Postgraduate Medicine*, 50:245–249, September 1971.
3 Ibid.
4 A. F. Brunswick and E. Josephson, "Adolescent Health in Harlem," *American Journal of Public Health*, 62 (supplement): 1–62, October 1972.
5 K. P. Blaker, "Comments on Suicide among College Students," in D. B. Anderson and L. J. McLean (eds.), *Identifying Suicide Potential*. New York: Human Sciences Press, 1971, pp. 21–22.
6 J. P. Chaplin, *Dictionary of Psychology*. New York: Dell Publishing Co., 1968.
7 B. K. Redman, *The Process of Patient Teaching in Nursing* (3d ed.). St. Louis: C. V. Mosby Co., 1976, pp. 9–10.
8 J. W. Vander Zanden and M. V. Vander Zanden, "The Interview," *Nursing Outlook*, 11(10):743, October 1963.
9 J. L. Bledsoe, "Your Four Communicating Styles," *Training*, 13(3):18–21, March 1976.
10 Chaplin, op. cit.
11 W. H. Weiss, "Motivation," *Training*, 12(9):41–43, September 1975.
12 R. Walsh and D. Soat, "How Trainees Learn," *Training*, 12(6):40–41, 52–53, June 1975.
13 Walsh and Soat, op. cit., p. 40.
14 Ibid.
15 Ibid.
16 Ibid.
17 *Family Study and Interviewing Guide—Health Professionals, Health Issues, and Family Study*, mimeographed, University of Colorado Medical Center, Fall 1977, p. 20.
18 R. V. Hall, *Basic Principles: Managing Behavior Series, Part 2*. Lawrence, Kansas: H&H Enterprises, 1975.
19 L. Walkup, "A Concept of Crisis," in J. E. Hall and B. R. Weaver (eds.), *Nursing of Families in Crisis*. Philadelphia: J. B. Lippincott Co., 1974.
20 L. Raths, M. Harmin, and S. B. Simon, *Values and Teaching*. Columbus, Ohio: Charles B. Merrill Publishing Co., 1966.
21 S. B. Simon, L. W. Howe, and H. Kirschenbaum, *Values Clarification*. New York: Hart Publishing Co., 1972.
22 "Counseling—What Does a Counselor Say?" Class handout, School Nurse Practitioner Program, Rutgers Medical School, 1975.
23 J. S. Hays and K. Larson, *Interacting with Patients*. New York: Macmillan Co., 1963, p. 22.
24 M. McClosky and P. Kleinbard, *Youth into Adult*. New York: National Commission on Resources for Youth, Inc., 1974.
25 Redman, op. cit., p. 57.
26 Ibid.
27 R. Byler, G. Lewis, and R. Totman, *Teach Us What We Want to Know*. New York: Mental Health Materials Center, Inc., 1969, p. 8.

The Adolescent
in the General Hospital

Anne Altshuler

Nurses in the hospital setting encounter some adolescents who have a wealth of experience with the health care system as a result of congenital defects or acquired chronic illnesses necessitating frequent and often lengthy hospital stays. Other adolescents are admitted for acute illness, injury, or elective surgery with little knowledge of or prior experience with either the hospital system or the role of being ill. Nursing intervention for both groups needs to be based on a thorough knowledge of and sensitivity to the normal developmental tasks being faced by adolescents, with support for maintaining healthy growth despite the disruptive impact of illness. This chapter presents nursing interventions that facilitate adolescents' adaptation to hospitalization in a growth-producing fashion, regardless of whether they are admitted for an acute health problem or for a chronic condition.

WHY HAVE A SEPARATE HOSPITAL UNIT
FOR ADOLESCENTS?

Although teenagers can receive excellent care in a variety of settings, such as an adult unit or a pediatric ward for children of all ages, there is much to be said for providing an area where hospitalized adolescents can be cared for as a group, with special attention focused on meeting their needs at this phase of development. While some authors recommend that adolescents be cared for on general pediatric units, I favor nursing action to admit adolescent patients to a teenage unit whenever possible.

Despite the fact that grouping patients according to age rather than diagnosis can put stress on the nursing staff, the advantages to the patients seem to warrant it. They are helped to see themselves as teenagers rather than as people with a diagnosis. They learn that they share many of the same interests and concerns. The peer group in the hospital can serve as a testing ground for acceptance by peers at home, can help the ill adolescent feel less isolated and alone in the problems he or she faces, and can provide a forum for role play and problem solving of common issues to be faced upon return to the community after hospitalization. With careful selection of staff members, appropriate design of the physical setting, fostering of peer support groups, and planning of a program attuned to teenage interests and needs, an adolescent unit can be an environment that contributes to development and adjustment. If a teenage patient is hospitalized among adults or younger children, many of the interventions described in this chapter can be implemented on an individual basis to assist the adolescent's adaptation.

WHO SHOULD BE ADMITTED TO THE ADOLESCENT UNIT?

When adolescents are to be hospitalized together in a specific area, decisions must be made about appropriate admissions to the unit. Ordinarily, the age range includes patients from 12 or 13 years old through high school graduation. Flexibility in application of this policy, rather than rigid adherence to age levels, helps avoid inappropriate placement of patients. A number of exceptions to the age rule need to be considered.

The retarded adolescent or young adult provides a special problem. Should a 22-year-old be hospitalized on an adult unit when developmental functioning indicates that he or she would most benefit from the program offered on an adolescent unit? What about the severely retarded 13-year-old who sleeps in a crib and needs to be spoon-fed like an infant? Such patients' influence on other adolescents on the unit needs to be considered. In some instances, the presence of retarded individuals on the unit may provide positive experiences both for them and for the more normal teenagers. It is not reasonable to ask the adolescent unit to accept all the retarded patients in the hospital, even though they may be developmentally at the level best served by that unit. A unit caring primarily for a retarded population is unlikely to meet the needs of normal adolescents. By the same token, retarded individuals cannot be automatically excluded from the areas serving the adolescent age group.

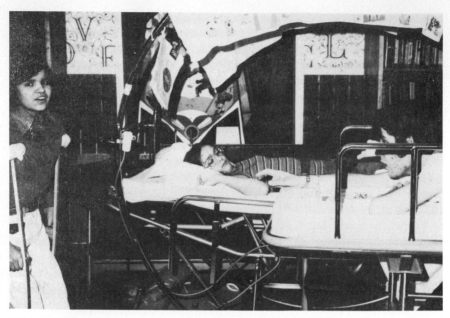

When nurses keep normal developmental tasks clearly in mind, they can better understand the impact of illness and hospitalization. (*Photo courtesy of Frederick Seidl and the* American Journal of Maternal Child Nursing.)

Valerie, age 21, had been hospitalized in the past for orthopedic surgery on the adolescent unit. Her intellectual functioning was that of a 4-year-old. Now returning to the hospital, she was again admitted to the teenage ward. She shared a four-bed room with three nonretarded adolescents. In traction for 3 weeks, she derived much enjoyment from watching the activities of her roommates, and they learned to be quite obliging about her needs. Although she had limited speech, clearly articulating only 10 or 12 words, she indicated a desire to join in teen group meetings, where she listened attentively and demonstrated appropriate responses of laughter and seriousness according to the topics being discussed. She participated in the unit craft and recreation programs on the level of her ability with such activities as coloring, cutting, and pasting. Valerie's roommates learned to value the contributions she could make and praise her achievements. Ordinarily, they might never have had this opportunity to share with a retarded person in such close proximity.

A second exception to the age guidelines arises when a chronically ill adolescent, used to frequent hospitalizations on an adolescent unit, reaches the age at which a patient would be admitted to an adult floor. Again, individual needs must be considered. It does not seem justified to place a 19-year-old dying of cystic fibrosis or leukemia on a new unit simply because he or she is beyond the age limit of a familiar ward where trust and rapport have been established over years of contact with the nursing staff. On the other hand, chronically ill young adults cannot continue indefinitely to return to a unit geared toward supporting developmental needs of a younger age group. They may need considerable help and support in making the transition to an adult unit.

> Paul, age 19, had been born with a myelomeningocele that left him with a severe handicap necessitating frequent and lengthy hospitalizations on an adolescent unit. As he grew older, he expressed many feelings of anxiety about future hospitalizations. Comments such as "When I'm 65, can I still come to the teen unit if that's what I want?" demonstrated his worry about his ability to face new hospitalizations in a different setting and his fears of being rejected by the staff people he had come to know and trust. The staff helped Paul to explore at length over several admissions the advantages and disadvantages of being hospitalized with adults rather than teenagers. They did not insist that he be placed on an adult unit, but showed understanding and sympathy for his feelings while supporting any moves he made toward increased independence. Eventually, Paul himself decided to plan admission to the adult orthopedic unit for a spinal fusion, reassured by promises of continued visits and support from the familiar staff members on the teen unit.

> Ken, age 21, had had numerous admissions to the teenage unit for treatment of cystic fibrosis over the past few years. He and his family now recognized that his condition was terminal. They and the medical and nursing staff planned together that Ken's admissions would continue to be to the teen unit. Ken and his family expressed satisfaction and relief that his final hospitalization would be among people whom they had come to know and feel confidence in.

Concerned debate on adolescent units is stimulated when inpatient care is needed for abortions, treatment of anorexia nervosa or other emotionally based illnesses, evaluation of major behavior problems, and detoxification for drug or alcohol abuse. Some units have found that they can absorb 1 to 3 teenagers with behavior problems or anorexia nervosa into the adolescent program without a great deal of disruption, but that additional patients with these disorders severely compromise the ability of the staff to provide an effective, safe, and meaningful program. Staff members may feel torn between the need to spend time with the emotionally disturbed young person and the concurrent expectations to carry on the many other demands of an acute-care medical-surgical unit. Few adolescent units have integrated young abortion patients into their programs; more often the approach has been to admit them to the regular abortion unit and work with that staff to help them serve the special needs of adolescents. Several adolescent units have experimented with admission of intoxicated juveniles. Further study is needed to determine the benefits and disadvantages for all concerned—the total group of patients, their families, staff members, and the overall unit program—of admitting these "atypical" adolescents to an adolescent unit.

The above examples make it clear that the nursing staff needs to be closely involved in planning with the admissions office about location of adolescents and young adults within the hospital. Reliance upon chronological age alone is not sufficient to meet individual needs. Whenever possible, the desires and preferences of the patients involved should be taken into account and their active participation in the decision solicited by the staff. The persons who are best able to weigh the needs of individual patients against the capabilities of the unit in order to make appropriate decisions about admissions are the adolescent unit nurses.

DESIGNING HOSPITAL CARE TO ACCOMMODATE AND ENHANCE DEVELOPMENT

When adolescents are grouped together on a hospital unit, the developmental tasks and characteristics of their age form the framework within which nursing care is given. Nurses can use their knowledge about development to create both a unit program and individualized nursing interventions that minimize disruptions of normal development and also provide new opportunities for further growth. Among the major developmental tasks of adolescence are the following:

1 Forming a clear individual identity
2 Accepting a new body image
3 Attaining emancipation from parents
4 Developing a personal value system
5 Achieving financial and social independence
6 Developing relationships with members of both sexes
7 Developing cognitive skills and the ability to think abstractly
8 Developing the ability to control one's behavior according to socially acceptable norms and to take responsibility for one's own behavior

Although illness and hospitalization can interfere with the accomplishment of these tasks, opportunities also exist to make the hospital experience into a period of learning, growth, and improved adjustment. This is an exciting challenge in the nursing care of adolescents.

Camille, age 13, was confined to a wheelchair because of a myelomeningocele. During a 6-week hospitalization for a spinal fusion she attended the twice weekly teen group meetings and joined in discussion with other adolescents on a variety of topics. Initially, she alienated others by her loud and whiny tone of voice as she complained about her lack of friends and about peer teasing at school. In time, she learned to modify her voice tones, to be able to listen to others about their problems and interests in addition to sharing her own, and to gain from the suggestions and feedback she received from the other teenagers. It appeared, on subsequent hospitalizations, that some of the gains she made had indeed carried over into her home and school situations as positive learning experiences that enhanced her ability to establish more satisfying peer relationships.

Predictable Problems of the Hospitalized Adolescent

When nurses keep adolescents' normal developmental tasks clearly in mind, they can better understand the impact of illness and hospitalization on adolescents and anticipate their likely responses. They are then able to support normal growth and adjustment. Regression is bound to take place in some areas of behavior when illness occurs. Acceptance, coupled with support toward new coping and growth, can help minimize the problem.

> Carol, age 15, began to scream and throw belongings around her hospital room after learning that chemotherapy for a tumor would cause her to lose her long, blonde hair. A nurse moved in rapidly to hold Carol, firmly telling her that she could not be allowed to injure herself or others or damage her room. She expressed understanding for Carol's feelings, but conveyed the expectation that Carol would have the strength to cope with this loss successfully and that the nurses and her family would be there to help her do so. Carol regained control of herself rapidly and expressed her sadness and distress through crying and talking about her feelings. She was later able to participate in purchasing a wig to conceal her temporary hair loss during treatment.

Adolescents can be expected to engage in testing to ascertain the limits of acceptable behavior. The staff needs to determine what rules are necessary for safety, welfare, and comfort of the patients and make these known, along with their rationale. Other issues where conflicts occur may best be handled by a collaborative problem-solving approach. When a staff member is drawn into a power struggle with an adolescent, the situation may rapidly deteriorate. It is important for the staff to keep in mind the normal developmental tasks and provide opportunities for patients and staff to participate together in problem solving and discussion. This approach may help adolescents feel that they have some control over their lives and that their needs, feelings, and sensitivities are valued and respected. When adolescents and nurses begin to work together to solve a problem, there is a much greater chance of satisfactory resolution than if they enter into a conflict with each other.

> Rich was hospitalized for regulation of his medications to gain better control of his seizures. Although only 14, he was over 6 feet tall. He felt that his local doctor and his mother had forced him to agree to the hospitalization against his will.

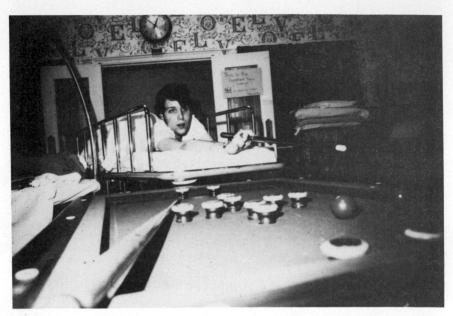

Recreation is a major need of hospitalized adolescents, particularly those whose mobility is impaired. (*Photo courtesy of Frederick Seidl and the* American Journal of Maternal Child Nursing.)

When the length of stay extended beyond the 4 days he felt he had been "promised," he reacted by periodically leaving the unit without permission and threatening to "blow up the hospital." The staff initially told Rich that if he left the unit again he would be restricted to his room. This caused even more belligerent behavior.

At this point, one nurse invited Rich to sit down with her in an empty conference room where they could talk privately and he could share his feelings. Rich repeated his angry threats. The nurse gave recognition to these feelings and showed by her continued calm presence that she was unafraid of Rich's size and words and was concerned for his welfare. As they talked, Rich gradually shared information about his life at home, the recent divorce of his parents, his dissatisfaction with school, his sadness at having seizures, his anger at the doctor for miscalculating the length of hospitalization, the difficulty of being separated from his friends, and his desire to learn to drive.

The nurse and Rich were able to work out a number of common goals. Rich was able to see his desire for a driver's license as an incentive for cooperating with attempts to regulate the medications so as to keep him seizure-free. The nurse and Rich paged the physician, and together they were able to gain a clearer plan for an early discharge. Rich sensed that his feelings were recognized and respected. His acting-out behavior ceased, and he cooperated well on the unit from then until discharge the next afternoon.

Separation anxiety, expected in young children, can often be a major problem for adolescents as well. Longing for the familiar people, surroundings, and activities of home is common. At a time when peers assume a major importance, having to be away from this vital support group poses a real threat. Especially in a large university medical center, patients may be far from home, friends, and family, and feel acutely the loss of familiar and cared-for support systems. Nurses can find ways to help adolescents maintain their ties with home through such measures as phone calls, letters, tape recordings, and liberal visiting policies that welcome peers as well as families.

> John, age 16, was hospitalized 200 miles from home for one month for orthopedic surgery. By special arrangement with the nursing staff, his best friend came to spend a weekend at the hospital. He brought his sleeping bag and spent Saturday night on the floor of John's hospital room. He ate his meals in the hospital cafeteria, and on one occasion purchased McDonald's hamburgers to share with John. The visit did much to boost John's morale and ability to cope with the separation from home. His friend was cooperative with unit policies and posed no problems.

PHILOSOPHY AND MANAGEMENT
OF AN ADOLESCENT UNIT

A hospital unit dealing with adolescents must make special efforts to create an environment in which teenagers feel safe, comfortable, respected, and encouraged to continue to grow in normal ways. Basic philosophical components need to include the following areas of emphasis:

- Teenage patients will be viewed in a context of the normal growth and developmental characteristics of this age group. Care will be designed to provide opportunities to support healthy development as much as possible.
- Teenage patients will be invited to be active participants in planning, implementing, and evaluating their care. Their assistance will be sought in gathering data about their lives at home and school, goals, concerns, knowledge of illness, and expectations of health care.
- Teenage patients will be recognized both as individuals and as members of families. Attention will be directed to enhancing good communication and understanding among family members. Ties with families who cannot visit regularly will be supported and maintained.
- Confidentiality and privacy will be respected. Information will not be shared unnecessarily without the teenager's knowledge and consent.

The rights of minors to seek (or to refuse) health care and treatment have more often come into question regarding outpatients than hospitalized children or adolescents, but the issues of informed consent and permission for procedures occasionally arise in the hospital.

Sally, age 14, was newly diagnosed with systemic lupus erythematosis. She needed a kidney biopsy to assess her renal involvement. Her mother signed the operative permit, but Sally refused to cooperate with the procedure, saying she would run away and would not have it done. The nurses and doctors gave her time to express her feelings of fear and concern over her new diagnosis and the changes it would impose on her life. Sally sought further clarification of the information to be provided by the biopsy and how it would be used in treating her disease. After one day, she announced that she now felt able to go ahead with the procedure. She signed the permission form along with her mother. With nursing support to facilitate her coping during the procedure itself, she was able to cooperate well and complete the biopsy with no further problem.

Bill, age 18, was born with a congenital defect and had undergone numerous surgical procedures. Now facing another operation, he was required to sign his own consent form for the first time. He described the tremendous sense of responsibility this requirement placed on him. He wanted to continue to have the opportunity to discuss the operation with his parents and his physician together before signing his permit. This group discussion was arranged, and Bill received the information and recommendations he felt he needed to make his decision wisely.

In most hospital situations, permission for treatment is the prerogative of the minor's parent or guardian, and, technically, an adolescent's consent is not required. Ethics, common sense, and caring, however, make it mandatory that the adolescent be an informed participant in his or her health care.

Admission and Patient Assessment

When a teenager is admitted to the hospital, the nurse must decide whether to interview the adolescent separately or with parents. If the interview is initially conducted with the parents and the adolescent together, important data about their relationship can be gathered through observation of their behavior as a family group. The nurse can check later with the parents to determine if there is any additional information they would like to share in order to make their child's hospital stay more comfortable and effective. The adolescent can also provide additional data in private discussion with the nurse and can continue to be involved in day-to-day data gathering and planning with the nursing staff. Some adolescents feel more at ease speaking with the nurse with the parents absent, especially if issues about smoking, use of alcohol or drugs, sexual activity and birth control, or conflicts within the family are problematic. Other teenagers are uncomfortable having the staff talk with their parents when they are not present and much prefer to participate in discussions together. The teenager's preferences can be solicited in making a decision.

The admission interview provides opportunities for answering the adolescent's and family's questions about the hospital and orienting them to the setting, people, programs, and routines they will encounter. At the same time the nurse can explain that information about teenagers' preferences and favored life-style can be of assistance in planning care in the hospital to be as comfortable as possible. Special attention will be given to data about areas that are particularly important in an adolescent's life. Information about functioning within the family, school, and peer group can provide a rough assessment of normal development and coping. The adolescent's understanding of his or her illness and expectations of the hospitalization and health care should also be included. The ways in which adolescent and family have utilized the health care system in the past, whether on a consistent basis or for crisis intervention, can help identify needs for later counseling or teaching. Review of eating, sleeping, elimination, rest, activity, smoking, drinking, and other behavior patterns can help identify further areas for later support or intervention. The nurse can share information about hospital routines and practices in each area discussed in the admission interview. Understanding of normal body functioning can also be assessed. The hospital nurse may have a unique opportunity to carry out health teaching at a time when teenagers are interested in the body and its functioning and are receptive to information and instruction. Adolescents are frequently unclear about their history of infectious childhood illnesses and immunization status. The nurse may use this topic, too, as an opportunity for helping the patient become more aware of and responsible for his or her own health care.

When an adolescent enters the hospital under emergency conditions, the bulk of the admission interview may need to be deferred, but the same information needs to be obtained at a later time. Without a sound, comprehensive data base, truly effective care cannot be given.

Necessary Unit Regulations

In the overwhelming array of complex and unfamiliar situations posed by the hospital setting, a set of clear rules and expectations is necessary for ensuring an environment conducive to effective care and maximal developmental function. The challenge for an adolescent unit lies in making rules that are clear, reasonable, and fair, sufficient to offer protection of the rights and needs of the group yet flexible enough to provide for differing levels of maturity and individual needs. Policies of the unit need to be made clearly known to staff, patients, and visitors through direct lines of written or verbal communication. The patients themselves may form a valuable resource group in helping to set up reasonable policies for the unit.

Guidelines for visitors need to allow for adequate quiet and rest for

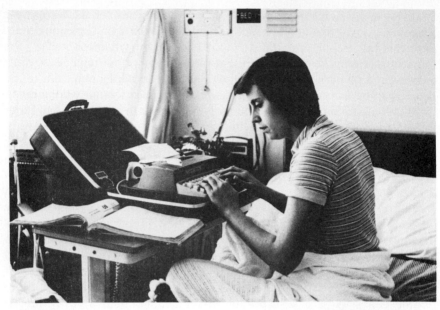

All feasible arrangements should be made to minimize the disruption that hospitalization makes in the teenager's daily life patterns and to make it as easy as possible for the young person to return to normal activities after leaving the hospital. This 16-year-old keeps up with her high school typing class while she is hospitalized. (*Photo courtesy of William Allen.*)

patients, time to carry out needed care, protection of patients from infectious diseases, and continued support from the ill adolescent's family and peer group. Unlimited or generous visiting hours avoid the overcrowding and upheaval that tend to result when visitors are restricted to a few hours a day. Visitors should be made aware of their responsibilities, the needed program of care, and special considerations required by the patient or other adolescents with whom they may have contact on the unit, such as need for special diets or a quiet environment. Most hospitals place limits on the number of people visiting a patient at one time, with special exceptions made in consultation with the nursing staff. Some hospitals welcome young friends and siblings, provided they have been carefully screened for infectious illnesses before entering the unit. Many benefits of visiting can be noted for both the ill adolescent and his or her healthy siblings and friends.

   Leaving the unit is another issue that must be worked out. Adolescents are increasing their independence and responsibility at home. They have widely expanding horizons. They take increasing responsibility for working at part-time jobs and traveling to and from school or other activities on their own. Restriction to one hospital room or even a specific unit is seen as a hardship and does little to promote normal developmental experiences. Nevertheless, the hospitalized adolescent needs to be available on the unit for doctors' visits, medications, treatments, and participation in the ward program. Some adolescent wards are fortunate enough to have access to the outdoors, providing opportunity for large-muscle movement and escape from the narrow confines of the unit. Other hospitals provide varied areas within the unit, such as a "teen room," recreation areas, or schoolroom. Still others provide for expeditions off the unit by allowing adolescent patients to eat their meals in the hospital cafeteria when they are able to do so, or to visit the gift shop, chapel, snack bar, or lobby.

Because of the differences in levels of illness, mobility, required care, and maturity, individualized decisions have to be made about the appropriateness of leaving the unit. All patients need to take seriously the responsibility for their own behavior so that they do not pose a danger to themselves or others. Arrangements may be made for a clear system for signing in and out at the nurses' station, including a statement of destination and expected time of return. Some hospitals provide their patients the opportunity to go outside of the hospital "on pass," with or without accompaniment. A physician's order and parental permission for minors are needed. Adolescents frequently speak of feeling imprisoned in the hospital. The ability to leave the unit from time to time may boost their sense of responsibility, independence, and freedom, and give them renewed energy to cope with the painful demands of illness and hospitalization.

Eating and mealtimes are important in an adolescent's hospital day. Hospitalization offers an opportunity for evaluation of the adolescent's knowledge of good nutrition, assessment of his or her current eating practices, and assistance in planning for a healthy, well-balanced diet to suit individual needs and preferences. Feelings of frustration, anger, and depression at being hospitalized and ill often become focused on the issue of food and result in numerous complaints about quality or lack or variety. Efforts can be made to make mealtimes in the hospital a pleasant, social occasion which teenage patients can share together as they are accustomed to doing at home and at school. Teenagers value the opportunity to select their own menus. It is often helpful for nursing personnel to offer some assistance in interpreting the menu for those with limited reading skills, or to seek modifications that will satisfy the adolescent patients' personal tastes as well as meet their nutritional needs.

Bedtime is apt to become a major issue on the teen unit as staff members try to settle a busy ward for the night and provide a quiet, sleep-enhancing environment, while the patients struggle with sharpened feelings of homesickness, an urgent need to talk, a desire for self-determination about bedtime, and an interest in the late movie on television. In few other hospital settings is it as likely for home routines and bedtimes to show as great a variation as on a unit accepting patients from 10 or 12 to 18 or 20 years old. Most adolescents are very understanding of the needs of younger or sicker patients for quiet or early settling for bed. Many teenagers like to read, listen to the radio, or watch television as they fall asleep. Often arrangements can be made to allow these activities to continue without disturbing others. The teenagers themselves are resourceful in planning ways to accomplish such arrangements. A TV or radio with ear plugs may be used so that it is inaudible to all but the listener, and night lights can allow reading without interfering with others' sleep. At times, the nursing staff will differ with the adolescent over reasonable bedtimes to ensure adequate rest. The goal is to provide opportunity for open discussion and problem solving and to avoid provoking a power struggle around rigid rules. It helps when unit expectations and needs are made clear from the start and are coupled with an open invitation for discussion of individual adolescent needs in relation to bedtime and sleep.

Smoking, in view of the evidence of long-term health risks, is difficult to condone in the hospital, particularly by the young. Nevertheless, hospitalization itself poses enough of a stressor for teenage patients without the added burden of having to relinquish a practice often viewed as a method of coping with anxiety. If smoking is entirely forbidden, it is likely to go underground. There are consequent safety risks for the smoking patient and for others on the unit when lighted cigarettes are hidden in wastebaskets or under the bedclothes. Teenage smokers need to be informed about the real risks to their health, especially if respiratory problems are involved in their illness or anesthesia is anticipated. They also need to know the dangers of smoking near oxygen and the discomfort caused to other patients. Safe times and areas for smoking need to be pointed out.

Dress is an important aspect of adolescents' life-style. As an adolescent struggles to form an identity, much of his or her self-image and self-concept may be tied up in dress. Through choice of clothing, adolescents convey to the world the outer image of the person they feel they are or want to be. Being required to dress in impersonal hospital attire may be especially threatening. Adolescents may also feel mortified at being restricted to nightclothes when others around them, such as visitors or staff members, are dressed in a more normal fashion. Confining adolescent boys and girls in close proximity and requiring them to wear nightclothes does not help them to control burgeoning sexual feelings. A teenage unit needs to work out an acceptable system for use, care, and storage of the adolescents' personal clothing that does not impose unreasonable expectations on a busy staff. Patients themselves can often take the major responsibility for caring for their own clothes if given minor assistance from staff or family members.

Educational programs can be part of the adolescent's hospital experience. Adolescents are at a point in their lives when they are open to new information and are eager to learn. Their cognitive development allows them to be active in problem solving. Nurses have a unique opportunity to help these patients to learn skills for dealing with a complex health care system that will serve them all their lives.

> Steve, age 15, complained that his doctor did not spend enough time explaining treatment rationale, plans, and progress to him on his daily rounds, during which he was accompanied by three or four other physicians and students. The nurse assisted Steve in making a list of his questions and discussed ways to let the doctor know of Steve's need for more information. Steve then used his bedside phone to call the doctor's secretary, and stated his desire to make an appointment with the physician. The next day the doctor set aside a half hour to sit down with Steve and discuss his concerns. Steve derived satisfaction from the fact that he had taken a major role in intervening in his own behalf in the hospital system.

Nurses can also make use of numerous daily opportunities on a hospital unit to talk with adolescents about the normal functioning of their bodies and clarify points of anatomy and physiology, nutrition, sexuality and sex education, differences in physical and intellectual development among people, and health care practices. Patients may have many questions about their own illnesses, medications, and treatment programs. Problem solving with the adolescent about how to deal with questions from peers and members of the community can also provide many opportunities for learning and can support social competence and self-esteem.

School forms a regular, vital part of the adolescent's life at home. Its continuation in the hospital provides some semblance of normal expectations and daily routine and conveys the message that all is not hopelessly changed. Many hospitalized teenagers worry about missed schoolwork or feel overwhelmed by the amount of material they think they will need to make up on their return home. Being "left back" at the end of a school year can be a major source of anxiety in terms of social relationships as well as academic progression. An adolescent hospital unit should work to provide a well-planned school program for patients hospitalized longer than a week or two or those who have had to face repeated hospitalizations that are disruptive of normal school attendance. Such a program may vary from hospital to hospital or city to city, and may range from a full-time school staff based on the unit to arrangements with the local school system for special inpatient tutoring on an individual basis. Nursing staff can assist by taking a careful admission history that includes data about schoolwork, planning with patients and families to meet school needs in the hospital and after discharge, and providing quiet, uninterrupted study time during the hospital stay.

Recreation is another major need of hospitalized adolescents. Teenagers at home are resourceful in finding ways to enjoy their free time, surrounded by their friends, with access to the outdoors, and with a variety of personal belongings and hobbies around them. The hospital environment limits all these opportunities, and boredom becomes a frequent complaint. Adolescents can make good use of an active recreational program to cope with their illness. Production of arts and crafts items to take home may be given long hours of concentrated attention by teenagers and help them to feel that they are spending their time in a worthwhile way. The pride in a completed project helps to boost self-esteem. Group games, programs, and projects help adolescents work together and enjoy the peer interaction so important at this developmental level. Recreational activities need to be available during both daytime and evening hours, seven days a week. Recreation, school, and nursing staff may wish to join together to collect and maintain a unit library of books, magazines, and records of interest to teenage patients.

Group meetings are another way of supporting healthy adolescent growth in a hospital setting. They provide an opportunity to develop a new peer group as a forum for learning, sharing common experiences, acting as a sounding board for problem solving, and testing out peer acceptance before returning home with changes in appearance that have resulted from injury, surgery, or treatment. Hospital staff members can keep in touch with the views, needs, and desires of the patient population through such meetings, and the teenagers can be actively involved as a group in helping to design the rules and policies of the unit.

The Staff

Nursing staff members for a teenage unit need to be selected for their comfort and skill in working with adolescents. They need to have sincere warmth and concern for growing people. They must be able to listen, support active moves toward growing independence, and understand behavior within a context of growth and development theory. Staff differences in terms of age, sex, and areas of special interest can be helpful in allowing teenage patients to relate to a variety of caring adults. Nurses need not strive to talk, dress, or act like teenagers in order to be effective. Adolescents want staff members around them who behave like adults while being able to listen to, respect, and support them as teenagers. The nurses need to clearly identify their own feelings, share them in an open and straightforward manner and help adolescents to recognize and handle feelings too. All the staff members serve as role models. Awareness of this fact can place special meaning on actions such as gathering adequate data before making decisions, being open to questioning about a planned course of action, and expressing anger or sadness in a way that is clear but not insensitive to the feelings of others. An adolescent unit is no place for the staff member who has difficulty around control issues and needs to adhere to rigid rules or to be always "in the right."

In addition to being experts in the care of teenagers, nurses on an adolescent unit may have to be knowledgeable and skillful with regard to well over twenty medical and surgical subspecialties. Rather than interacting with one set of physicians, they often must relate to numerous teams. This can lead to a hectic pace on a busy unit. The situation provides a stimulating atmosphere of continual learning, but it can also produce feelings of being overwhelmed by demands for knowledge and expert practice in such a wide variety of areas. Such a setting may be especially difficult for the new graduate who is just mastering the skills and roles of nursing practice. A valuable quality in staff members is the ability to tolerate busy situations in a fairly calm manner.

The ideal medical director of an adolescent unit is a physician specializing in adolescent health care. When this arrangement is not possible, it is helpful to have access to consultation from such a specialist.

When school staff is based in the hospital setting, it is appropriate and desirable that the teachers participate in unit conferences, help plan a unit milieu that places value on the continuation of schoolwork, share information, and plan for the optimal care of individual patients. Where the hospital does not have its own teacher, the nursing staff needs to make the primary effort to contact individual teachers for special conferences, consultations, and planning and evaluation sessions.

Religious needs of adolescents are frequently overlooked, yet religion is a primary focus in some teenagers' lives and a major support in coping with illness. Information about religious beliefs and practices should be solicited early in the hospital course and, where appropriate, chaplaincy services should be sought. Often, local church youth groups are eager to be helpful by regularly visiting adolescents who must cope with a lengthy hospitalization far from home.

Social workers available to an adolescent unit must be skillful in communicating both with adolescents and with parents or family groups. There is also much opportunity for social workers and psychiatric staff to meet regularly with the other disciplines working on an adolescent unit to explore psychosocial issues of care, air staff feelings, and plan sound methods of intervention for troubled patients and their families.

The Physical Facility

A physical setting that offers support to the kinds of programs described above can be carefully planned with a new hospital building. It can also

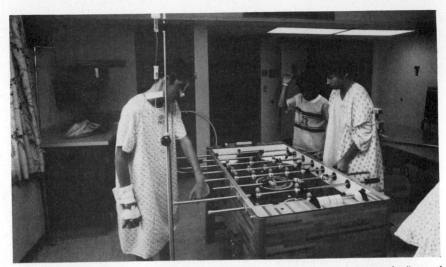

Peers and shared activities greatly help hospitalized teenagers to decrease feelings of isolation and cope effectively. Personal clothing should be permitted for all patients whose condition permits. Hospital gowns are depersonalizing, and bed clothing (nightwear) is considered by many adolescents to be embarrassing, demoralizing, or sexually provocative. (*Copyright © 1980 by Anne Campbell.*)

be developed from existing facilities. A commitment to excellence in the care of adolescents can mold a creative, workable program in a wide variety of settings.

The unit needs to be of a size that is economically feasible, usually between 18 and 36 beds. Rooms may have 1, 2, 3, or 4 beds. Double rooms are often cited as ideal, but variety allows for flexibility to meet individual needs and preferences. Room assignments can be changed as patients progress along an illness continuum and require varying amounts of quiet, privacy, or activity and peer interaction. Within their rooms, teenage patients have a special need for space for their belongings and freedom to make their living space an extension of themselves. Bulletin boards or wall spaces allowing for display of meaningful posters, cards, poems, etc., are very important. Bedside telephones help an adolescent maintain normal contacts with the family and peer support group at home. Television and radio help the adolescent pass the time and keep in touch with the outside world. These items are especially important to the adolescent in isolation.

Bathrooms are very important to teenagers with their newly developing bodies and sense of modesty. Ill teenagers, like all others, value privacy and access to mirrors. Wheelchair-accessible bathrooms enhance independence in toileting functions for many hospitalized adolescents and save them much worry and embarrassment. Beds, including those in single rooms, need curtains to screen the bathing teenagers from physicians on rounds and others who might unwittingly open the door at the wrong moment. Teenagers need a way to wash their hair even when they are confined to a wheelchair, cart, or bed. Access to a low sink or tub or spray hose can make the task immeasurably easier.

Conference rooms are helpful in providing additional privacy for interviews or discussions with patients or families. A teen room, however small, provides a different kind of needed privacy in furthering the opportunity for patients to gather together away from adults. It can be elaborately equipped with jukebox, pool table, Ping-Pong equipment, pinball machines, and stereo, or it can be much simpler. The importance of the teen room lies in the fact that it is the teenagers' own place, a haven from intrusive procedures and the other impingements of the hospital world. (Treatments, rounds, and similar intrusions should *not* be permitted in the teen room.)

School and recreation programs work best when they have adequate space. School and recreation facilities may be shared, if necessary, to justify the need for this space and demonstrate full and effective use of it. For example, the game room or schoolroom may also serve as sleeping space for parents who stay overnight.

Hospitalized teenagers speak clearly of their need for access to the outdoors and of their longing for the feel of sunshine, wind, rain, and snow. The sight of trees, grass, and sky helps them to touch base with the real and familiar world. Going outside is not merely a luxury for the adolescent confined to the hospital, but a major support in the ability to cope with prolonged confinement and immobilization. Nurses have to talk with adolescents about this need and be advocates in their behalf by making it an issue as plans for new hospitals or new units of existing institutions are developed. Where easy access to the ground floor is not available, rooftop areas might be developed as a second-best alternative.

SUMMARY

This chapter has suggested ways to create an environment within a general hospital setting that will be helpful to ill adolescents. Expert nursing entails keeping in mind the developmental tasks of adolescence and providing opportunities for movement toward their attainment.

BIBLIOGRAPHY

Altshuler, Anne and Ann Seidl: "Use of Teen Meetings to Facilitate Coping with Illness and Hospitalization," *MCN: The American Journal of Maternal-Child Nursing*, 2(6):348–353, November-December 1977.

Blake, Florence G.: "Immobilized Youth: A Rationale for Supportive Nursing Intervention," *American Journal of Nursing*, **69**:2364–2369, November 1969.

Denyes, Mary J. and Anne Altshuler: "Illness: The Adolescent," in Gladys M. Scipien et al., eds., *Comprehensive Pediatric Nursing* (2d ed.). New York: McGraw-Hill Book Co., 1979.

Fine, Louis L. : "What's a Normal Adolescent?", *Clinical Pediatrics*, **12**:1–5, January 1973.

Hofmann, Adele D., R. D. Becker, and H. Paul Gabriel: *The Hospitalized Adolescent: A Guide to Managing the Ill and Injured Youth*. New York: The Free Press, 1976.

Lindheim, Roslyn, Helen Glaser, and Christie Coffin: *Changing Hospital Environments for Children*. Cambridge: Harvard University Press, 1972.

Schowalter, John E. and Ruth D. Lord: "The Hospitalized Adolescent," *Children*, **18**:127–132, July-August 1971.

Wear, Elise T. and Patricia Blessing: "Child with Cancer: Facilitating the Return to School," in Barbara Peterson and Carolyn Kellogg, eds., *Current Practice in Oncologic Nursing*, Volume I. St. Louis: C. V. Mosby Co., 1976.

Chapter 13

The Adolescent in a Rehabilitation Setting

Rosemarie B. King
Susan M. Strawn

> *"Just as I was brave enough*
> *to reach out of my cocoon," said*
> *the caterpillar, "it turned into*
> *a chair with wheels.*
> *"Be brave, I was told. So*
> *I was brave. But inside, I was*
> *afraid," he whispered.*
> *". . . is a butterfly who can't*
> *fly still a butterfly?"*
> *"Come," said the owl,, "I will*
> *help you find out. . . . "**

Nina Herrmann, Chaplain,
Rehabilitation Institute of Chicago

A small number of adolescents enter the rehabilitation setting with a temporary disability such as multiple fractures. More often, though, the adolescent rehabilitation patient is one who has a permanent or progressive disability that requires prolonged hospitalization and results in altered physical function. Permanent disability, unlike a condition that may be serious but is temporary, threatens socioemotional development.[1]

*Reproduced by permission of the author.

Inasmuch as the physiologic alterations associated with disability and rehabilitation are similar to those of an adult with a comparable lesion, they are not the focus of this chapter. Rather, an attempt is made to define the special needs of the adolescent with a physical disability and to describe the attributes of the setting and personnel necessary to meet those needs.

PHILOSOPHY AND OBJECTIVES
OF ADOLESCENT REHABILITATION

Rehabilitation may be defined as the process of relearning the activities involved in everyday living.[2] For adolescents, who are already struggling with physical changes, sexual awareness, and identity crisis, the imposition of physical disability is quite traumatic and disruptive of development. Rehabilitation is a formidable challenge for an adolescent. He or she must relearn the basic skills ordinarily taken for granted, such as feeding, dressing, and hygiene, and must learn or relearn the social, vocational, and avocational skills necessary for a meaningful life.

Rehabilitation begins when either physical trauma or disease renders the adolescent disabled. It is not possible to say when the process ends, for optimal goals most often are achieved long after discharge from the rehabilitation setting. Implementing and integrating newly learned activities into one's life is a long-term challenge to be met by the youngster after returning home. The objective of the rehabilitation effort is to help the young person select a feasible and satisfying life-style and to assist him or her in preparing to assume it. Efforts are directed toward helping adolescents learn to do for themselves, not at doing for them.

The initial treatment plan centers around meeting the immediate physical and psychological needs of the disabled person. Early involvement of family and close friends is crucial, for the teenager's ability to cope with the condition is greatly affected by the attitudes of those closest. Consequently, a critical task of the rehabilitation team is to help the youth's family and friends reconcile their feelings about the disability. It is not enough merely to help the adolescent relearn the tasks of daily living, for these will be of little value if the teenager cannot be accepted by family and friends.

A strong philosophical belief in client determination of goals and active participation in moving toward attainment of those goals is necessary. Efforts at rehabilitation cannot succeed unless the young person himself or herself is heavily committed to goal attainment and assumes responsibility for self-care. Adolescents, with their natural developmental drives toward self-assertion and self-determination, usually respond well to encouragement to participate in decision making and directing care. The nurse may often need to help ancillary staff (and others) understand youths' efforts to direct their care and assert control over their environment, since these actions can be misinterpreted.

The young person's feelings of self-worth are basic to optimal attainment of goals. Indeed gains made during the rehabilitation process will soon be lost if they have developed solely because of external motivating factors and not because the adolescent is able to internalize feelings of worth. The nurse can foster positive self-regard by taking time to listen, by recognizing and giving encouragement for even small successes, and by demonstrating understanding and acceptance of regressive behavior and grief.

The ultimate goal of the rehabilitation team is to equip adolescent and family with the knowledge and skills necessary for the adolescent to achieve optimal functioning in order to live a useful and satisfying life on his or her terms and those of the family. Achievement of long-term goals hinges largely on commitment to maintaining integrity of the body.[3] It is not necessary that adolescents be able to do their own care, but it is essential that they be well enough informed about their condition and any possible complications to effectively direct others to provide care.

ATTRIBUTES OF THE REHABILITATION SETTING

Many authorities in the care of acutely ill adolescents advise that a separate unit of the care facility be devoted to the adolescent age group.[4] Segregation by age is also desirable for youths in a rehabilitation setting. Adolescents in rehabilitation, like other adolescents, need freedom to be themselves, express themselves, and be with age-mates. The noisy exuberance characteristic of this age makes separation from adult patients desirable.

At the time a new patient is admitted to the setting, both adolescent and family should be oriented to the physical layout of the unit as a matter of routine. An overview of the programs offered should be given. Unit rules and regulations and staff expectations, including attendance at scheduled therapy sessions, should be explained.

The nursing assessment at admission enables the nurse to formulate goals and establish a plan of care that will facilitate the adolescent's adjustment to the new setting. In addition to physical needs, the assessment should identify the patient's and family's goals; their knowledge about current treatment regimens; the teenager's perceptual and language deficits, ability to carry out activities of daily living, interaction with peers, use of nonprescription drugs and alcohol, educational level, and previous sexual experiences; information that has been given the young person about the condition and prognosis; health education to date; and pertinent information about the family unit.

Room assignments must be the prerogative of the nursing staff. The value of peer contact and the need to share feelings and experiences that occur during rehabilitation make it advisable to avoid private rooms in most situations. Thus, compatibility of roommates is important since roommates are a major source of support for each other. The busy therapy day followed by visiting hours and recreational trips often leaves only the after-bedtime hours for sharing and reflecting upon personal matters with a peer.

Bright rooms with space to hang posters, cards, etc., are recommended. Street clothing is far more supportive of rehabilitation than are institutional garments, so it is advantageous to have laundry facilities on the unit. When possible, the youngster can assume responsibility for care of clothing. Recreational space for table games and active sports is important. Classroom space and a few quiet areas for study and time alone are essential. A nourishment area that allows patient access to a refrigerator and hot plate is a good idea, since teenagers are well known for their sudden hunger pangs after cafeteria hours. A group dining area enhances social exchange and promotes a sense of community that is quite therapeutic. For the youth who is easily distracted or who is embarrassed when starting self-feeding, an alternate area should be available.

In general, there should be few restricted areas. Curiosity about what goes on in the usually restricted areas is unavoidable. There are obviously disadvantages to having patients moving freely throughout the unit, but we have also found some distinct advantages. Often allowing a youngster to answer the phone and do minor clerical work can bolster confidence. On rare occasions, this arrangement has been set up with the vocational counseling department in order to evaluate certain skills.

LEGAL AND ETHICAL CONSIDERATIONS

Because of the length of time involved in rehabilitation, the staff, especially the nursing staff, frequently encounters many of the same problems that parents would deal with if the adolescent were at home. It is not possible to completely avoid drug and alcohol use, for example, and patients frequently stay out on pass beyond the prearranged time for their return. Since the majority of adolescents are legally minors, the staff has the responsibility of closely monitoring behavior and activities. Both youths and parents should be informed on admission of hospital regulations governing alcohol and drug use, passes, attendance at therapy sessions, and the consequences of violating the policies. The adolescent should be informed that, even though parents may give permission for the adolescent to go on pass without them, the nurse will need to know with whom he or she is going and where. The adolescent should also know that if the circumstances are questionable or additional approval seems advisable, the parents will be contacted. Though tedious at times, these regulations are necessary to guarantee the adolescent's safety and to assure parents that their child is receiving adequate supervision.

Staff must be aware of the need for maintaining confidentiality. To do so is difficult at times, because the nature of the program requires that parents be actively involved. If the youngster does offer private information that staff feel the parents should know, the situation should be discussed with the youth before parents are informed. Whenever possible the adolescents should be encouraged to talk with their parents themselves, with the option of having a staff member present.

Since parents are not generally present daily, as they might be if the youngster were in an acute care setting, the staff must be conscientious about keeping the family informed about changes in their child's condition and plans that are being made. Too often parents are surprised with new information when they come to visit. The need for special consultants, tests, equipment to be purchased, and so forth, should be discussed with parents in advance. Because many third-party payers do not assume expenses for certain therapies and equipment, it is especially important that parents be involved in decisions regarding such costs. Encouraging parents' attendance at therapy sessions and conferences helps keep them informed and alleviates some of their anxiety. A quick phone call between times to share information is an important courtesy. Again, the adolescent should be informed when staff are consulting with parents.

PERSONNEL

Most adolescents undergoing rehabilitation require the services of a physiatrist, nurse, social worker, child psychologist, and physical and occupational therapists, and many need a speech pathologist. The nature of the disability and the adolescent's goals determine the extent to which still other professionals are involved and at what stage they enter the adolescent's program. The youth who was planning to attend college or get a job may need vocational assistance. The youngster still in school should have the opportunity to continue those studies in the hospital setting. The severely disabled adolescent may need the expertise of biomedical engineers. Complex adaptational problems often require a chaplain or psychiatrist.

Patience, maturity, and a desire to work with adolescents are prerequisites for staff members. The ability to be consistent about expectations and limit setting is also important. Consistency among team members is vital if there is to be effective communication and if the young person is to develop trusting relationships with therapists.

Nursing staff, professional and ancillary, spend more time with the patient than other members of the team do. It is to the nursing staff that the patient returns at the end of the day. As coordinator of the patient's overall program, the nurse assesses the youngster's physical and emotional needs, establishes a plan of care, does health teaching, and evaluates the young person's ability to integrate newly learned skills and knowledge into his or her daily routine.

Ancillary nursing staff members are a rich source of invaluable information about how the patient is progressing. Because of their intimate everday involvement with the patients, they not only are well aware of each youngster's current physical condition but also are frequently the persons adolescents approach when they want to talk about what is happening to them. The nurse needs to collaborate with ancillary staff, both in order to gather information from them to incorporate into the nursing care plan and to assist them with their feelings and difficulties which they encounter in their work with the disabled adolescents. Team conferences allow the registered nurse and the ancillary staff time to problem-solve together and work collaboratively to develop a plan that will best serve the patient's needs.

THE IMPACT OF DISABILITY

Many adolescents in a rehabilitation program have not experienced disability or significant illness before, and many have never been hospitalized. Others, whose disability is congenital or was acquired at an early age, have had long-term experience with their disability and many have undergone numerous hospitalizations. Depending on their previous experiences, congenitally or long-term disabled adolescents may present maladaptive behavior. Adjustment to disability depends to a great extent upon the family's reaction and acceptance of the child's condition. Parental reactions of overprotection, guilt, or rejection can contribute to the teen's being fearful, guilty, or overly dependent upon parents. Long-term disability in the congenitally disabled may also be accompanied by resentment of persons who are able-bodied.[5] Even those youths who have coped well with a disability through childhood are likely to experience psychosocial difficulties as adolescence approaches and progresses. At this time, they become increasingly aware of the effect of their disability on peer acceptance, physical activities, and their future life.[6] It is imperative that the health care team maintain contact with and actively seek information from patient and family about their understanding of the youngster's disability and its implications. This assessment allows accurate planning of long- and short-term goals and forms the basis of ongoing instruction and counseling.

The sudden onset of progressive or permanent disability requires a change in self-concept. Alterations such as motor deficits; diminished cognitive function; amputation; and bowel, bladder, or sexual dysfunctions are serious threats to body image and self-esteem. These threats and persons' reactions to them are likely to be especially intense in adolescence since beauty, physical prowess, and conformity to peers are primary concerns.

Mourning, which is associated with any loss, is part of the painful process of revising the self-concept. The first stage of the mourning process is denial, which occurs as a healthy and natural defense to ward off the anxiety and despair that accompany awareness of the meaning of the loss. Denial that persists is harmful; it leads the young person to perceive parts of the therapy as unnecessary and hence raises barriers to full participation in his or her rehabilitation. Examples are the youths who refuse to learn to use an upper extremity orthosis because "my hands will be okay," or decline to learn to give themselves a bowel-program suppository because "I won't need this when I go home." The professional's task is, without abruptly removing the needed defense mechanism of denial, to nudge the adolescent gently forward by focusing on current needs. The youth can be helped to understand that his or her body has special requirements now because certain dysfunctions are present now.

As denial begins to break down in the natural course of the mourning process, and awareness of the permanence of the loss and its repercussions intensifies, depression, anxiety, and anger surface.[7]

A 17-year-old male, quadriplegic from a motorcycle accident, was initially treated with halo traction. He actively participated in his rehabilitation and talked enthusiastically about all that he would be able to do when the traction was removed. Following removal of the halo, when his unrealistic expectations for restored function did not come true, his behavior changed markedly. He refused medications and therapy and wanted to stay in bed with his door closed.

The adolescent equates being different with being worthless and no longer being someone that others can care about.[8] These feelings are frequently aggravated by the isolation which occurs as peers and special boyfriends or girlfriends begin to withdraw.

A 15-year-old female with traumatic brain damage resulting in hemiparesis and aphasia openly expressed concern over whether she would ever be "normal" again. She dwelt only on her deficits. One night, she wept bitterly as she told the nurse how alone she felt. Although deficits were minimal at the time of discharge, she continued to need supportive psychologic counseling.

Suicidal ideation is not unusual during the depression accompanying severe disability. In time, and with support, most youths once again find reason to live.

Depression is often disguised as critical, angry remarks directed at staff members and others close to the adolescent. Such behavior can alienate personnel, peers, and family just when they are most needed by the youngster. Understanding staff will help the adolescent to talk out feelings and will listen to the meaning rather than the content of the displays of anger. Expression of anger is necessary if the individual is to be helped from turning anger inward. An enormous amount of the adolescent's energy can be tied up in controlling his or her emotions, so recognition of tension buildup and acknowledgement of frustrations, disappointments, and sadness are essential parts of care. The adolescent who loses control in an angry outburst or in tears will likely feel ashamed, and will need to be reassured about the normalcy of this behavior.

Physical methods of coping with tension and anger are limited by immobility, and adolescents who have been accustomed to dealing with anger by walking away or participating in some other physical activity may express their anger verbally.[9] Uninformed, insensitive staff who personalize a youth's angry behavior and expect the youth to act "grown up" may engage in power struggles that cannot be resolved without someone's losing face. When sullen and angry behavior is understood as a normal grief reaction, staff become better able to intervene and allow the teenager to talk about his or her feelings if and when desired; or, at least, they can understand the anger and avoid making an issue of the behavior.

Professionals must realize that the process of mourning can linger for some time. Seldom has the youth fully resolved this grief by the time of discharge from the hospital. Recently, a 19-year-old female, who became paraplegic a year and a half ago, described how her response to her loss fluctuates: "It's like a burning coal until something ignites the coals, and then it's a fire—but it's always there." Intense awareness of loss was reactivated as she undertook to live independently and to begin college.

A fundamental strategy for assisting during the period of depression is to be aware of the adolescent's difficulty in expressing feelings and to let the adolescent know that these feelings (and the desire to express them or not) are respected. Those young people who are unable to verbalize their feelings may respond to someone's just sitting with them, or perhaps acknowledging that they seem "down." Staff may tend to avoid the depressed youngster because of their own discomfort. However, at this stage of the adolescent's grief small attentions such as trying a new hair style or combing a young man's hair before his girl visits are particularly therapeutic. These activities help adolescents feel "special" at a time when they believe that no one cares. It is important also to help parents, siblings,

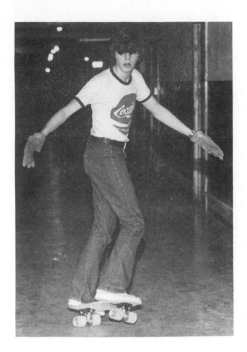

Physical activity and mobility play central roles in most adolescents' normal everyday activities and seem to be very important in their coping. When a teenager becomes immobilized by illness or disability, anger and/or depression readily result. (*Copyright © 1980 by Patricia Yaros.*)

and peers understand what the adolescent is experiencing and why he or she is unsociable and depressed. Typically, these significant persons don't know what to say or how to act; they are afraid of harming the patient physically and emotionally and may appear rejecting when, in fact, they are fearful. The disabled tend to focus on all that is lost, but efforts to help them to recognize assets and potentials that remain can substantially bolster their self-esteem. A sense of accomplishment stemming from taking an active part in decision making and mastering tasks also helps to alleviate depression.

The provision of realistic information about matters of concern can do much to alleviate anxiety and depression and to promote self-esteem, for the future is seldom as dark as the newly disabled adolescent supposes. Young people with spinal injuries are understandably distraught by bowel and bladder incontinence, for example, and should have early reassurance that bowel retraining programs and catheter regimes can be expected to succeed in excellent regulation and to eliminate "accidents." Persons with spinal cord lesions also express a variety of concerns about the effect their disability will have on sexual function. Information and counseling appropriate to age and experience should be given. It is important that females know that women, regardless of the level of their lesion, are able to have intercourse and to conceive and deliver a healthy infant. For males, erection is possible if the lesion does not involve the sacral segments or cauda equina, but fertility is markedly reduced regardless of the level of the injury.[11] It is often the nurse who can best deal with these and other concerns, since nurses help the adolescent to manage many intimate body functions and usually develop a relationship of trust with the adolescent.

Eventually, youngsters who have mourned successfully become able to overcome depression and care about themselves. Good adjustment is characterized by adolescents' coming to accept and value themselves as they are—someone who has lost or damaged a part of his or her body but remains a whole person.[10] Those who do not think positively about their bodies are likely to develop future complications that result from self-neglect.

EFFECTS OF DISABILITY ON DEVELOPMENTAL TASKS

Identity formation is widely recognized as the primary developmental task of the adolescent years. Conformity in dress, activities, and mannerisms within the adolescent group lends security while the teenager struggles toward an adult identity.[12] Isolation of the disabled youth from peers should be avoided, not only to reduce depression but also because involvement with peers is so necessary to the development of self-definition.[13] The philosophy of care should foster peer support by welcoming friends from outside the hospital to continue to be part of the patient's life. Weekend and evening passes are necessary to allow the youth to resume activities with friends.

During adolescence physical attractiveness is highly valued, so a visible physical alteration is a threat to self-esteem and is interpreted as a barrier to attracting the opposite sex. Activities such as athletics or dancing, which formerly enhanced the young person's self-image and also provided social contacts, are seen as inaccessible. Disability in adolescence interferes with the young person's attempts to define a heterosexual role, including dating and thinking about an eventual marriage partner. Assisting the youngster in learning early that disabled persons do indeed date and marry can be quite helpful to psychosocial development. With help, the adolescent will eventually be able to focus on qualities beyond the physical alteration which contribute to a masculine or feminine self-image.[14] This is a necessary step if the youngster is to help others get to know him or her and see beyond the disability.

Because of their heightened awareness of sexuality and their self-consciousness, adolescents find it especially difficult to undergo such experiences as physical examinations and bladder and bowel procedures. Provisions for privacy and tact when discussing personal care are courtesies that must be extended to adolescent patients.

The educational and vocational plans typically central to adolescent development are interrupted by disability. The inability of many educational institutions to accommodate disabled persons adds to the adolescent's handicap by limiting contact with peers as well as preparation for employment, preparation for further education, and choice of college. Vocational evaluation and planning are essential aspects of rehabilitation, especially for the late adolescent, if education and skills for a work role are to be obtained. Vocational counseling assists the youth in exploring realistic work and/or school options.

Dependence upon others for personal care contributes to feelings of inadequacy and is especially difficult for the mid-adolescent to accept at the point of emancipation from parents.[15] Hospital personnel must exercise care not to contribute unnecessarily to the young person's feelings of being inadequate and out of control by their failure to explain what they are doing and to involve the teenager in decisions and conferences.

> A 14-year-old female with severe juvenile rheumatoid arthritis began to refuse evening care and to quarrel and swear at staff. After a short time, no one wanted to work with her. When her nurse explored the situation with her, the nurse learned that the staff did not consider when and how she wanted care given and the fact that she wished to complete care early so that she could stay up later with the other patients. Staff and patient thereafter conferred briefly together to plan care at the beginning of the shift.

THE FAMILY

Rehabilitation of a family member cannot occur successfully without involvement of the family unit, since adequate adjustment of the young person depends at least in part on the family's acceptance of the disability and their ability to relate to the patient.[16] Both parents need counseling and frequent encouragement to meet their own needs and to attend to the needs of the patient's siblings. Parent group discussions can be a vehicle for encouraging parents to share and resolve feelings of guilt, depression, and anxiety. They may also help the family solve many of the problematic aspects of financial planning, home care, and arranging for the adolescent's education. Meeting and observing parents who have coped successfully can be enormously encouraging and may even establish a bond of mutual support that will endure long after the hospitalization. The fact that the family employs the same defense mechanisms as the patient to deal with loss and goes through the same grief sequence is often overlooked by professionals.[17] Assessing the family's strengths and resources, as well as previous methods of coping with crisis, enables the rehabilitation team to intervene more adequately.

Attendance at staff conference keeps the family abreast of progress and allows time for discussion with the entire team. It is important to remember that parents need support to allow their disabled child the freedom and independence he or she must achieve.

RECREATIONAL NEEDS AND ACTIVITIES

Adolescents need to know early in the rehabilitation program that they will be able to share in many of the same activities they enjoyed previously. A variety of individual and group activities that encourage self-expression and promote a sense of achievement as well as relaxation should be available to the teenager. Activities should include relatively quiet and passive forms of recreation, such as listening to music and watching television; medium-range pursuits, like cards, board games, and arts and crafts; and more vigorous activities, such as basketball, bowling, swimming, horseback riding, and fishing.[18]

The disabled youth becomes restless and bored as easily as the nonhandicapped adolescent and has the same needs to work off energy. For this reason, a recreation program offering a wide range of activities in and out of the rehabilitation setting is recommended.

The recreational therapy program assumes special importance when the adolescent first becomes able to leave the hospital. Both youth and family can be helped over their fears about the youth's leaving the protective environment of the hospital by participating in short excursions in the company of recreational therapists and other patients who have similar problems. These experiences are invaluable in bolstering self-confidence not only about physical mobility but also about dealing with the inevitable stares from the public. Adolescents and their families learn quickly that it is not difficult for a person confined to a wheelchair to ride in a car. They become aware that more and more public facilities are accessible to the handicapped, and the young person begins to see that he or she can still go to ballgames, movies, restaurants, and on shopping trips.

Since many of the recreational outings from the hospital last only a few hours, youngsters are frequently able to participate in out-trips long before they are ready to go home for a weekend pass. Disabled adolescents usually fear exposure to nonhandicapped persons and sometimes demonstrate their fear by avoidance of outings. The degree of a patient's willingness to participate in out-trips may be an indicator of success in dealing with the disability. The youngster may be working hard in therapies and relating well to peers and staff on the unit; however, if he or she is not participating in recreational outings, it is likely that the youngster is not coping as well as the staff may otherwise have thought.

DISCHARGE PLANNING

Adequate discharge planning is essential to ensure maximal success of the rehabilitation effort. Each professional member of the rehabilitation team shares in the preparations for the patient's leaving the hospital. Much of the responsibility, however, rests with nursing and social service, who handle referral to and coordination with community agencies. Multidisciplinary team conferences help to clarify discharge responsibilities. The adolescent and the family members, of course, also participate fully in planning for discharge.

The care routines used in the hospital should be simplified and otherwise adapted to fit schedules and resources in the home. Thoughtless planning can result in a physically dependent youth's being discharged on an every-two-hour turning schedule which interrupts youth and family's rest, whereas teaching the patient to sleep prone would have allowed four to eight hours of uninterrupted sleep.

Of course, patient education must be paced, and planning toward discharge must begin soon after admission, because the necessary amount and complexity of learning and preparation cannot be accomplished quickly. Family attendance at therapy sessions helps family members learn care skills and increases their confidence.

Weekend passes are an essential part of the preparation for going home. They enable the nurse, the patient, and the family to identify problems that arise around the patient's being at home, and to begin problem solving before the adolescent goes home permanently. In complex situations, where the family's ability to manage for an entire weekend is not assured, starting with a single day or night pass decreases anxiety.

Advance help to anticipate problems can enable the adolescent and family to avoid many crises that might otherwise occur. Consider the frustration that can arise, for example, when toilet transfers are taught and bathroom equipment is ordered before anyone discovers that the bathroom door is too narrow to admit a wheelchair. It is not economically feasible for most families to move to housing especially designed for disabled persons or to make extensive architectural changes, so the team must anticipate the need for structural adjustments and help the family plan accordingly. If a predischarge home visit by the rehabilitation nurse is not possible, it is important that parents bring in door and room measurements so problems about the adolescent's mobility at home can be dealt with before discharge.

Near the time of discharge, the recreational therapist can assist the adolescent and the family in locating suitable community recreational agencies. The identification of accessible recreational facilities is an important part of discharge planning, because the job of meeting leisure needs, if left solely to the family, can become a major problem.

Occasionally, because of the complexity of an adolescent's care requirements or because of psychosocial dynamics within the family, the patient may be discharged to a residential school or nursing home rather than to the family home. Obviously, in such situations, it is necessary for the rehabilitation nurse to work with the receiving agency. It is helpful for a staff member from the receiving facility to attend a predischarge conference and to attend therapy sessions or otherwise be instructed as necessary about the adolescent's care prior to discharge. Staff in the placement agency may blame families for not taking their children home unless given adequate information and opportunity to discuss their feelings related to the placement. These reactions can contribute to the family's already existing guilt.

It is the unusual adolescent with a newly acquired disability who does not require a referral to a community health nursing agency, whether the adolescent is discharged home or to an institution. Often, several agencies may be involved if needed services, such as counseling or social work services, are not available within the nursing agency. Home health aide services, although frequently temporary, can help greatly in smoothing the transition to the home. Communication between the community health care agency and the rehabilitation team is critical to maintain coordination and effectiveness of care after discharge.

The hospital team's assurance to the patient and family that hospital personnel will remain involved is frequently helpful in allaying anxieties. Follow-up must be individualized so that the patient at high risk to develop complications is seen early after discharge and on a regular basis.

CONCLUDING REMARKS

The long-range success of an adolescent's rehabilitation program depends on many factors, as has been discussed above, but the adolescent's motivation and the environmental supports available are among the most important. A plan that is not based on the *youngster's* goals, or that does not take into account the youngster's and family's strengths and limitations, is very likely to fail. Economic and psychosocial resources within the family and the community must be identified and utilized to support the adolescent's and family members' coping and to sustain the progress that has been achieved during the hospitalization phase of rehabilitation. Even the best-planned rehabilitation program will have little enduring success unless provision for long-term follow-up is adequate and appropriate adjustments are made as the young person's coping patterns, physical condition, and development change with the passage of time.

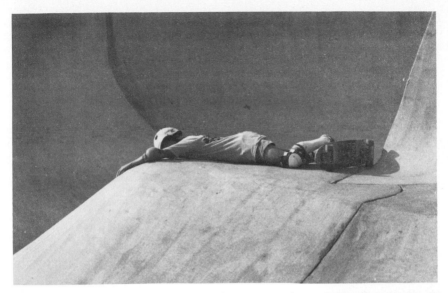

Preventive intervention directed at individuals, groups, and communities is a yet underdeveloped aspect of nursing care. Immunization and safety programs aimed at preventing disability need greater attention in the adolescent age group than they have received. (*Copyright © 1980 by Anne Campbell.*)

Rehabilitation nursing needs to extend its influence into the larger social arena. Unfortunately, societal attitudes and practices, although changing, still present many barriers to disabled persons' full function and development. Inaccessible public facilities and transportation are a hindrance to independence and productivity, as well as a constant source of demoralization and annoyance. Appropriate residential facilities for those youths unable to return home are rare, so they too often have to be admitted to nursing homes where there may be no companions in their age group or programs to assist them in their continuing development. Innovative programs which allow the disabled to manage their lives independently are needed. Programs providing shared attendant services or financial assistance for full- or part-time home care would allow many young people to remain in their communities with their families.

Prevention of disability must be addressed to a greater degree than it has been in the past. Nurses in almost all practice settings can do much to educate young people about accident prevention and to organize school or neighborhood safety programs to reduce the incidence of disability resulting from, for example, automobile and diving accidents. Once a disability has occurred, however, efforts must be focused on the prevention of complications, readmissions, and disintegration of the youth's support system. Prevention at either level can be done only by extending nursing and the other health care services into the community.

REFERENCES

1 A. Mattson, "Long-Term Physical Illness in Childhood: A Challenge to Psychosocial Adaptation," *Pediatrics*, **50**:801–810, November 1972.
2 N. Martin, "Nursing in Rehabilitation," in I. L. Beland and J. Y. Passos (eds.), *Clinical Nursing: Pathophysiological and Psychosocial Approaches*, 3d ed. New York: Macmillan, 1975.
3 Martin, op. cit.
4 Society for Adolescent Medicine, "Characteristics of an Inpatient Unit for Adolescents," *Clinical Pediatrics*, **12**:17–21, January 1973.
5 Mattson, op. cit.
6 A. Hofmann, R. Becker, and H. Gabriel (eds.), *The Hospitalized Adolescent*. New York: The Free Press, 1976.
7 J. Nemiah, "Psychiatrist and Rehabilitation," *Archives of Physical Medicine and Rehabilitation*, **38**:143, 1957.
8 M. Gunther, "Psychiatric Consultation in a Rehabilitation Hospital: A Regression Hypothesis," *Comprehensive Psychiatry*, **12**:572–584, November 1971.
9 J. Siller, "Psychological Situation of the Disabled with Spinal Cord Injuries," *Rehabilitation Literature*, **30**:290–296, October 1969.
10 B. Wright, *Physical Disability: A Psychological Approach*. New York: Harper & Row, 1960.
11 E. Tarabulcy, "Sexual Function in the Normal and in Paraplegia," *Paraplegia*, **10**:201–208, 1972.
12 E. Erikson, *Identity, Youth and Crisis*. New York: W. W. Norton and Co., 1968, pp. 128–133.
13 L. Fine, "What's a Normal Adolescent? A Guide for the Assessment of Adolescent Behavior," *Clinical Pediatrics*, **12**:1–5, January 1973.
14 Wright, op. cit.
15 Hofmann, Becker, and Gabriel, op. cit.
16 R. Davis, "Family of the Physically Disabled Child: Family Reactions and Deductive Reasoning," *New York State Journal of Medicine*, **75**:1039–1041, June 1975.
17 L. Shellhase and F. Shellhase, "Role of the Family in Rehabilitation," *Social Casework*, **53**:544–550, November 1972.
18 J. Pomeroy, *Recreation for the Physically Handicapped*. New York: Macmillan, 1964, pp. 19–32.

BIBLIOGRAPHY

Blake, Florence: "Immobilized Youth: A Rationale for Supportive Nursing Intervention," *American Journal of Nursing*, **69**:2364–2369, November 1969.
Browse, N. L.: *The Physiology and Pathology of Bedrest*. Springfield, Ill.: Charles C Thomas Co., 1965.
Chodoff, Paul: "Adjustment to Disability: Some Observations in Patients with Multiple Sclerosis," *Journal of Chronic Disease*, June 1959.
Crate, Marjorie: "Nursing Function in Adaptation to Chronic Illness," *American Journal of Nursing*, **65**:72–76, October 1965.

Diamond, Milton: "Sexuality and the Handicapped," *Rehabilitation Literature*, **35**:34–40, February 1974.

Dillon, Ann: "Nursing Care of the Patient with Multiple Sclerosis," *Nursing Clinics of North America*, **8**:653–664, December 1973.

Drew, Nancy: "How to Cope with Speech Defects," *Nursing 74*, **4**:20–21, February 1974.

Fowler, Roy, and Wilbert E. Fordyce: "Adapting Care for the Brain-Damaged Patient—Part I," *American Journal of Nursing*, **72**:1832–1835, October 1972.

———— and ————, "Adapting Care for the Brain-Damaged Patient—Part II." *American Journal of Nursing*, **72**:2056–2059, November 1972.

Freeman, Roger: "Psychiatric Problems in Adolescents with Cerebral Palsy," *Developmental Medicine and Child Neurology*, **12**:64–69, 1970.

Gardner, Richard: "Psychogenic Problems of Brain Injured Children and Their Parents," *Journal of the American Academy of Child Psychiatry*, **7**:471–491, 1968.

Henderson, Gloria: "Teaching-Learning for Rehabilitation of the Spinal Cord Disabled Individual," *Nursing Clinics of North America*, **6**:655–668, December 1971.

Hirschberg, Gerald, Leon Lewis, and Patricia Vaughn: *Rehabilitation: A Manual for the Care of the Disabled and Elderly*, 2d ed. Philadelphia: J. B. Lippincott Co., 1976.

Ladicu, Gloria, et al.: "Studies in Adjustment to Visible Injuries: Evaluation of Help by Injured," *Journal of Abnormal Social Psychology*, **42**:169–192, 1947.

Licht, Sidney (ed.): *Stroke and Its Rehabilitation*, Baltimore: Waverly Press Inc., 1975.

Norsworthy, Edith: "Nursing Rehabilitation After Severe Head Trauma," *American Journal of Nursing*, **74**:1246–1250, July 1974.

Chapter 14

Free Youth Clinics

Patricia S. Yaros

Within the past several years, many hospital outpatient services have been criticized as outmoded, cumbersome, and unresponsive to the needs of the ambulatory patient population. Such clinics have been seen by some as facilities for the destitute and terribly ill where people spend hours waiting in cavelike corridors to become "practice patients" for students of the health professions. The mass of paperwork, stark environment, and impersonal attitudes of personnel add to the quinine reputation. A vanguard of consumer groups and health practitioners has sought to organize innovative and responsive outpatient health care services that are not necessarily tied to the hospital domain. Joining in this attempt has been the free youth clinic movement.

This chapter describes how free youth clinics have evolved and examines reasons why adolescents have found them appealing. Recommendations for establishing developmentally sound adolescent health care in the free clinic setting are presented.

HISTORY

The birth of the free youth clinic occurred during the sixties, when "Tune in, turn on, drop out" was the watchword of youth. In the mecca of San Francisco and in cities and college towns across America, thousands of young people drifted onto the streets. These youth had more to give one another than love, flowers, and drugs. They had VD, hepatitis, and many other medical and psychological problems that "establishment" health care services could not or would not deal with. Moreover, the young people would not deal with the establishment. Alternative health care was imperative, and so arrived the concept of free youth clinics.

The first free clinics built upon an expanded meaning of the word *free*. One meaning was the economic one, of course. Free clinics were not just for those who could pay nothing or only part of the cost of their health services; they provided care for *everyone* without cost. But *free* also meant free from hassles, i.e., free from rules that often limit the availability or acceptability of care. In addition, *free* was also used in the sense that all clients in a free clinic were considered to be "free people," and no one judged them for the practices whose consequences brought them to the clinic. Implementing these ideals became both the pain and the pride of the free youth clinic movement.

The history of free youth clinics, like adolescence itself, has been full of "storm and strife." The Haight-Ashbury clinic was formed in 1967 as a drug emergency care center when acute overcrowding and intensive drug use occurred among the naive youth population of San Francisco.[1] However, the broad range of health needs of this population soon became apparent, and the clinic expanded its staff to offer more comprehensive services. To maintain standards acceptable to professional and public review was an initial and ongoing concern of this clinic and those that followed. In addition, the same problems that establishment clinics have in keeping their doors open, especially the problem of financing, have kept most free youth clinics in a precarious situation.

The future of almost 300 clinics now functioning across the United States cannot be assured. In the past, approximately 50 clinics have shut down. They succumbed, in varying degrees, to the hazards of trying to be "all things to all people" with a minimum of financial resources. Many also had failed to cultivate the necessary broad community support and endorsement of the health professions. Those clinics that survived learned many lessons that have since been shared in national conferences. Also, with great caution, the federal government has appraised the health care provided by free youth clinics and has provided a portion of support through Law Enforcement Assistance grants and some public health monies.

The free youth clinic movement has survived, partly because it promoted women's clinics and clinics for many kinds of minorities. These clinics were quick to take up an approach to health care that assured anonymity and equality for "special" clients. But another reason youth clinics have survived and flourished is that the health and developmental needs of adolescence have been uniquely served in the free clinic atmosphere.

DILEMMAS FOR ADOLESCENTS
IN TRADITIONAL HEALTH SETTINGS

The attraction of adolescents to free clinics is no doubt related to the general difficulties they encounter in obtaining health care from standard providers. Adolescents may seek alternative health care services because of the scarcity of health professionals who are knowledgeable about adolescent development or because of the lack of health care environments in which they feel comfortable. Additionally, their trust in community health care agencies is not enhanced when they encounter the legal barriers used to prevent the majority of youth from obtaining care without parental permission (whether or not there are parents). These issues have all been implicated in the alienation of young people from such health agencies as physicians' offices, outpatient clinics, and even emergency services.

No adolescent is comfortable in a pediatrician's office with diapered toddlers and rash-covered first-graders. Being accompanied by Mother only intensifies a teen's perception of being treated like a child. The caricature of the smiling pediatrician who still offers a 13-year-old a lollipop, saying, "You're not too old for this, are you?" is based on reality. It is understandable that an adolescent would seek an alternative for help with health problems.

Changing doctors is often not a satisfactory solution. Just as the pediatrician may view the adolescent as a youngster, the internist may also miss the essence of adolescent problems by judging the teenager only by his or her adult traits. Adolescents are often not the only ones who are uncomfortable about their presence in a physician's office; office personnel, including the professionals, frequently feel ill at ease and unequipped to deal with patients in the teen years.

Public health agencies and adolescents experience many incompatibilities. If the health department has no screening or care programs in the after-school hours, teens have little access to its services. If an adolescent does come in without a parent, the agency may be unable to provide care. Laws governing health care for minors are confusing, unstandardized, and crippling to many agencies. (An expansion on this topic will follow later in the chapter.) The consequence for the adolescent is a cynical view as to who is the "public" served by the public health departments. The teen then sees the need to find "underground" communications as to which agencies bend the rules and which are hard-liners.

The laws concerning parental consent are geared toward ensuring parental responsibility for a young person's health. However, in many states there is no leeway in the law to provide any kind of health information to a teenager without a parent's permission. Not only are such controversial matters as contraceptive education and abortion counseling denied to an adolescent unless parental approval is obtained, but even nominal health information is denied. A teenager who goes as far as to give a history before being informed that he or she cannot receive care may find that the information is not held in confidence; the health professional may feel obligated to inform parents of the situation whether or not the adolescent sees that as acceptable. Such disclosures can easily contribute to mistrust of authority and health agencies in general.

The free clinic movement sought to narrow this gap in health care by means that particularly appealed to young people. Free clinic organizers were pioneers in liberalizing parental consent laws and creating the category of adolescent called the *emancipated minor*. Free clinic organizers also saw the need to make the youth clinic environment as comfortable and nonthreatening as possible. In a free clinic one is likely to see a waiting area that does not prohibit sitting on the floor, health care providers who make it plain that they are there to help and not to call in parents or police, health professionals who are knowledgeable about the world of today's teenager, and few, if any, white-coated authority figures.

Youth clinics were quick to recognize two other factors that were appropriate for their kind of adolescent care. The teenager's sense of immediacy about his or her problems is recognized by the use of a walk-in, no-appointment arrangement in most free youth clinics. Also, teenagers' generally poor financial situation is acknowledged in most clinics by the provision of free care for those who cannot pay anything and the requesting of donations from anyone who can pay something to help keep the clinic going. This writer has witnessed donations from some adolescents that far exceeded what they would have had to pay for the same service in any other health agency. Such donations may be accompanied by a statement of trust and belief in the services of the free clinic. This type of sentiment, expressed without the characteristic cynicism of teenagers, can be taken as another indication of the success of such a health care service.

ESTABLISHING A FREE YOUTH CLINIC

Assessing Support

When free clinic programs across the country are examined, it becomes apparent that few, perhaps none, were developed according to a com-

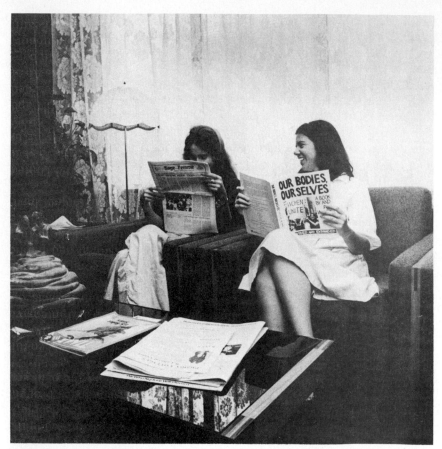

An effective feature of free clinics and other kinds of alternative health care facilities is that they are designed to meet young people's needs and preferences with regard to hours, fees, confidentiality, accommodation of minors, decor, educational materials, walk-in appointments, and kinds of health problems treated. (*Copyright © 1980 by Anne Campbell*.)

prehensive plan. In most cases, as one element of a program (such as staff, money, or a building) became available, decisions were then made about the next step. However, anyone undertaking to establish a youth clinic, free or otherwise, must pay particular attention to the forces that will hinder or support such an endeavor. This assessment must be made before any definitive planning occurs, or a great deal of effort may be wasted.

Persons planning a free youth clinic must recognize what is involved in promoting a change in any aspect of health care delivery, especially in such a controversial area as free services. Public health agencies and the medical, nursing, and pharmaceutical professions must be apprised of the move and shown how such a clinic in their community will be advantageous to all. Strategies for doing this vary according to the professional group being approached, the composition of the youth population to be served, and numerous other circumstances, of course, but the overriding objective is to develop incentives for all the professions to support the clinic. Unless such support is obtained, insurmountable barriers may be encountered later. Furthermore, it is obviously beneficial to the clinic to include representatives from the major health disciplines on the clinic staff; communication and cooperation, as well as comprehensiveness of services, are fostered in this way.

Innovative and responsive adolescent health care should be the general goal of free clinic planning. In achieving this, however, planners may have to deal with the traditionalism of some members of the health disciplines. Some physicians and nurses may be able to envision only the traditional physician-dominated practice in an ambulatory setting. The stereotyped arrangement in which a physician and nurse are assigned to an examining room and patients are ushered in and out is not the best approach for a youth clinic. The staff can be encourged to look at a more flexible organization of services that utilizes professionals in their broadest functions. The physician need not be the only one who ''sees'' the patient, and in fact many patients can more advantageously see other staff members instead.

Many pharmacists now have the ideal training to counsel and evaluate persons with drug problems. Social workers have counseling and teaching skills that often fit in with teen emotional and health problems. Nurses, depending on their background, may function at all levels of assessment and intervention in the health care of adolescents. Nurse practitioners in many free clinics take responsibility for a large part of the clinic services, particularly those parts of health care that utilize practitioners' assessment, counseling, and teaching skills.

Obtaining the support and participation of all relevant health disciplines is the prime factor in beginning a successful free youth clinic. The ''connections'' each discipline has for providing volunteer professional services as well as donating funds and equipment make the youth clinic a community effort in a short time.

Services Offered Depend on the Clientele

The particular services included in the clinic's program must be selected to fit the needs of the population of adolescents who will utilize the facility. Some differences are to be expected in the frequency of certain adolescent problems in an inner-city area, for example, as opposed to a college town. It is crucial that free youth clinic organizers know their potential clientele well in terms of ages, sex ratio, socioeconomic background, drug usage, and other health vulnerabilities.

Types of personnel and arrangements for referral are determined in accordance with the kinds of patients who use the clinic. In most if not all settings, the professional staff should include both physical and mental health generalists. If there is a need in addition (or instead) for specialists in, for example, gynecology or drug abuse, the clinic must either find ways of bringing in persons with this expertise or find acceptable referral resources. Philosophically, it is difficult for a free clinic to refer patients out to agencies that supposedly were not acceptable or available to the adolescents in the first place. But the organizers need to remember that trying to be all things to all people is clearly a prescription for failure in a free youth clinic.

Many towns and cities have a large transient adolescent population that for various reasons is difficult to accommodate in the facilities serving residents. Transient youth have many difficulties obtaining health care, not only because they lack residency but also because they often do not have money or any verifiable legal status. In many states teens can be picked up as runaways, so they often stay away from establishment health care agencies except the emergency rooms (which they may overcrowd in certain seasons). Being treated in an emergency room may be impossible if the teenager has no money at all.

The transient teen population is usually constituted largely of counterculture adolescents, a group who do not endear themselves to mainstream health professionals and agencies. However, because of their lifestyle, they may have especially aggravated health problems. They usually live in vans or camp out, and their poor hygiene and poor nutrition make them good candidates for a number of communicable diseases. The likelihood that they will not get follow-up care for minor problems makes them vulnerable to subsequent major complications. This population heavily utilizes the services of a free clinic, and the clinic must be prepared to deal with the particular problems of transients.

The permanent adolescent residents of an area usually constitute the greatest portion of the client load of a clinic. If they are very young adolescents who are not using the local pediatricians for health care, then they are probably in the free clinic for help that they wish to keep secret from their parents. This can be a rather risky situation for a clinic, depending upon the state laws, and no matter how well such occurrences are handled there may be irate parents at the door.

In a college town where the infirmary service is limited or unpopular, a free youth clinic attracts college-age young people. Usually there are no problems with parental consent because college youth are old enough to be accorded adult legal status. However, all manner of health problems may be encountered in this group; generally psychological problems predominate. Teens are vulnerable to severe depression and possible suicide, particularly in this older age group and in the college or university life-style. A free youth clinic in a college town may see the need for a suicide and crisis intervention center to be associated with the youth clinic.

Most free youth clinics have found that the majority of health problems brought to them result from drug use or sexual encounters among teens. These problems include "bad trips" and poisonings related to drugs, and venereal disease, other genitourinary disorders, abortion, and pregnancy connected with the sexual freedom adolescents have claimed for themselves. The second largest group of problems teens bring to free clinics is respiratory ailments such as flu and severe colds. Victims of severe accidents usually go to an acute care facility, but the many minor accidents that are so common among adolescents comprise the third largest health problem category free clinics encounter. Psychological problems rank fourth. Free youth clinics need not be able to handle every one of the problems teens bring to them, but they should have an active referral system they can trust to meet the challenge.

The Environment of a Free Youth Clinic

Nowhere is more vigorous attention paid to the health care environment and personnel than in the free youth clinic movement. Most free clinics intend to be hassle-free and seek to create an environment that does not alienate the group they wish to serve. This goal is accomplished in different ways, but most clinics take their cues from the youths themselves. If young people are involved in the planning, they can assist in designing appealing facilities and selecting personnel.

Adolescents respond favorably to an environment in which they have choices: choices about where, how, and whether to sit; whether or not to join a VD discussion group; whether or not to watch short films about health or social subjects. If some or all of these activities are offered to adolescents in a free-choice atmosphere, they usually engage in them and learn from them. Waiting time may seem shortened by interesting activities.

The physical setting of any adolescent clinic needs to reflect the life-style and interests of its client population. Decor need not be elaborate, for it can easily be overdone. The young people who participate in the planning can often serve as the decorators because of their expertise in the current social world of adolescents. Themes change periodically, and the music and decor of the clinic can be changed accordingly. The comfort of the facility is not usually a prime concern except that the environment should be welcoming and flexible, not stiff or sterile.

To set up a hassle-free procedure for caring for patients in a clinic is not easy. However, successful clinics have used a triage system that has the advantage of finding out each client's problem as he or she comes in and letting the patient know immediately whether the clinic can deal with that problem. This triage system has an additional advantage of taking care of any preliminary lab work or examination before the patient sees the primary examiner. A few clinics have blanket protocols that move the patient quickly through routine procedures and then leave plenty of time for discussion, counseling, and teaching related to the teen's presenting problem.

It is obvious that an important part of a free youth clinic's effectiveness depends upon caring, concerned staff. When one recognizes that an adolescent may have few other resources for health care, it is apparent that a youth clinic needs to provide the nonjudgmental and respectful atmosphere youth need and deserve. Starched white uniforms and numbered patients do not belong in a free youth clinic. High regard for each adolescent's personal freedom and right to privacy should be part of every clinic's *operating* practice, not simply the rhetoric of the practice. Provision of confidentiality, however, is sometimes difficult because legal constraints and inflexible governmental rules may invite compromise.

The Legal Constraints on Free Youth Clinics*

The movement toward giving more adult rights to minors has been especially forceful in the area of adolescent health care. Nearly every state in the country has enacted legislation in the past 12 years to allow defined groups of minors to consent to some or all of their health care.[2] These laws have recognized that many adolescents are able to give a valid informed consent. This legislation can also be said to be a response to the fact that many adolescents are engaging in activities that have serious health consequences and that they conceal from their parents.

The new laws have tried to deal with the question of who has the right to sign consent for a young person's health care. In the past (in most states and even now in a few), health care was treated as a contract, and as a minor the young person could not legally sign for care. Further, health professionals were vulnerable to assault charges if they examined a young person who was not legally eligible to consent to care. Fortunately, the trend toward more realistic and responsive legislation is continuing and there seems reason for hope that soon all states will recognize the problems in adolescent health care and clarify the laws.

The concept of the emancipated minor is one with which everyone

---

*This section refers to the general status of the law at the time of publication. There will undoubtedly be changes in the laws related to the rights of adolescent minors in the future. Because of the constant changes in these laws, only a general overview is provided here without a detailed listing of the status of these laws in each state. Persons who have an interest in the legislation binding in a particular state are directed to that state's attorney general or the local and state health departments.

caring for adolescents should be familiar. Narrowly defined in the past to include only married teenagers, those in the armed forces, and teens without any family, the term has broadened in scope in the last few years. Free clinics have been in the forefront of helping to clarify the emancipated minor concept in the law because they deal with minors who do not fit the old definitions exactly but are acting in their own behalf in every area except health care. The law varies among states; health professionals working with adolescents who may qualify under the liberalized laws need to know the law for their state.

Laws concerning health care related to sexual behavior and drug abuse vary greatly across the country. Some health professionals have broadly interpreted the emergency-care laws for treating minors without parental consent to encompass contraceptive care and drug counseling and treatment. Obviously this practice jeopardizes the health professional, who may be taken to court if a parent wishes to test the issue.

The greatest legal risk for nurses, physicians, and other professionals in a free clinic setting, however, is their professional liability as practitioners. The cost of malpractice insurance is usually borne by the individual, for few free clinics use federal grant money for that purpose.[3] Health care professionals who supervise nonprofessional volunteers, as many in free clinics do, should be especially aware of their liability for the errors of those with little training.

CONCLUSION

The full impact of free youth clinics on the American health care scene has not yet been fully realized. The clinics have existed with tenuous support and uneven standards of practice. The professionals who contribute their time to them are experimenting in a break from tradition. It is to be hoped that some of the reforms free clinics have pioneered will be seen as good health care by other public and private health care agencies. Even if this movement dies out and few free clinics remain, it will have stood as a precedent for a future time when health care is made available to people who cannot obtain it from traditional sources.

REFERENCES

1 H. Creighton, *Law Every Nurse Should Know*, 3d ed. Philadelphia: W. B. Saunders, 1975, pp. 278–279.
2 A. D. Hofmann and I. R. Shenker, "Medical Care of Adolescents and the Law," *New York State Journal of Medicine*, **70**:2603–2611, 1970.
3 D. Smith, "Runaways and Their Health Problems in Haight-Ashbury during the Summer of 1967," *American Journal of Public Health*, **59**:2046–2050, 1969.

BIBLIOGRAPHY

American Academy of Pediatrics, Committee on Youth: "A Model Act Providing for Consent of Minors for Health Services," *Pediatrics*, **51**(2):293–296, February 1973.

Smith, D. E., D. J. Bentel, and J. L. Schwartz (eds.): *The Free Clinic: A Community Approach to Health Care and Drug Abuse*. Beloit, Wis.: Stash Press, 1971.

Chapter 15

School Health Programs

Judith B. Igoe

During adolescence at least four major developmental tasks have to be completed. These are: (1) achieving a stable identity or self-image; (2) adjusting to an adult sexual role; (3) establishing independence from the family unit; and (4) making a vocational or career choice.[1] Any school health program of merit will be so designed as to facilitate the accomplishment of these goals.

WHAT COMPRISES A SCHOOL HEALTH PROGRAM?

There are three principle areas of activity that are usually involved in a program of school health. First, *health education*, which is the process of providing learning experiences that are positive and change the understanding, attitudes, and behavior of students, resulting in preventive health measures and the maintenance of individualized health. Second, *health services* are important. These are procedures that are carried out by health professionals and others to appraise, promote, and maintain the health of students. Finally, *environmental health*: Efforts at school to

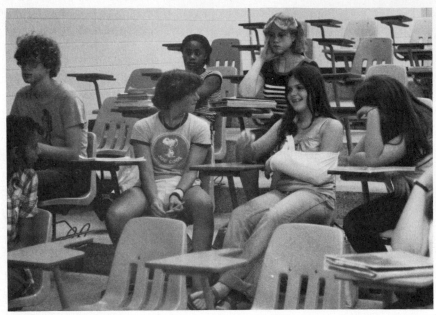

Assessment of the health needs of the student population must precede the planning of programs for health education, direct health service, or environmental school health. These members of a regular public school class demonstrate the presence of traumatic injury, dental bracing, and scoliosis bracing. Observation, interview, and review of records would reveal other problems and their incidence and help identify program priorities. (*Copyright © 1980 by Anne Campbell*.)

provide physical and social conditions necessary to maintain physical as well as mental health and safety of students fall into this category. Although these three spheres of activity may interact, and are most effective when operating compatibly, each may operate alone and still benefit the health of children in school. However, identifying all these as activities to be included among the school's objectives provides the greatest potential for impact on adolescent health.

Planning for the school health program should begin with a needs assessment to determine (1) the health conditions which exist among the adolescents enrolled in the school and (2) the resources already available within the community to handle these problems. This evaluation process should also determine the extent to which adolescents actually seek out the health services and education available to them. (Frequently, this age group avoids contact with health personnel unless serious health problems exist which require attention.) The environment of the school should not be overlooked during this assessment period. Frequently, vending machines filled with high-fat, high-carbohydrate foods; industrial arts workrooms improperly designed for safety around dangerous power tools; and poorly maintained bathrooms present the greatest hazards to health in junior and senior high schools. To complete the assessment of need for a school health program and the determination of the type of program which could meet these needs, the evaluator must consider the quality of the existent health education curriculum. Unfortunately, the majority of junior and senior high schools in this country have no organized program of health education despite legislative efforts in many states to mandate this type of curriculum offering.

Failure to document the need for particular aspects of the school health program, though a customary practice in the past, will today seriously jeopardize the future existence of the program. Severe budgetary restraints now imposed on schools have forced school administrators to eliminate those programs within school having little apparent relevance to the adolescent's learning and growth. School nurses, therefore, must pay particular attention to the development of a program of school health which is consistent with the health problems of the students. Moreover, an ongoing plan for program evaluation must be maintained in order to justify the necessity for continuing school health services and education.

SCHOOL HEALTH SERVICES FOR ADOLESCENTS

Services available as part of the school health program may be both group and individualized activities. Mass screening programs are well suited to evaluating vision, hearing, and growth, and identifying dental conditions, skeletal deformities, high blood pressure, and cardiac conditions. Individualized services include first aid; physical exams; neurological evaluations; and lab procedures such as throat culture, urine or blood tests, and tests for pregnancy and venereal disease. Health counseling is another individualized service requested frequently by adolescents.

Adolescents who seek health services at school should find an environment in which privacy is assured. Frequently the ready availability of the school clinic will motivate adolescents who have previously not availed themselves of health services in the community to consult the school nurse. However, if the clinic is no more than one room in which several students are simultaneously evaluated and treated, the adolescent in need of care or counseling may stay away out of fear of embarrassment and breach of privacy.

As school health services are provided to adolescents, every opportunity should be used to involve them directly in their own health care. The school nurse should request the adolescent to complete his or her own health history form. Decisions related to health planning following a health evaluation should be jointly shared by adolescent and nurse, with the adolescent encouraged to assume as much responsibility as possible for the maintenance of his or her health. This is especially important because the majority of health problems facing adolescents require the adoption of preventive health measures rather than passive receipt of intervention provided by the nurse.

The school nurse who manages a busy junior or senior high school clinic will soon identify a group of adolescents who repeatedly come to the clinic with complaints of illness and injury. Close investigation of these complaints usually reveals no serious physical difficulty. However, the astute school nurse will quickly identify this behavior as symptomatic and take the necessary steps to identify the cause. The need for health counseling among adolescents is paramount and it is important that the nurse consider this possibility with these adolescents who might be aptly labeled "the worried well."

One should not overlook the potential benefits of the school clinic as a mini–career education center for those adolescents who are interested in health as a career. In numerous school clinics, adolescents fill the role of health clerks through work-study programs. While it is important in these instances to guard against the possibility that adolescent patients coming to the clinic will worry about a peer's learning of their personal health problems, the situation can be properly handled in a well-planned period of orientation and training for the health clerk. The types of responsibilities assumed by health clerks include: assisting with mass screening programs, performing clerical duties, taking short health histories from adolescents complaining of injury and illness, giving basic first aid, and helping adolescent patients complete health history forms. Additional services provided by adolescent health clerks involve orienting new patients to clinic procedures, explaining and clarifying health care plans, and, in some instances, doing health counseling.

HEALTH EDUCATION FOR ADOLESCENTS

Individualized health teaching for adolescents has been described in detail in Chapter 11. What remains to be said here is to reemphasize the importance of direct involvement of adolescents in their own learning, and the importance of gearing educational efforts to their interests and concerns. A semester-long high school course, in which students learn (and teach others) to be participatory health care consumers, will be described.

Organized classroom instruction in health education varies from school to school in this country. However, there is a definite need in all schools for the nurse to be intimately involved in the development of the health curriculum because, frequently, no other health professional is in direct, regular contact with the school. Unfortunately, the health education curricula in schools are usually outmoded, dully repetitive of earlier learning, and relegated to the last period of the day. Teachers may be ill prepared to teach health in a meaningful way and, consequently, the school nurse is often helpful in a consultant role. More recently, values clarification programs and self-help classes for adolescents have appeared in some schools, and have been well-received complements to the rest of the health curriculum.

The school nurse who is interested in improving the school's health education program may find help with this task by contacting the state departments of health and education and by visiting with health professionals in community adolescent clinics.

An Example of Participatory Health Education for Adolescents

A pilot health teaching project to prepare adolescents to be health consumers represents the joint efforts of health professionals from the University of Colorado Medical Center (faculty and medical and nursing students) and adolescents and teachers from the target school district, Adams County, Colorado, District No. 14. The program shows high school students how to take an active role in their relationship with a health professional and in their own health care, and then allows the adolescents to work with other youths. It encompasses a self-help health education program in the classroom environment and active participation in health education at a summer school health clinic, for which the adolescents are paid.

Preliminary efforts began in 1976 with planning sessions involving representatives from the University of Colorado Schools of Nursing and Medicine and from Adams City High School, and members of the teaching staff for the school district's Career Education Center. Consultation was sought from Tri-County Health Department, the Public Health Center for the county, and the state department of education. The program employs a coordinator who has had previous experience in youth involvement as well as curriculum development expertise. The coordinator formalizes the curriculum from recommendations of the planning committee. Enrollment in the course is open to all junior and senior students in the high school.

The course, one semester in length, emphasizes the concept of the "participatory health consumer," i.e., the adolescent as a partner in his or her own health care. The University of Colorado School Nurse Practitioner Program has previously identified the preferred type of behavioral interactions between the health consumer and health professional. The goal is that the health consumer:

1   Ask questions for the purpose of clarification and improved understanding
2   Personally communicate information about his or her own health

3 Acquire pertinent health information simultaneously with the delivery of service
4 Participate in the decision-making activity related to the consumer's own health at the time health services are rendered
5 Assume responsibility for certain tasks related to the maintenance of health

The planning committee for this health teaching project uses this stated goal as a reference point. But the program reflects the joint planning and involvement of representatives of all three groups (adolescents, teachers, and health professionals), and, therefore, other parameters evolve. The course objectives of the health education program state that the adolescents will

1 Exhibit an increased frequency of behaviors designated as the "participatory health consumer" role
2 Achieve an understanding of self-help information in the area of health for the purpose of improving their judgment and self-confidence related to health matters
3 Participate in clinically situated learning experiences to clarify the relevance and application of classroom instruction to their daily living habits
4 Learn useful health screening procedures
5 Gain knowledge and skill in the recognition and management of minor illnesses and emergencies

The self-help health course is designed to accommodate 30 high school students in their junior and senior years and is comprised of two phases. The first is classroom-centered learning about self-help skills to evaluate illness and wellness, including a 4-week period of practice with the school nurse and health clerk at the school clinic. In the clinic, the adolescent works directly with younger children in providing first aid, taking health histories, and participating in health screening activities. The second phase follows in a summer school health clinic, where 600 children and adolescents from the school district receive preventive health care evaluations from experienced school nurses who are enrolled in the University of Colorado School Nurse Practitioner Program under the supervision of pediatricians. The students in the self-help program design and operate the health education center in the clinic and perform initial health screening services (e.g., vision, hearing). For their efforts, the adolescents are paid.

The following list of study topics is indicative of the curriculum:

- Health and Illness—Definitions and Characteristics
- Health and What It Means to Me
- The Present Role of Health Consumers—The Need for Change

- The Roles of Different Health Professionals—What You Can Expect
- Compliance versus Noncompliance
- Decision Making—Your Right and Responsibility and Your Health
- Communication Skills (including information on how to ask questions)
- Health Services and Agencies—What's Available and Where
- Adolescence—What's It All About? (developmental tasks of this age)
- Health Hazards and You (stress, drugs, fatigue)
- Maintaining Your Own Health (nutrition, rest, exercise, relaxation techniques)
- Health Evaluations—What's Involved and Why (preventive health care and sick care evaluations)
- History Taking (overall health history—"present illness" history as a guide to assessing the seriousness of a health complaint)
- Physical Examination Skills
    Height, weight, temperature, pulse, respiration
    Blood pressure
    Vision screening
    Hearing screening
    Use of the otoscope
    Skeletal evaluation
    Mouth and throat evaluation (including dental)
    Skin inspection
- Minor Illnesses—How to Assess and Manage
    Upper respiratory infections
    Headache
    Gastrointestinal disturbances
    Skin rashes (acne, communicable disease, scabies)
- Evaluation of Available Health Services
- Effective Conflict Management Involving Health Professionals and Consumers
- Drugs
    Over-the-counter
    Prescription
- A Reference Library for Health—Guides for Selection of Health Information Texts
- Planning for the Health Education Center
    Growth and development of children ages 5 to 12
    Interviewing skills
    Principles of learning
    Development of health education materials

Specialized teaching techniques are utilized in an effort to enhance learning in the self-help course. For example, value clarification techniques prove useful to students as they struggle to realize the personal meaning of health for themselves. Role playing is also effectively utilized to reenact previous experiences in health facilities as the adolescents attempt to identify new approaches for dealing with health systems and professionals. Actual practice in history taking and performance of demonstrated physical examination procedures (e.g., vision screening, plotting heights and weights on growth graphs, etc.) is emphasized to assist students in integrating their new skills and knowledge. The course instructor (project coordinator) consistently role-models the participatory health consumer role and positively reinforces the related behaviors as they are demonstrated by students. A series of case presentations involving minor health problems is the focus of group discussions. For these sessions, the discovery method of instruction prevails in order that students can perfect their own problem-solving skills. Closely intertwined throughout the entire course is the consistent use of teaching methods and role development strategies designed to improve the adolescents' concepts of themselves and to increase their self-confidence. Development of personal characteristics of this kind is most important if these adolescents are to succeed in utilizing the information and skills gained from the self-help course.

To prepare these students to function effectively in their health education center at the clinic, the self-help course also incorporates specific instruction related to the development and operation of the center. Responsibility for these arrangements rests with the class and the project coordinator. University of Colorado Medical Center faculty are available to assist students in developing the necessary understanding, knowledge, and skill to work with children ranging in age from 5 through 12 years as well as with their own age group. In this regard, an audiovisual educational program about the growth and development of school-age children is used. Furthermore, the adolescents learn to use the *Guide to Participatory Health Behavior*, which is a chart from the University of Colorado Medical Center that designates a developmental profile, health interests, and suggested ways to involve children and adolescents in their own care. Additional help and instruction from the state department of education health educator assist the high school students with the actual development of learning materials and experiences for use in their health education center. Finally, representatives from the school district's Career Education Center work closely with the program coordinator in arranging salary support for the adolescents during their period of clinical practice in the health education center.

The following descriptions explain the way in which students enrolled in the self-help course function in their health education center at the clinic.

Role of the Adolescent Health Worker and the Elementary School Child in the Clinic   Prior to the clinic appointment for a child of elementary school

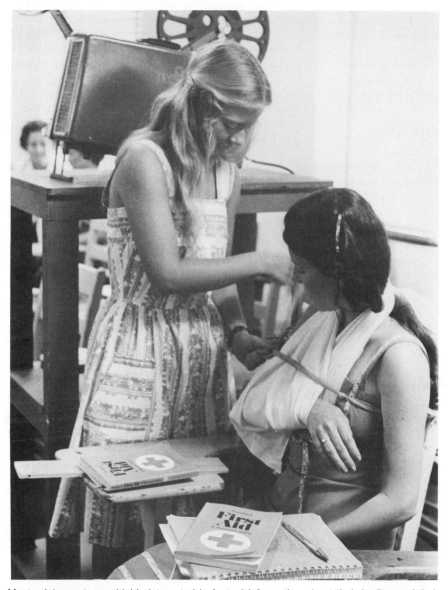

Most adolescents are highly interested in factual information about their bodies and their health; too often overlooked in health education, however, is preparation for the role of health care consumer. (*Copyright © 1980 by Anne Campbell.*)

age, the self-help class mails out information in comic-book form to the child about the clinic and the child's role as a health consumer. Parents are also informed by letter of the clinic philosophy to involve children in their own health care.

Upon arrival at the clinic, children are assigned to a member of the self-help class, who initially goes over the materials the child received in the mail and answers any questions which arise. Next, the adolescent health worker accompanies the child to an exhibit area in the health education center. Here the child finds a series of instructional booths presenting health information and activities of interest to children of different ages. The child is allowed to select the booths he or she wishes to see. As they visit the booth, the adolescent health worker works with the child by providing assistance in understanding the material contained within the booth and encouraging the child to become involved in this learning experience.

Once the child has finished touring the exhibit area, the adolescent directs him or her to another area of the health education center in which initial health screening (vision, height, weight, etc.) is done by the adolescent worker with supervision. The teenager continues to encourage the youngster to ask questions and to practice being a participatory health consumer. The adolescent health worker, having completed the screening, presents the child with a personal health record book in which to record the findings. Following this the adolescent assists the child in recording in this health booklet whatever health history the child knows about herself or himself.

At the end of this activity, the adolescent reunites parent and child and takes them to the area of the clinic used for evaluations. Parents have the option of accompanying their children through the education center or attending a parents' class conducted by the staff of the School Nurse Practitioner Program. Finally, the adolescent introduces parent and child to the school nurse practitioner, who proceeds with the evaluation. The adolescents spend approximately one hour with each child in the health education center.

Role of the Adolescent Health Worker and the Adolescent Patient in the Health Education Center   Prior to the clinic appointment, the adolescent patient receives information about the clinic and about the patient's role as a participatory health consumer. In addition, adolescents receive a health history which they are asked to complete and bring with them at the time of their appointment.

The adolescent health worker assigned to the adolescent patient accompanies the adolescent to an exhibit area (separate from the one for younger children) in which films, videotapes, audio-cassettes, and resource persons from the community are available to provide health information on such topics as venereal disease, breast self-examination, drugs, sexuality, and depression. It is felt that the adolescent health worker is helpful as co-counselor in regard to these subjects. Adolescent health workers are responsible as well for orienting the adolescent consumer to the existence of the Adolescent Hot Line (a telephone counseling service for adolescents with problems); Tele Med (a telephone service which provides information to the community about numerous health topics); and the various Denver-area agencies specializing in health and social services for adolescents.

Later, the adolescent health worker does the initial screening (vision, blood pressure, etc.) and presents the adolescent with a personal health record. The worker spends time helping the adolescent patients to identify areas of concern they wish to discuss with the school nurse practitioner. As is true with the younger children, the adolescent health worker accompanies the adolescent patient to the examination room and handles the introduction to the school nurse practitioner.

This educational program is designed to enable adolescents to become partners in their own health care and to teach younger children and peers similar skills. As yet, it is too soon to be able to measure the program's effectiveness. Informal observations, however, indicate that this is an extremely meaningful health teaching experience for everyone involved.

HEALTHFUL ENVIRONMENT IN SECONDARY SCHOOLS

Many nurses have succeeded in improving their schools' environment by enlisting the help of the environmental health department of the local public health agency. A variety of public health regulations exist with respect to school health, and it is important for school nurses to familiarize themselves with these policies. Furthermore, the local health department can often assist in the evaluation of the school's environment.

The student council in some schools has been extremely helpful in development and implementation of an environmental health plan within school. In one school, the student council was instrumental in convincing the owners of the vending machines to stock fruit and juices rather than candy bars and soft drinks.

QUALIFIED SCHOOL HEALTH PERSONNEL

Most school health personnel are school nurses. Some of these nurses are highly qualified to work with adolescents and their health problems. Other nurses, although interested in adolescents, may find they lack the skill and knowledge necessary for working effectively with this age group.

Preparing School Nurses

Recently the Society for Adolescent Medicine has developed a curriculum guide to help prepare physicians to provide the highest quality of adolescent care.[2] Although this guide is not specifically directed at the educational needs of nurses, the increasing tendency for medicine and nursing to share a number of skills related to health care delivery makes it appropriate to suggest that school nurses working with adolescents require similar knowledge and skill. The society supports this position.

The curriculum guide is presented with three levels. Level I is an introductory unit providing for a basic understanding of adolescent growth and development and common health problems, and should be covered during undergraduate years. Level II is designed to secure skills for managing common problems of adolescents, and is geared to students in their senior year or beyond the basic training. Level III is designed to develop leadership abilities in teaching and research as well as in providing expert patient care, and is intended for those individuals who have finished their basic training and wish to obtain postgraduate training. The curriculum objectives for the first two levels follow and should guide nurses working with adolescents in determining their own educational needs:

Level I

Objective 1   An introduction to adolescent growth and development, emphasizing normal physical and psychological changes of puberty.

Objective 2   An understanding of the common disorders of adolescents, including growth deviations (obesity, delayed puberty, short stature, etc.), school underachievement, and common behavioral problems.

Objective 3   An understanding of the common causes of morbidity and mortality during the adolescent period. A review of the common causes of illness and death in this age group, emphasizing prevention.

Objective 4   Introduction to the social, cultural, and political influences upon adolescent behavior and development.

Objective 5   Introduction to interviewing and history-taking skills used with adolescent patients.

Objective 6   Introduction to the physical examination of the adolescent.

Objective 1E (elective)   Experience in adolescent and family counseling.

Objective 2E   Advanced experience in adolescent medicine.

Objective 3E   Additional electives in subspecialty areas could be offered, such as adolescent gynecology (including experiences in family planning centers), adolescent learning problems, and the handicapped adolescent (depending on resources available).

Level II

Objective 1   Knowledge of normal physical, emotional, and psychological development of adolescence, including an understanding of the interactions of psychological and physical development.

Objective 2   Knowledge of social, cultural, and political influences upon adolescent development and behavior.

Objective 3   Skill in interviewing adolescents and their parents.

Objective 4   Understanding of adolescent sexuality.

Objective 5   Experience in family counseling.

Objective 6   Knowledge of community resources serving adolescents (e.g., schools, social agencies, "free" clinics, drug centers).

Objective 7   Ability to perform an adequate physical examination on adolescents.

Objective 8   Diagnosis and treatment of diseases and medical problems common in, and peculiar to, adolescence.

Objective 9 Diagnosis and management of adolescents with psychological, school, and social problems.

Objective 10 Ability to make appropriate organic and psychological referrals out of the adolescent clinic.

School Nurse Practitioner Program

To make high-quality health care more readily available to children, school nurses are obtaining additional education to expand their present roles and are becoming school nurse practitioners so they can provide diagnostic, therapeutic, and preventive health care; health education; and environmental health supervision. In consultation with physicians, these nurses, unlike other school nurses, are capable of performing these important health services:

1 They may develop a health history, including identification of a preventive health behavior profile for a child and his or her family.

2 They may perform physical, common neurological, and psychosocial examinations.

3 They are qualified to make primary diagnoses of childhood diseases and injuries.

4 They may, in collaboration with physicians and other health and school personnel, initiate and modify treatment plans for children.

5 They can teach children the skills necessary to become participatory health consumers and to assume greater responsibility for their own health care.

Several studies have concluded that, in the delivery of comprehensive health care for school children, school nurse practitioners have proven more effective than other kinds of school nurses.[3] Some reasons for these conclusions:

1 School nurse practitioners devote a larger portion of their time to thorough, extensive appraisals of health problems.

2 School nurse practitioners manage a significantly greater proportion of health problems without referral to others.

3 School nurse practitioners exclude only half as many children from school due to illness or health problems, thus reducing school absences.

4 School nurse practitioners counsel parents with sharply focused recommendations as to the health care attention required.

5 School nurse practitioners provide twice as much direct patient care as other school nurses.

6 School nurse practitioners are likely to triple the usual number of daily contacts with parents to discuss emotional, physical, learning, or other problems of students.

7   School health aides, teacher aides, and parent volunteers are an important asset in permitting school nurse practitioners to practice their expanded role.

SUMMARY

School health encompasses the delivery of health services, health education, and the provision of a safe and healthful environment. Adolescents are particularly in need of an effective school health program as they frequently fail to seek health care elsewhere except in times of emergency or illness. The school health program requires well-qualified personnel, including school nurse practitioners. The school clinic may often serve as a site for career development for those adolescents working as health clerks who are interested in health as a profession. Because of the importance of health to adolescents, the school program is of great interest to many adolescents.

REFERENCES

1   David Smith and Edwin Bierman, *The Biologic Ages of Man*. Philadelphia: W. B. Saunders, 1973, p. 143.
2   I. R. Shenker et al., "A Curriculum Guide for Adolescent Medicine. By the Committee on Education, Society for Adolescent Medicine," *Clinical Pediatrics*, **16**(6):516, June 1977.
3   Judith B. Igoe and Henry K. Silver, "Improving Health Care in the School Setting," *Nurse Practitioner*, September/October 1977, p. 7.

Chapter 16

College Health Programs

Peggie J. Moyer

College health programs have typically, in the past, been viewed as second-rate services provided in obsolete facilities by retired physicians and incompetent nurses. Over the past decade there has been a change. Administrators of colleges and universities have found that quality health programs are demanded or at least highly desired on their campuses. Students have provided much of the impetus for change. Their demand for a voice in decision making has pressured many college administrators to upgrade campus health services and facilities. Students and their parents recognize that the student years represent a major investment of time, money, and energy, and that ready access to high-quality health services is a protection of that commitment.

It is surprising, perhaps, but the availability of health care for young adults, particularly college students, has been far from adequate. Access to services has been limited because (1) students are basically young and thought to be completely healthy, (2) their health care needs are not seen as urgent by persons unfamiliar with adolescent health, and (3) their financial resources are often limited by parental control. A high-quality college health program is important, for it has the potential of

1   Detecting and reducing the effects of some debilitating disease conditions
2   Maintaining the health of persons engaged in highly demanding and significant endeavors
3   Preparing citizens concerned about the health and well-being of their community
4   Educating persons about health and maintenance of health

As with the colleges themselves, there is considerable variety in the size of facilities and the scope of services in college health programs. Some health services operate from one small office staffed by a nurse whose functions consist of triage and referral, first aid, and health education. In contrast to that kind of setting are those college health programs that operate large outpatient clinics in addition to providing the traditional hospital services, and employ a full complement of highly trained physicians and nurse specialists. Some college health programs are associated with medical centers or medical schools, while others are in isolated areas and are the only source of medical care for the student. Regardless of size or location, a good college health program is dependent upon

1   Adequate funding for its operation
2   A facility that allows for efficient functioning of staff
3   A staff that can produce quality patient care
4   Institutional support
5   Skillful management and administration of the health care program

High-quality health care is an important service to provide to students, but good college health programs do not just happen. The excellence of health care is largely dependent upon having a nursing staff that can produce quality patient care. To provide a high level of care is the responsibility of the college administration; to demand it is the right of students; to produce it is the obligation of health professionals.

CHARACTERISTICS OF THE CLIENTELE

Although the age range of students attending college is considerable, the great majority of students are young adults, and it is the purpose of this chapter to discuss components of college health nursing that focus on meeting the health needs of that age group. To best meet those needs it is important for the nurse to understand the developmental tasks of young adulthood, the typical factors motivating young adults to attend college, and the impact of the college setting on young people.

Developmental Tasks

Establishing one's personal identity and sharing oneself in intimate relationships are the major developmental tasks of this age group. Attainment of these tasks involves detachment from the family, selection of an occupation, development of a value system and ideology, and establishment of peer group roles and sex roles. According to Sheehy, there are two impulses at work during this period. One is "to build a firm and safe structure for the future by making strong commitments"; the other is "to explore and experiment, keeping any structure tentative and therefore easily reversible."[1] The nurse who understands and is sensitive to these developmental tasks has a head start on being able to facilitate the care of students who come to the health facility. The frustrations of dealing with developmental tasks and conflicting urges can result in health problems as diverse as attempted suicide, unwanted pregnancy, obesity, homosexual crisis, ulcers, depression, and alcoholism, to list just a few.

Motivation

Understanding students' motives for attending college can be helpful in understanding a student's health problem or response to a health problem. Not all students go to a college or university because of great interest or desire. Some are there because of parental pressure or what they perceive as societal expectation, or because they are seeking a mate. Others are sent by a sponsoring group, e.g., governmental agency, professional association, business concern, or ethnic group. Some students have come with clear-cut goals and the ready resources of intellect and finances but with little enthusiasm for the educational process. Others are highly motivated but frustrated by limited ability or resources. Some students are determined to prepare themselves for an occupation but are overwhelmed or confused by career choices.

The effects of motivation on health are often reflected in the way a student uses a college health facility. The commitment to meet educational goals is so great for some students that they fail to care for themselves properly and seek treatment only when they feel it is an absolute necessity. This kind of student may, by self-neglect, compound a health problem and further compromise his or her academic goals.

Such was the case for Elizabeth, who failed to appreciate the early warning symptoms of fatigue and refused to treat her diagnosis of mononucleosis seriously. The result was severe liver damage that required her to drop out of school for a year.

The problem was quite different for Greg, a junior, who was following in his father's footsteps by majoring in business. Greg suddenly began making frequent visits to the health center for a variety of problems, all of which were minor. On one visit, the nurse asked Greg how he really liked school. Greg admitted that he had wanted to become a social worker, but that he knew his father was counting on his taking over the family business. This discussion led the nurse to suggest that Greg consult with one of the health center's mental health specialists so he could get some objective, professional assistance in exploring his dilemma.

Impact of the College Setting on Health

Nurses should also be aware of the ways the college setting may affect the health and well-being of students. The college campus can be an impersonal and hostile environment for young people unaccustomed to being uprooted from family and friends, and having to prove their ability to faculty, to a new set of peers, and to the community left behind. Depression and loneliness are very painful problems for many students. Peer pressure often strongly influences the choices young people make about their activities. Experimentation with alcohol, other drugs, and sex, frequently the result of peer influence, may lead to serious health problems. Suicide and accidents are major killers of young adults, and all health professionals should be concerned about college students' special vulnerabilities to these tragedies while under pressure from other students to participate in hazardous activities.

STUDENT INVOLVEMENT IN THE OPERATION OF THE HEALTH FACILITY

Most college health centers are funded by health fees paid at the time students pay tuition. Students frequently demand that, since they must support the college health center, they want to have an influence in its operation and programs. Students, as consumers, should be involved in developing policies and programs, since it is their welfare and their needs that the program should be designed to serve.

Working with the consumer may be a frustrating task; frequently, it takes a lot of time to educate students to cost factors, availability of health personnel, and standards and legal requirements. However, failure to involve students, particularly in these times, may prohibit their support of health issues on campus. Further, failure to educate the young consumer becomes failure of the educational institution to prepare skillful and knowledgeable participants in community decision making. Students make many valuable and responsible contributions to policy and procedure, as will be described in later sections of this chapter.

EMPLOYEE SELECTION

In many college health centers, students are involved in interviewing and evaluating candidates for employment. This practice demonstrates to prospective employees that the student consumer has a voice in the functioning of the health center and that the health center accepts accountability for selecting practitioners who relate well to the student group. It further serves to help educate students about the various qualifications, viewpoints, availability, and salary expectations of health professionals.

The orientation of nurses new to college health begins with the initial employment interview. This interview provides an opportunity not only to evaluate a nurse's potential and ability for a job, but also to assess his or her attitudes about patient care, consumer involvement, and controversial health issues, such as sex education, availability of contraceptive services, mental health care, specialty clinics, and health fee versus fee for service.

Some of the questions that help students (and, of course, others) assess a nurse applicant are: What attracts you to college health work? What expectations do you have of students? How would you encourage student participation in the operation of the health center? In what priority would you list the services a health center should provide? How will working in this facility help meet your personal and professional goals?

The employment interview should also help orient a prospective employee to the institution's expectations regarding standards of performance and attitudes about providing care. Public relations problems in college health centers often arise when a receptionist exhibits a surly attitude or when a staff member has a condescending approach to patient care. Students want to feel that they are going to a place where they will be treated with personal and professional concern, where their rights to privacy and confidentiality will be respected, and where high-quality care is always available within a reasonable time. The health center is expected to select the staff necessary to meet this consumer goal.

OUTPATIENT CARE

Student input, through a student health advisory council, can be of valuable assistance to the administrative officers of the health facility in determining the priority and the scope of services. Generally, students place emphasis on the availability of efficient outpatient services. Outpatient care is more economical to provide than hospital care. Appropriately utilized, outpatient services reduce the incidence of debilitating illness, thus conserving the financial, physical, and mental resources of the student, the family, and the institution. The goal of the outpatient nursing program is to help students stay in school and minimize the effect of illness on their ability to achieve their educational goals.

The interest, motivation, and intellectual level of student outpatients offer the nurse an opportunity to examine with them their health habits, health values, the consequence of these habits and values to their future

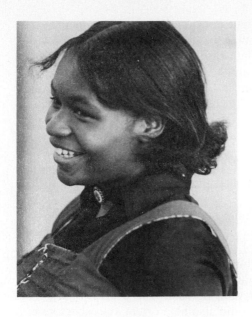

The consumers of student health services are a valuable advisory resource about policies, priorities, and procedures of the college health service and its programs. (*Copyright © 1980 by Patricia Yaros.*)

well-being, and the students' desires to make changes that might improve their future health. The college health nurse must be prepared to be questioned by students. Students frequently inquire about the source of information the nurse or the physician offers; study the literature about their illness, medication, or therapy; debate about their symptoms or diagnosis; challenge the effectiveness of their medication; and question the clinical management! For example, at one college health center, patients were asked to state the reason for their visit and one student wrote, "I had a cold three weeks ago. Last week you said it was an allergy. It is worse now after taking your pills. I need a new diagnosis." Effective college health nurses make time for questions and have the skills to help students learn more about their physical and mental health.

The American College Health Association recommends that provisions be made for seeing outpatients both by appointment and on a walk-in basis. Usually students, like other patients, are most satisfied when they can be seen by appointment rather than having to wait for long, undetermined periods of time. On the other hand, a large number of health problems of active young adults are unpredictable and sudden in origin. There must be an opportunity for students who have such problems to be seen promptly rather than deferred for some time until an appointment may be available.

Sexual Health

Students' educational needs related to sexual health are considerable. There are numerous ways in which nurses can participate in educational efforts to help students become more knowledgeable and, thus, more responsible for their sexual health. First, however, it is important for college health nurses to understand their feelings about contraception, abortion, venereal disease, and sexual practices. Many students are victims of poor judgment and misinformation, the results of which may be shattered egos, impotence, gonorrhea, or unwanted pregnancy. These students need help to explore the alternatives for dealing with an unwanted pregnancy, relief of suffering from the pains of rejection and guilt, and assistance in sorting through the confusion that sometimes accompanies sexual experimentation. Working with these problems in either an educational, curative, or preventative way calls for nursing approaches which are sensitive and knowledgeable and which do not ridicule the student.

During the past decade women have especially been vocal about the expectations they have for health care. Until the early 1970s, most college health programs had limited gynecological services or none. This situation is now the exception. Smaller college health programs that cannot provide comprehensive gynecological services do provide many educational services regarding female health. The larger programs employ gynecologists and nurses with special preparation in gynecological nursing. In most college health centers, female students are encouraged to have yearly gynecological examinations and are taught breast self-examination for early cancer detection. They are provided with services, not lectures or condemnation, if they have problems with venereal disease, unwanted pregnancy, or vaginitis, or if they seek contraceptive advice or help.

Residence hall programs, in which students can interact with several multidisciplined professionals who are comfortable discussing aspects of sexuality, can help provide students with a greater awareness of the issues and responsibilities related to sexual activity, knowledge of educational and health resources, and an opportunity for value clarification. Professionals from medicine, mental health counseling, social work, religion, sociology, law, home economics, and nursing are among those that can be valuable participants in these discussions. Commonly such groups discuss such topics as these:

1 The difference between responsible and irresponsible sexual activity
2 The consequences of irresponsible sex
3 The games people play
4 The impact of religion on sexual behavior
5 The barriers to sexual adequacy and fulfillment
6 The effects of changing sex roles on sex, marriage, and child rearing
7 The legal considerations of confidentiality, venereal disease, abortion, marriage, divorce, unusual sexual practices, or rape

Much of the value of such programs is the interaction that takes place among students and between students and the health professionals.

Nurses should participate in and promote other activities that help meet the educational needs of students as they relate to sexual health. At no cost, or minimal cost, the nurse can make available brochures and pamphlets that have been developed by various agencies and organizations. The American College Health Association has developed several pamphlets particularly appropriate for the young adult in the college setting ("What You Should Know about Contraception," "Sexual Dysfunction—An Aspect of Being Human," "Drug Use during Pregnancy?" and "Love Means Taking Care—What You Should Know about Venereal Disease"). Other activities might include developing educational displays; providing conferences on aspects of sexuality; promoting classes on female health; utilizing the college newspaper, radio, and television to acquaint students with health resources; and providing articles on protection from venereal disease, the considerations of abortion, etc.

Specialty Services

A service frequently requested by students is a weight control and weight reduction program. Although concern about appearance and not health is the major motivation for this request, once students are enrolled in a weight control program, they begin to learn new concepts of health and begin to develop habits that will protect their future health. There are many health benefits to be accrued from this type of program. If the student is successful in weight reduction, the risk of cardiovascular problems associated with obesity is reduced. Self-concept is enhanced, which frequently improves interpersonal relationships and mental health. Nurses can provide or promote weight control programs. They can also work with food service personnel on campus and in sororities and fraternities to provide a food selection that enables students to properly reduce or maintain their weight. Other appropriate nursing activities include working with students from the department of home economics (or other interested persons) to develop a campaign to provide healthful food in vending machines; placing bulletins and placards in such places as campus bulletin boards and buses to promote healthful eating habits; and providing articles for the college newspaper about the consequences of obesity and the available resources for students afflicted with this health problem.

Dermatologic services are also a special need of the young adult. Many college health centers cannot afford a full-time dermatologist but make limited services available on a contractual basis. For young adults, the psychological aspects of skin problems are as important as the physical ones. If a student's severe acne responds well to treatment, perhaps his or her self-concept need not be the concern of the health professional;

but the nurse must carefully observe behavior to identify those students who need the help not only of a skin specialist but also of a mental health specialist.

Mental Health Services

> Sound emotional health is recognized widely as being essential if full use is to be made of both individual and institutional resources in expanding the horizons of students and achieving the educational goals of the institution. It is through integration of thought, feeling, and action that students and others can release the full vigor of their critical and creative facilities and develop a robust response to environmental stresses. Each institution has an opportunity—indeed, an obligation—to see this period of continuing change and remarkable flexibility in the lives of students as a rich opportunity to promote the development and synthesis of personality functions and relationships which will form the basis of continuing creative personal growth. It is important, therefore, that every institution make available for students, through either its own or extramural resources, appropriate skilled professional assistance in coping with the emotional facets of their personal and social lives during this critical period.[3]

College health nurses are challenged to provide health care that is supportive of the emotional growth and well-being of the young adult, as well as providing appropriate physical care. Nurses need to be keenly aware of their abilities and limitations for helping students with mental health problems. The skillful nurse can help students evaluate their behavior, explore their feelings, identify their frustrations, and clarify their values—or the nurse can refer the student for help. Above all, it is important that college health service nurses be able to recognize mental health problems and guide the student to some appropriate source of assistance. Many potentially disabling emotional difficulties can be corrected if they are promptly identified and skillfully treated.

Frequently, students need considerable support and encouragement to accept referral to a mental health service. Some are less reluctant to seek help if they can be part of a group, rather than if only individual therapy is available. For that reason many mental health programs provide group sessions. Groups usually are organized around a particular focus, such as (1) growth groups, in which students explore their thoughts about themselves, their relationships with others, their feelings about parents, their concerns about their futures, etc.; (2) couples groups, in which married or single couples explore the nature of their relationships; (3) stress groups, where students (particularly graduate students) examine their responses to stress situations and explore alternative ways for coping with stress; and (4) groups for divorcees, where students explore their feelings about their divorces and search for positive ways of adjusting to the consequent changes in their lives. Some students may need individual counseling and therapy.

INPATIENT SERVICES

Most colleges have found it necessary to provide some type of bed care for students. Inpatient services vary among institutions from temporary day care to complete general hospital care, including surgery. Most college health centers provide intermediate bed care and refer their patients to general hospital facilities for more intensive medical care and surgery. Inpatient care within the college has several advantages. It provides for students who are too ill to be in their regular living quarters but not in need of hospitalization. It facilitates the removal of students with a communicable disease from an environment where the infection is likely to be quickly shared with others. A college inpatient center allows students who need bed care to maintain relatively close contact with classes and the academic setting; this is especially helpful to students with mild emotional problems. Finally, an inpatient unit for college students is more likely than a facility for the general population to provide a staff that relates well to the special needs of young adults.

Nurses staffing the inpatient unit of the college health center must be as perceptive of the needs and characteristics of student patients as nurses who work in the outpatient services, previously discussed.

One nurse, Ms. T., left college health nursing because of her difficulty in adjusting to the changing "permissiveness" of the college health center. A male student, admitted for a lengthy hospitalization because of a back injury, offended Ms. T. by taping some posters (of questionable taste) to the wall around his bed. Her response was to refuse to give the student his medications until he removed the posters. The patient refused. Ms. T. complained to the director of nursing, who explained that Ms. T. was obligated to provide the patient his medication and suggested ways that were more appropriate for dealing with the patient's behavior. Ms. T. felt that she could demand that the patient conform to her rules of behavior and, when her actions were not supported, she resigned. What she failed to see was that she had an opportunity for significant dialogue and interaction with the student.

Another nurse asked the patient if he would remove the posters because other people found them offensive and because tape would mar the walls if left there too long. She continued to talk with the patient and found he was both anxious and angry about his illness, was concerned about the need for surgery, and was concerned about whether or not he could continue in school and whether or not he was going to have a permanent disability. Later, the patient removed his most objectionable posters; the nursing staff found "replacements," and, soon after, there developed a more supportive climate for the patient's hospitalization.

EDUCATION FOR HEALTH

The American College Health Association recognizes that one of the most important objectives of a college health program is "the development of a resource for influencing the health behavior of students, both as individuals, and as active participants in the community."[4] Each contact the student has with a nurse should be an example of high-quality care, and no opportunity should be missed to help students understand more about their health, their health problems, and ways to maintain or attain health. A female student with recurrent cystitis needs to understand the importance of properly taking her medication, the need for a high fluid intake and personal hygiene, the importance of voiding after sexual intercourse, the advantages of cotton underclothing, and so forth. The future health of a student with early hypertension may be related to how well health professionals help him or her understand the potential seriousness of present symptoms.

Young adults are eager to know more about themselves. This developmental trait makes health education a necessary and effective component of a college health program. Health fairs are an interesting way of exciting students about health, alerting them to new health concepts, making them aware of new technology, and providing them with useful health information they can take home with them.

Health forums dealing with such issues as drug use and abuse, food fads, smoking, depression, abortion, homosexuality, etc., can stimulate the interest and intelligent concern of the entire campus community. Many colleges have general courses on personal and community health through which students develop an understanding of the dynamics of bodily functions and the interrelationship of human beings and their environment. These classes also increase awareness of community health problems, health issues, and individual responsibility to community health. Nurses should know about these resources and help promote their development if they are insufficient.

As mentioned before, many health-related agencies and organizations have developed health information materials appropriate for distribution to college students. Some college health centers, working in conjunction with student groups or through individual staff effort, have developed their own materials. Working with students can be especially valuable in selecting brochures which have student appeal, in evaluating the interest and need for the information, and in determining the most effective means for distributing the materials. On one campus, students decided that taping bulletins to the stall doors of dormitory toilets would provide interesting reading material for a captive audience. The material was changed often and received much favorable comment. Journalism or other communications students help by preparing articles for the college newspaper, radio spots, slide/tape or film presentations, bulletins, brochures, and posters. The benefits of getting students involved in these activities are that students learn more about health, become acquainted with health professionals, and provide a valuable service that is well accepted by the students to whom the activities are directed.

College health centers can also sponsor small group discussions in dormitories, sororities, fraternities, the student union, and other appropriate settings in which significant health concerns can be explored. Students need to understand the consequences of improper drug use, the dangers of alcohol, the research findings on the use of marijuana, etc. These are sensitive subjects, and students can be greatly helped by opportunities to talk freely without fearing reprisal, and to talk with professionals who come with facts and supported opinions rather than moral judgments. Students need to feel that they will not be labeled drug users, alcoholics, etc., because they have attended a session. Health education is not a luxury service of a college health center, it is a necessary component of any high-quality college health program. The health industry and educational system have an obligation to help consumers stay healthy and to help them be intelligent users of health resources.

VOLUNTEER PROGRAMS

To maximize the availability of health resources, some college health centers have established effective volunteer programs. A properly managed volunteer program can have significant benefits for a college health center. Volunteers recruited from the community help create a closer bond between "town and gown." Not infrequently, a volunteer becomes an advocate for the health center and increases the community's understanding of the health problems and needs of young adults on a college campus.

Volunteer programs frequently are the responsibility of the nursing department. Experience indicates that the dependability of volunteer help is greatest when the coordinator for the program is a volunteer rather than a college employee. It is this person's responsibility to schedule the staffing of volunteers and to arrange for replacements when there are absences. It is essential that the volunteer coordinator work closely with a designated staff person so that the volunteers are selectively screened and provided with appropriate orientation. Volunteers are seen by the patient as staff members, so it is important to have a system for evaluating volunteers. The confidentiality of medical and personal information about patients must be thoroughly understood by volunteers; they must also know the policies and procedures of the health center pertaining to their work.

When volunteers or paid student health aides are recruited from the

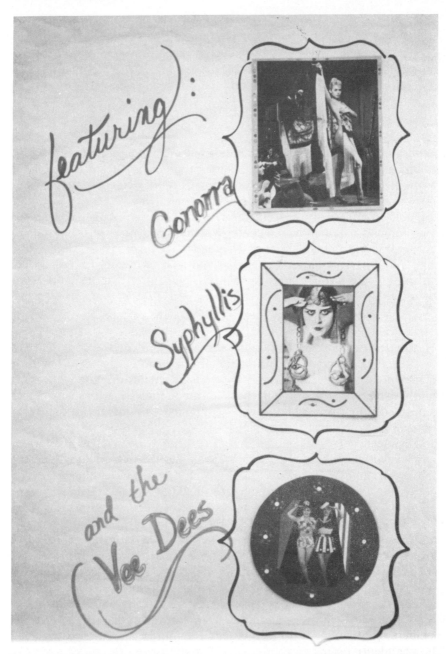

featuring:

Gonorra

Syphyllis

and the Vee Dees

Student-designed health education programs and informational materials, such as this part of an announcement for a venereal disease information session, generally have a flair that elicits response from the other young people for whom they are intended. (*Photo courtesy of the University of Georgia Health Service.*)

student population, discretion must be used to select students who work well with staff and who do not use their position as a volunteer for personal benefit. If initial care is taken to develop the volunteer program, considerable financial savings can be realized, and an effective public relations program for both the institution and the community can also result.

NURSE PRACTITIONERS

Several educational programs have been developed to prepare nurse practitioners for college health work. These programs are designed to expand the skill and knowledge of registered nurses so they can assume increased responsibility in the delivery of primary health care. Nurse practitioners are able to effectively and efficiently manage large numbers of patients who come to a student health center with clearly defined health problems. Nurse practitioners and other new categories of health professionals offer a potential savings in personnel cost and tend to increase the quality of a center's care through more specific assignment of responsibility.

ETHICAL CONSIDERATIONS

Health professionals in college centers *must* protect the confidentiality of student information. Students have been critical of student health facilities in the past because staff too freely shared information with faculty and members of the administration. This breach of ethics has caused students to be distrustful and has kept unknown numbers of them from obtaining health care.

In most centers the only information that may be given to institutional officials without a student's permission is that the individual was seen at the health center and the date and time of the visit. The established ethical codes consider all other information confidential between the health center and the student. Information should be released *only* with the specific written authorization of the student. Certain departures from this principle are indicated in the case of minors, and under circumstances involving threat to the public health or distinct danger to the student or others if the information is *not* shared. Laws vary from state to state, especially in areas of confidentiality, minority rights, informed consent, reportable diseases, and abortion services. Nurses need to be aware of the legal regulations governing their practice with college students. The ethics of health care in colleges are discussed at length in the American College Health Association's *Recommended Standards and Practices for a College Health Program.*[5]

It is important that the health center maintain a reputation for confidentiality [of student information] so that . . . students with personal problems will feel free to seek help without fear of dissemination of the information. There should be no intimation at any time that seeking such help from the health service will result in any action which may lead to disciplinary action on the part of the institution. . . .

For the health service to be cast in the role of disciplinarian, or even to appear to assume this role, is in opposition to its purpose and is contrary to the principles of medical ethics. Matters of felony should be reported in accordance with state laws. In other disciplinary matters, as part of the management of a problem, the health professional may counsel the patient to report the matter or to take action, but the therapist's primary responsibility remains to the patient and not to any institution.[6]

STUDENTS WITH SPECIAL HEALTH NEEDS

While there are many similarities among young adults with regard to their health needs, there is also, of course, great variety. Handicapped young people with good intellectual ability have been encouraged to attend college. Often the availability of adequate health care can be a determining factor in their opportunity to complete their educational goals. Foreign students are another group who require special consideration. College health nurses must be prepared to deal with cultural differences, differing expectations for health care, difficulties in communication, and situational problems which are often quite challenging.

Alex, a young foreign student, had been sent to the United States by his government to study agricultural economics. He was overwhelmed by the largeness of the college campus, isolated, and extremely lonely because there was no one on campus who spoke his native language. Alex was brought to the health center one evening by some students who found him sitting alone in the basement of the library muttering and crying. The health center was able to locate an interpreter and to provide a supportive climate for Alex. It was determined that Alex had a severe emotional problem that made it impossible for him to continue in school. The question then was what to do with Alex. He was financially unable to pay for private care and ineligible for public funding. He wanted to return home, but it was felt that until his health improved he could not travel alone. He did not have money for travel fare, neither did his family, and it was difficult working through bureaucratic governmental agencies to find assistance. Eventually help was found to return Alex to his home, but the circumstances of his illness called for resourceful intervention by the health care team.

Minority groups also have expressed a need to know that the health center has staff professionals that they can relate to, preferably persons of their ethnic background. When this is not possible, the staff have an obligation to assess their effectiveness in providing health care to minority patients and take the necessary steps to provide these patients with health care that is well received.

REFERENCES

1 Gail Sheehy, *Passages: Predictable Crises of Adult Life*. New York: E. P. Dutton and Co., 1976, p. 86.
2 American College Health Association, *Recommended Standards and Practices for a College Health Program* (3d rev.). Evanston, Ill.: ACHA, 1977, p. 6.*
3 Ibid., p. 8.*
4 Ibid., p. 13.*
5 Ibid.
6 Ibid., pp. 32, 34.*

BIBLIOGRAPHY

American College Health Association: *Recommended Standards and Practices for a College Health Program*, 3d rev. Evanston, Ill.: ACHA, 1977.
————: *The Development of Health Programs for Junior Colleges and Colleges*, Rev. 1977.
Chinn, Peggy L.: *Child Health Maintenance*. St. Louis: C. V. Mosby Co., 1974.
Helms, Donald, and Jeffrey S. Turner: *Exploring Child Behavior*. Philadelphia: W. B. Saunders Co., 1976.
Levey, Samuel, and N. Paul Loomba: *Health Care Administration: Managerial Perspective*. Philadelphia: J. B. Lippincott, 1973.
Redman, Barbara Klug: *The Process of Patient Teaching in Nursing*, 3d ed. St. Louis: C. V. Mosby Co., 1976.
Sheehy, Gail: *Passages: Predictable Crises of Adult Life*. New York: E. P. Dutton and Co., 1976.
Yaros, Patricia S.: "The Adolescent," in Gladys M. Scipien et al. (eds.), *Comprehensive Pediatric Nursing* (2d ed.). New York: McGraw-Hill Book Co., 1979.

*Quoted with the permission of the *Journal of the American College Health Association* from Volume 25, Special Issue, March 1977.

Substance Abuse
Treatment Settings

Dee Williams

The treatment and rehabilitation of young people who abuse drugs is a community concern. It requires the involvement of a wide variety of community organizations, agencies, and individuals, and multiple treatment modalities must be available if a community is to succeed in its efforts to aid the adolescent drug abuser.

In some areas, the already existing health, counseling, and educational facilities have tailored their services to include intervention with drug-abusing adolescents. "Rap houses" may offer free drug analysis, peer counseling, professional counseling, and referral for appropriate drug abuse intervention. Free clinics (see Chapter 14) may deal with drug abuse in the course of treating other problems of young people. Schools may create peer counseling programs which are available to students with drug problems. Detoxification units can be established in hospitals and clinics that already function as treatment resources within the community. Crisis centers may advertise a telephone hot line to deal specifically with the problems of young people.

If a community is unable to meet the needs of its drug-abusing adolescents through existing facilities, then new ones are needed. Specialized programs for the treatment of substance abuse in adolescents include detoxification centers, residential care facilities, maintenance programs, self-help groups, and counseling programs, each of which will be discussed in this chapter. The purpose of this discussion is to describe the overall treatment programs and the settings in which treatment and rehabilitation are provided to adolescents, rather than to instruct the reader about specific nursing problems and interventions. However, since facilities and services obviously must be planned in accordance with the needs of the clients, some description of withdrawal syndromes and related problems is included.

DETOXIFICATION CENTERS

Detoxification is the physiologic process of reducing the toxicity of a substance. Time is the key factor in this metabolic process, and little can be done to accelerate or retard detoxification. Medical supervision is unnecessary for adolescents who are detoxifying after abuse of most of the psychoactive drugs. Persons who are physically dependent on alcohol and/or barbiturates are exceptions to this generality.

Withdrawal from alcohol or barbiturates may be accomplished in a conventional hospital setting in communities where no special detoxification center exists. Some hospitals have adolescent units and can accommodate adolescents there for the withdrawal process (see Chapter 12 for discussion of the advisability of admitting detoxification patients to adolescent inpatient areas). Some communities have responded to their need for a drug withdrawal program by establishing special detoxification centers, usually housed separately from the local hospital. Such facilities generally are available to persons detoxifying from any type of drug, and intensive medical and nursing supervision are provided for those with alcohol or barbiturate dependence.

Detoxification centers need to offer a broad therapeutic program that includes regularly scheduled group meetings (both therapeutic and educational), individual counseling sessions, nutritious meals (see Chapter 5 for a discussion of the special nutritional requirements of adolescent drug users), free time, family involvement, and an effective process for ensuring follow-up treatment after discharge from the facility. Drug use in general, not just withdrawal, should be discussed. The environment should be geared to the needs and developmental characteristics and tasks of adolescents. For example, the decor should permit informal interaction. Staff members may be more effective if they wear casual street clothes rather than uniforms. While adolescents in the initial phases of withdrawal may not feel well enough to participate, activities such as television, games, records, and crafts need to be available for those who are interested.

Alcohol Withdrawal

Alcohol withdrawal is more severe and life-threatening than withdrawal from narcotics or barbiturates. The withdrawal syndrome (described in Chapter 6) is generally of shorter duration but greater intensity for adolescents than for adults. The detoxification process lasts about three to five days, but complete recovery from delirium tremens can take up to three weeks.[1] Each alcohol-dependent youth should have a physical assessment upon admission. If traumatic injury is suspected, x-rays should be taken. Blood work should include liver and kidney function analyses, blood glucose measurement, a check for electrolyte balance, and screening for infectious organisms. Treatment during detoxification consists of drug therapy, correction of fluid and electrolyte imbalances, and supportive measures. Drug therapy is initiated with the objective of preventing or minimizing delirium tremens. If the alcohol-dependent adolescent has had severe diarrhea or vomiting, oral or parenteral fluids and electrolytes are given. Supportive measures include rest, counseling, treatment of other health problems, and diet therapy.[2,3]

Barbiturate Withdrawal

The barbiturate withdrawal syndrome (described more fully in Chapter 6) resembles withdrawal from alcohol and may include convulsions and acute psychosis. Phenobarbital and pentobarbital are the most frequently used medications for the treatment of barbiturate withdrawal. A stabilizing or maintenance dose of these drugs is given for two or three days, after which the daily dose is gradually reduced at a rate which does not precipitate severe withdrawal symptoms. Withdrawal may take as long as two weeks. Fluid and electrolyte replacement may be necessary. The adolescent benefits from general supportive therapy such as diet management, rest, and the treatment of any physical complications or illnesses.[4]

Some detoxification centers are prepared to care for adolescents who have taken overdoses of drugs. Barbiturate overdose may result from repeated large doses taken within a short period of time, from the combining of significant quantities of short- and long-acting barbiturates, or from mixing barbiturates with other drugs such as heroin or alcohol. The barbiturate overdose victim is usually comatose; shock may be present or may develop later. Care requirements may include assisted ventilation; intravenous therapy to counteract electrolyte imbalances, hypovolemia, and hypotension; gastric lavage, forced diuresis, and/or dialysis to speed detoxification; and such general supportive measures for comatose patients as skin care, prevention of corneal damage, etc. Barbiturate overdose may be complicated by respiratory infection, pulmonary edema, atelectasis, aspiration, urinary tract infection, and severe bullous lesions of the skin.[5]

Narcotic Withdrawal

Although repeated, regular use of narcotics may produce physical dependence in the abuser, the withdrawal syndrome (described in Chapter 6) is usually not life-threatening and can be managed in a nonmedical setting. There are two accepted methods of narcotic withdrawal: abrupt abstinence ("cold turkey") and methadone withdrawal. Heroin is the most widely abused narcotic, and for that reason the discussion here will pertain to heroin. Unless otherwise indicated, however, statements also apply to morphine.

In the abrupt withdrawal process, the abuser simply endures the discomforts experienced. Some take medications for relief of various symptoms: for example, chloral hydrate for insomnia, a muscle relaxant for cramps, an antiemetic for vomiting. Symptoms usually last about 4 to 10 days.[6]

Methadone withdrawal involves the substitution of methadone for heroin and a gradual reduction in dose so that withdrawal symptoms are prevented or at least minimal. Detoxification is complete in 4 to 10 days.[7] Methadone maintenance programs are discussed below.

Detoxification centers may treat adolescents for narcotic overdose. Overdose results from use of a particularly potent batch of the drug, from use of a dose in excess of his or her reduced tolerance by a person who has recently withdrawn, or from suicide attempt. The needs of patients who have overdosed with narcotics are similar to those of persons with barbiturate overdose, discussed briefly above.

Amphetamine Psychosis and LSD "Bad Trips"

Detoxification centers may be called upon to treat young people experiencing amphetamine psychosis or hallucinogen-related "bad trips." The administration of large doses of amphetamines for several days may result in hallucinations, paranoid ideation, and impulsive, sometimes violent, behavior. Most amphetamine abusers learn to accept these paranoid symptoms, expecting them to disappear after sleep and detoxification. Occasionally someone becomes distraught enough to seek relief or comes to the attention of a helping organization. Hospitals have used diazepam (Valium) to calm amphetamine abusers. This is not usually necessary and may even reinforce users' belief that people are trying to harm them. In a safe environment with a trusted person to provide reassurance, the amphetamine abuser is likely to sleep. This reassurance and supervision can occur in a drug detoxification center, in a youth-oriented rap house, or in the home of a friend. The person working with the user can be a family member, a volunteer or professional counselor, or a friend. Sleep may last for several days before the user awakens feeling hungry, fatigued, and depressed. These feelings may continue for several weeks of abstinence. Suicidal thoughts and behavior may result if the depression is severe.[8]

"Bad trips" are usually associated with LSD use but may result from the use of any of the hallucinogens. The user begins to feel anxious, paranoid, and confused. Perceptual distortions produced by the drug become frightening. The adolescent may believe he or she is "going crazy."[9]

Administration of chlorpromazine (Thorazine) will end the LSD trip and has been used for this purpose in hospitals. However, increased incidence of suicide is associated with this method of treatment. The recommended method of treatment for bad trips is the "talk down" approach. The user should be placed in a room with minimal stimuli. One person, preferably someone the adolescent already knows and trusts, stays with the user for the duration of the trip. If this is not possible, two people may alternate if the adolescent is comfortable with both. The intervening person should assure the user that the experience is drug-related and will end. The user should be encouraged to describe his or her perceptions. The intervening person should present the adolescent with pleasant images to think about. If, after 8 to 10 hours, the user seems no better, it may be assumed that more in-depth treatment is needed. The adolescent should then be referred to a psychiatric facility (it is possible for LSD use to precipitate a psychotic episode in a susceptible individual).[10,11]

RESIDENTIAL TREATMENT PROGRAMS

The two types of residential care facilities most commonly used for the treatment of adolescent drug abusers are halfway houses and therapeutic communities.

Halfway Houses

A halfway house provides a structured, drug-free, live-in environment for the adolescent drug abuser. Most facilities are administered by public or private agencies and are staffed by professional and paraprofessional counselors. Most programs require the adolescent to have completed withdrawal prior to moving into the house. Residents are required to go to school or to work, to be responsible for their own activities of daily living, to participate in the upkeep of the house (e.g., cleaning up, doing yard work, making repairs), and to participate in scheduled treatment programs. Treatment may include group therapy, individual therapy, educational groups, and/or family therapy. Though staff do provide structure, the adolescents are basically responsible for themselves.[12]

Adolescents may enter halfway houses specifically designed for drug abusers or they may be admitted to programs that deal also with adolescents who have various emotional problems. It is not usually beneficial to place an adolescent in a halfway house facility designed to treat adults. A halfway house is an especially appropriate choice for adolescents who would benefit from either temporary or permanent separation from their families. Lengths of stay vary but usually do not exceed three to six months. At the end of that time the adolescents must either return to their families or function independently outside the halfway house.

Therapeutic Communities

Although the therapeutic community as a concept originated in work with the mentally ill, the term also describes a mode of residential treatment specifically for drug abusers. Synanon, founded in California in 1958 by Charles Dederick, a recovered alcoholic, served for many years as the prototype for all therapeutic communities for drug abusers.* Predicated on the idea that drug abusers cannot abstain from psychoactive substances in a drug-oriented society, Synanon created a drug-free subculture. Drug abusers accepted into the program enter a new "family." They are expected to participate in treatment, work and/or go to school, and live in the therapeutic community. Synanon does not claim to prepare the recovered abuser for return to society, because this seems synonymous to them with a return to drug use. Instead Synanon has homes in which recovered abusers live, businesses in which they work, and ongoing treatment to help them maintain abstinence.[13]

Several other well-known therapeutic communities, including Daytop Village and Phoenix House, have been developed following Synanon's basic treatment philosophy but with one major difference. These more recently developed programs do have reentry of the recovered abuser into society as their long-term goal. Admission criteria vary but therapeutic communities are quite selective. Most programs require that the applicant demonstrate some degree of motivation for change. Some therapeutic communities have detoxification facilities to treat the newly accepted resident during withdrawal. Others require that the abuser be drug-free on admission. Programs are generally divided into phases. New residents remain under strict supervision until they graduate into the second phase of the program. Gradually earning increasing privileges along with increasing responsibility, residents work through succeeding program phases. Graduation may take up to two years.[14]

The major treatment modality in most therapeutic communities is the group encounter in which attitudes, values, and interpersonal relationships are examined and critiqued. Individual counseling, vocational guidance,

---

*The fact that Synanon has recently been implicated in extreme sociopolitical activities has brought its status as a model into question, however.

educational groups, and family involvement may also be included in the total treatment approach.[15]

Originally, therapeutic communities were administered by former drug abusers, many of whom had also graduated from a therapeutic community. Because of the belief that the recovered abuser was in a better position to understand the resident than was a professional counselor, in most programs professionals were involved only in an advisory or consultative capacity. However, some therapeutic communities have more recently come to value professional counselors as equals in the treatment of drug abusers and are utilizing a combination of staff.[16]

The effectiveness of the therapeutic community approach to the treatment of drug abusers is not assured. Charles Dederick is quoted as having said that Synanon is probably suitable for only 1 out of 10 drug abusers. It appeals mainly to single, more dependent, young abusers. Though Phoenix House and Daytop Village publish impressive statistics on recovery (up to 85 percent), these figures often reflect the percentage of *program graduates* who maintain a drug-free life. That is, these figures do not include persons who drop out of treatment before graduation, and it is known that the longer a drug abuser remains in treatment, the greater is the chance of abstinence.[17]

MAINTENANCE PROGRAMS

The two drugs that are frequently used in the rehabilitation of drug abusers are disulfiram (Antabuse), used as an incentive for abstinence from alcohol, and methadone, which is used in the maintenance of physically dependent narcotic abusers. A third group of drugs, the narcotic antagonists, is being considered as a possible adjunct for the future treatment of narcotic abusers. The use of any medication to treat adolescent drug abuse should be viewed as only one part of the rehabilitation process.

Disulfiram Therapy

If there is a sufficient blood level of disulfiram, the person who then drinks becomes violently ill. Disulfiram inhibits the complete metabolism of alcohol in the body and produces a buildup of acetaldehyde, a toxin. The alcohol-disulfiram reaction is experienced as a pounding headache, flushing of the face, fall in blood pressure, nausea, vomiting, diarrhea, heart palpitations, perspiration, dizziness, anxiety, and confusion. The intensity of the reaction varies with the disulfiram blood level, the quantity of alcohol ingested, and the individual person's sensitivity.[18]

Disulfiram may be taken by oneself, as any other medication might be, or it may be administered in a supervised program. Disulfiram clinics are often one of the services offered by detoxification centers, alcohol

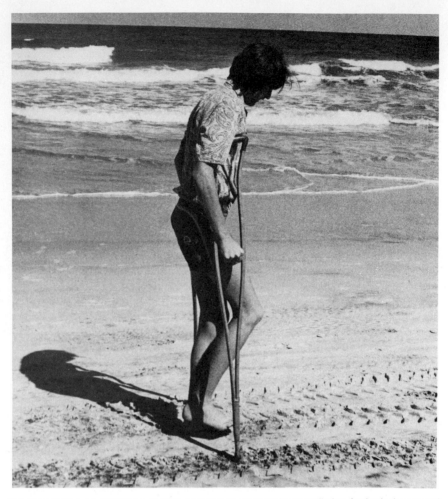

Treatment and rehabilitation of drug abusers must include remediation for both the mental and the physical health problems that have contributed to or resulted from the abuse. (*Copyright © 1980 by Anne Campbell.*)

halfway houses, and mental health centers. In some communities local resource people such as pharmacists, ministers and public health nurses monitor patients' disulfiram regimens. The purpose of the supervision is to help ensure that the abuser takes the medication.

Alcohol abuse among adolescents has only recently begun to receive serious attention from those concerned with its treatment. For this reason it has been somewhat uncommon to find an adolescent participating in disulfiram therapy. There are at this time, however, no published contraindications for the drug's use with young people. As the awareness of teenage alcohol abuse grows, so may the use of disulfiram as an adjunct form of treatment.

Methadone Maintenance

Methadone is a synthetic narcotic introduced in the United States after World War II. In 1964 Dr. Vincent Dole and Dr. Marie Nyswander began researching the use of methadone to maintain those persons physically dependent on other narcotics, particularly heroin. Their major rationale for maintenance programs rather than withdrawal came from the clinical observation that an abuser's drug craving following withdrawal frequently resulted in renewed heroin use. At low doses methadone blocks the symptoms of heroin withdrawal and prevents drug hunger. At higher doses it also blocks the effects of heroin if the abuser takes heroin in conjunction with the methadone.[19]

In addition methadone can be legally acquired, it is taken in a single daily oral dose, it is inexpensive, and in therapeutic doses it does not result in alterations in perception or consciousness. Such merits eliminate the necessity of the heroin abuser's involvement in a criminal, unproductive, and unhealthy life-style for the sake of drug procurement and use. On the other hand, opponents of methadone maintenance programs argue that methadone is a narcotic, that the abuser is still "addicted" to a drug, that it does not solve any underlying emotional problems, and that it does not guarantee the return of the abuser to a socially acceptable lifestyle. Methadone maintenance is obviously not "the cure" for narcotic abuse, but it seems to be one of the reasonable approaches to treatment.[20]

The use of methadone is strictly controlled by both federal and state statutes. The Dole and Nyswander program serves as the prototype for most other maintenance regimens. Initially the abuser is given small divided doses of methadone, approximately 10 mg twice a day by mouth. The amount is adjusted to individual response to prevent the occurrence of withdrawal symptoms. This dose is gradually increased over four to six weeks to a maintenance level of 80 to 120 mg per day in a single dose. This initial phase of treatment occurs in a hospital or in a medically supervised outpatient facility. Once the maintenance dose is reached, the client returns daily to the methadone clinic until he or she demonstrates sufficient motivation and responsibility to be allowed to take home several days' supply of the drug for self-administration. The frequency of clinic visits is gradually reduced as the client progresses in treatment.[21]

Numerous side effects have been reported by persons on methadone maintenance regimens. These include constipation, sleep disturbances, increased perspiration, muscle cramps, and sexual dysfunction. Persons taking methadone should not be given pentazocine (Talwin) for pain, because it blocks the effects of methadone and may precipitate narcotic withdrawal symptoms. Methadone overdoses have resulted in death, usually following accidental ingestion by young children. (The drug is frequently mixed in an orange-flavored liquid which may be mistaken for juice.) Withdrawal from methadone takes longer than withdrawal from heroin but is not necessarily more uncomfortable.[22]

The safety and effectiveness of methadone maintenance for narcotic abusers under 18 years of age is still in question. Therefore, certain restrictions apply to its use with adolescents. Since December 15, 1972, methadone maintenance for persons between the ages of 16 and 18 has been permitted only after at least a two-year history of narcotic abuse and at least two unsuccessful efforts at withdrawal. Parental consent must be obtained before persons between 16 and 18 are admitted to maintenance programs. Adolescents below the age of 16 may be detoxified with methadone but not maintained on it. Detoxification cannot take longer than three weeks and may not be repeated until at least four weeks after the last withdrawal period.[23]

Narcotic Antagonists

The use of narcotic antagonists in the treatment of narcotic dependency is now under study. Such drugs, when taken on a maintenance basis, attenuate or abolish the effects of narcotics and prevent the development of physical dependence. If a person on an antagonist maintenance regimen uses narcotics, both the reinforcing pleasures of the narcotic use and the fears of withdrawal are absent.[24]

The narcotic antagonists currently available are not practical for maintenance programs, however. Nalorphine (Nalline) has a duration of action of only a few hours. Naloxone (Narcan) is relatively weak when taken by mouth so the dose must be greatly increased. It is also expensive. Some of the narcotic antagonists can produce a physical dependence of their own which, following abstinence, results in a mild withdrawal syndrome. Cyclazocine is effective when taken orally but produces unpleasant side effects. It seems, therefore, that the use of narcotic antagonists in a maintenance program represents a possible form of treatment for narcotic abuse, but an effective and desirable antagonist has yet to be developed.[25]

SELF-HELP GROUPS

The best known self-help group in the world is Alcoholics Anonymous. Founded in the United States in the 1930s, A.A. is based on the premise that the person best able to help an alcoholic in efforts to maintain sobriety is another alcoholic. A.A. is the most effective program known for the treatment of alcohol abusers. Meetings are held as often as possible during each week, with the format varying from group to group. Some group meetings are open to all interested persons, and others are "closed," with attendance limited to alcoholics. Because of an increasing awareness of the problems of adolescent alcohol abusers, some A. A. chapters have started groups particularly for young people. Related groups sponsored through A.A. include Al-Anon, which is particularly designed for spouses and other persons who are closely involved with an alcoholic, and Al-Ateen for adolescents who have alcoholic parents. Other self-help groups, including Narcotics Anonymous, have been formed following the principles and format of A.A. Narcotics Anonymous is not well known and is not available in most areas.

COUNSELING

Counseling services form an integral part of most treatment programs for drug abusers, whether the programs are offered in detoxification centers, residential treatment facilities, or hospital or mental health clinic outpatient services. The purpose of the counseling is to aid the adolescent in exploring alternatives to drug abuse, increasing problem-solving skills, and accepting responsibility for his or her behavior. Services may be rendered by peer counselors, paraprofessional counselors, or professionals.

Peer counselors who work with adolescent drug abusers are young people who receive basic training and supervision from professionals. Such adolescents may or may not have had firsthand experience with psychoactive drugs. The basic rationale for the creation of peer counseling programs is that drug-abusing adolescents may be more receptive to peer influence than to adult intervention. Peer counselors may be available through school guidance programs or through youth-oriented public or private agencies. They may see adolescent drug abusers individually or, in conjunction with a professional counselor, may participate in group sessions.

Paraprofessional counselors are usually adults who have been formally trained in basic counseling skills. Many community colleges offer associate degree programs to prepare paraprofessional counselors. These counselors may or may not have had experience themselves with drug use or abuse. They, too, are supervised by professional counselors. Paraprofessional counselors are frequently employed as staff members of residential treatment facilities. They may also work with individual adolescents through mental health centers.

Professional counselors are those who have earned a college degree in a counseling-related field such as social work, psychology, nursing, or rehabilitation. Such persons may work with adolescent drug abusers in residential treatment facilities, mental health centers, or private practice settings. Depending on the training of the professional and the needs of the adolescent, the professional counselor may see the drug abuser in individual therapy, group therapy, and/or family therapy. Professional counselors may also work with peer counselors or paraprofessional counselors in any of these treatment settings.

CONCLUSION

The treatment of adolescent drug abusers is a complicated process. There is no single treatment modality or setting that meets the needs of all young people. Combinations of several approaches must be available if care is to be maximally effective for any particular adolescent. There is ample opportunity, among the diverse practice settings, for interested and qualified nurses to become involved in the treatment of adolescent drug abusers and to contribute to the effort to provide services needed by this segment of the population.

REFERENCES

1   P. K. Burkhalter, *Nursing Care of the Alcoholic and Drug Abuser*. New York: McGraw-Hill Book Co., 1975.
2   Ibid.
3   F. G. Hofmann, *A Handbook on Drug and Alcohol Abuse*. New York: Oxford University Press, 1975.
4   Burkhalter, op. cit.
5   Ibid.
6   Ibid.
7   Ibid.
8   Hofmann, op. cit.
9   Burkhalter, op. cit.
10 Ibid.
11 Hofmann, op. cit.
12 Burkhalter, op. cit.
13 O. S. Ray, *Drugs, Society, and Human Behavior*. St. Louis: C. V. Mosby Co., 1972.
14 Hofmann, op. cit.
15 H. J. Cornacchia, D. J. Bentel, and D. E. Smith, *Drugs in the Classroom*. St. Louis: C. V. Mosby Co., 1973.
16 Ray, op. cit.
17 Burkhalter, op. cit.
18 Hofmann, op. cit.
19 Ibid.
20 Burkhalter, op. cit.
21 Hofmann, op. cit.
22 Burkhalter, op. cit.

23 C. E. Baker, Jr., *Physicians' Desk Reference*, 31st ed. Oradell, N.J.: Medical Economics Co., 1977, p. 976.
24 Hofmann, op. cit.
25 Ibid.

BIBLIOGRAPHY

Brecher, E. M.: *Licit and Illicit Drugs*. Boston: Little, Brown and Co., 1972.
Phoenix House Foundation, Inc.: *Phoenix House Five Year Report*. New York: Phoenix House Foundation, November 30, 1972.

Adolescents in Mental Health Counseling Centers

Carol J. Dashiff

Outpatient counseling centers abound in both the private and public sectors, but programs are seldom specifically oriented to the particular needs of adolescents even though a number of adolescents may be among the clientele. This chapter describes the characteristic counseling needs of adolescents who are seen in the author's private nurse-therapist practice. The practice setting and its operation are described, as are therapeutic approaches used and the rationales for them in such a setting.

ADOLESCENTS IN COUNSELING CENTERS: PROBLEMS AND APPROACHES

The most common reasons that adolescents come for counseling stem directly from the developmental tasks of the age period, which are described in detail elsewhere in this book. The developmental characteristics of adolescents, identified by several theorists from different but compatible perspectives, form a useful framework for assessing and intervening in adolescents' problems: Each young person needs to develop a secure sense of identity,[1] a sense of idealism,[2] self-esteem,[3] and constructive methods of self-expression. These areas are not mutually exclusive but overlap and influence one another to a considerable extent. Successful development in any of these categories enhances development in the others, and deficiencies in one sphere leave the other areas vulnerable. While every adolescent is expected to struggle somewhat within each of these areas as part of the normal developmental process, there are some young people who because of previous experiences are at special risk, as discussed below.

Sense of Identity

The adolescent with a poor sense of identity is likely to demonstrate indecisiveness, contradictory or conflicting values and standards, an absence or deficiency of interest areas, and a tendency to be suggestible but not to carry through in implementing plans advised by others. Such a poor sense of "who one is" derives from repetitive experiences of disapproval, which prevent the integration and acceptance of various parts of the self. The overwhelming fear of disapproval places the adolescent in a position of dependency wherein he or she is unable, because of self-mistrust, to assert aspects of the self except when another will initiate the activity and assume responsibility for the consequences. This adolescent perceives experimentation as dangerous. A counselor who is quick to advise, inconsistent about the recommended approach, and uninvolved with the client offers little security to such a teenager. The therapist's goals should be to facilitate the development of a sense of independence, awareness of self, and a healthier pattern of self-identification.

Idealism

A certain amount of idealism is to be expected in adolescence. Cognitively the adolescent is developing the ability to conceptualize and consider things beyond the range of current possibility.[4] The growth of idealism is a developmental process that is likely to go awry in the absence of hope. Adolescents suffering from developmental disturbance in this area present with extreme cynicism, sarcasm, and/or depression. These clients doubt the therapist's intentions and motives, fear exploitation, and are sensitive to agency or bureaucratic deficiencies but feel hopeless about their own or others' ability to improve things. This attitude derives from a sense of powerlessness and a resentment of those in authority because of their perceived past abuses of that authority where the adolescents have been concerned.

Therapists must be careful not to confirm the clients' belief system by engaging in conscious or unconscious bribery or bargaining. Neither should therapists abuse their authority by relinquishing it. A need of the therapist to be liked will be viewed by these clients as an unfair attempt to divest them of their negative but "powerful" affect. The therapist's approach should be oriented to encouraging the verbal expression of negative affect without agreeing or disagreeing with the client's viewpoint. It is necessary to temper the use of humor, for humor is readily misperceived as ridicule. The therapist must also be careful not to allow the client's "rebelliousness" (demonstrated by lateness and missed appointments) to evoke reciprocal anger and avoidance, which will only confirm the client's suspicion that the therapist was not to be trusted anyway. As the relationship between therapist and adolescent progresses, it becomes possible to help the young person develop a sense of powerfulness and restored hope and idealism through more active and constructive behaviors.

Self-esteem

Pronounced fear of rejection and failure is most often a reflection of long-standing parental devaluation, which leaves the adolescent both sensitive to rejection or failure and without the necessary support to learn from these experiences. Adolescents with these fears need to develop skill in problem solving, identifying and selecting alternative courses of action, and implementing them with support. The therapist should identify and point out the client's strengths and build on them. With middle-class adolescents of normal intelligence, cognitive approaches such as transactional analysis or rational-emotive therapy are helpful for intervening in self-defeating patterns of thought and behavior.

The growth of self-esteem in adolescence is closely tied to peer relationships. The intimacy that develops with same- and opposite-sex peers is an attempt to see oneself through another's eyes and to affirm one's sense of self.[5] Isolation from peers for any reason during adolescence leaves teenagers with a fear of being different from others and of being strange in their thoughts, feelings, and behavior. Socially isolated young people are also fearful of being left out and unable to assert themselves with those they perceive as socially more mature than themselves. The resulting self-doubt contributes to further isolation and feelings of worthlessness.

Body image is another area that is closely linked to the development of self-esteem. The physical changes of adolescence and their psychologic ramifications can readily lead to feelings of strangeness about oneself. Social isolation or social rejection—so that the adolescent either is deprived of clear reference points such as the appraisals of peers or receives negative appraisals—intensifies feelings of strangeness and inadequacy.

Counselors must realize that their own relationships with adolescent clients cannot take the place of relationships with peers, and the counseling objective should be to place the clients in a group setting with age-mates.

Exploration of adolescents' feelings about their appearance and adequacy should be sensitively undertaken. It is not appropriate for the counselor to suggest to young women that they lose weight, wear makeup, and dress more femininely; nor is it appropriate for the counselor to engage in "masculine" repartee with young men (for example, insinuating that a client's good golf score may have been caused by his driving from the women's tee). This kind of response attacks adolescents' developing sexual identity and diminishes their self-worth.

To aid in assessing body image, the therapist may request that clients draw pictures of themselves. This approach is particularly useful with young or withdrawn teenagers. Older adolescents usually are able to talk about their body image if the therapist is sensitive to and pursues cues that are offered, such as a statement by a client that she resembles her father rather than her mother. In instances in which parents have repeatedly commented about the adolescent's appearance, it is best not to focus on the parental remarks in the initial interviews unless a complaint, cue, or comment is offered by the adolescent.

Feelings of inadequacy may also arise from lack of information, which prevents the adolescent from feeling competent about behavior and decisions. Common areas of ignorance are sex and drugs, hence assessment of the adolescent's knowledge of sexual function and drugs should take place in the initial interview, and both topics should be discussed in subsequent sessions. It is helpful with young adolescents (and others as indicated) to devote at least one session to the discussion of sexual changes, feelings, and functions. Research with female adolescents has demonstrated that opportunities for constructive affective learning about sexuality are often absent.[6]

Self-expression

Adolescence is a time of experimenting with a variety of modes of self-expression. Tensions are created by new sexual and aggressive feelings as well as physiologic changes and the increased demands of society and parents. Many times these tensions are expressed, particularly in early adolescence, in impulsive actions. As adolescence progresses, it becomes necessary to integrate energies in a more adaptive, much less impulsive way.

Many adolescents who come to counseling demonstrate action-oriented patterns of self-expressive behavior that have increased rather than decreased their anxiety. Conflicts with parents or legal authorities are common, with charges including shoplifting, running away from home, and self-destructive involvement with drugs and sex.

Acting-out behavior usually evolves from a variety of background factors, including feelings of frustration, helplessness, deprivation, and anger. In many instances acting-out patterns of self-expression are influenced by parental role modeling, as in the following examples.

> Marla, age 15, was brought to counseling because her mother was concerned about a recent incident of shoplifting and suspected that the girl was "promiscuous and involved with drugs." She complained of her daughter's lack of commitment to household responsibilities. In the second session Marla's recently divorced mother disclosed that she herself had been involved with a man for the past three months and during this time had spent at least four evenings a week at his apartment while the children remained home alone.

> Janet, a 14-year-old with well-developed secondary sexual characteristics, came to the initial session with her parents, who were upset because she had run away from home after attending a drinking party against their instructions. In the second session it was revealed that her father's behavior in response to the discovery that his daughter had run away had included breaking into her locked room, throwing her belongings around, and smashing pictures on the wall.

Deviant behavior may be acted out because of the role assigned by the family. An adolescent may be the scapegoat of conflict that exists between the parents but is communicated only indirectly, through the child. More direct communication is perceived as dangerous to the marital relationship. "Amorphous communication" occurs when rules are only vaguely stated yet accompanied by high parental expectation.[7] The parents find various ways to perpetuate the behavior for which they criticize the adolescent.

> An 18-year-old dropped out of college near the end of her first term because of difficulties in completing her assignments. Her parents criticized her for being too dependent on them, yet they arranged for her to move into a house across the street from them when she left college. As she attempted to assert herself more independently by asking to borrow the parents' car to buy her own groceries and attend ballet lessons, her mother became more solicitous and insisted on shopping for or with her and driving her to her lessons. Significantly, the parents did not interact with each other in the initial family session, and it was revealed in the second session that family members were discouraged by the mother from expressing negative affect because she feared that such expressions would cause the father to have a second heart attack.

Frequently all the family members experience feelings of deprivation. These feelings can be picked up by an astute therapist who observes nonverbal communication.

> Mr. F sat across the room from his wife, who had chosen to sit on a vacant sofa. The adolescent daughter sat in a chair between her parents but at a

distance from each. Mrs. F began to tell her perception of the problem but became tearful. The daughter and husband remained silent. Mrs. F made repeated attempts to elicit help by asking Mr. F and their daughter to verify her account of their situation, but she received no verbal response from either.

Acting-out is a mechanism for maintaining one's autonomy. As such, it is a reaction to rigidly imposed restrictions. It is a plea to be regarded as an individual. When the adolescent is burdened with a chronic illness and at the same time isolated from a support system, noncompliance with the medical regimen may be the only way to express anger about the system.

A 17-year-old woman, a diabetic, lived in her own apartment alone and was employed full-time. In her therapy group the therapist repeatedly held her up to the other group members as an example of "good adjustment." She never shared any problems of her own in the group, for each time she presented a cue it was disregarded by both the therapist and the members. She was eventually hospitalized in a coma precipitated by medical noncompliance.

A counselor who intervenes with young people who act out must be well in control of his or her own sexual and aggressive feelings. A therapist who winks and otherwise flirts with adolescent clients only adds to their fear and confusion. Therapists must be careful not to enter into competition with same-sex adolescents. The long-range goal is to help the teenager manage tension and the energy generated by anxiety in a more constructive manner. The short-term means to achieving this objective is to facilitate verbal expression of feelings. It is important for the resolution of the underlying conflict that negative feelings not be the only focus. Schneiderman and Evans[8] suggest that the therapist should help the family members become more aware of their loving feelings for one another so that self-esteem can be increased. The result is the facilitation of safe verbalization of aggressive feelings and a decrease in acting-out behavior.

Another technique that is helpful in remedying acting-out situations is to devise a contract specifying in behavioral terms what each family member may be expected to do for the specified period of time. The frustration that prompts an adolescent to act out may result from unclear expectations or conflict over some limit or rule that the adolescent feels is unfair.

An adolescent who had recently run away from home was told she had to be home by dark on school nights. No leeway was permitted for special occasions at school. The mother stated she wanted to know where her daugh-

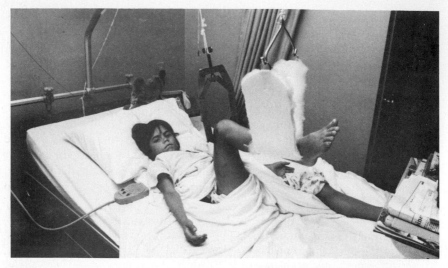

Isolation from peers, body image disturbance, lack of information, and curtailment of self-expression are among the detriments to self-esteem, idealism, and identity that can contribute to mental health problems in adolescence. (*Copyright* © *1980 by Anne Campbell.*)

ter was and to have her arrive home safely. The father stated that he felt the deadline was necessary because of the adolescent's poor school performance. The adolescent could see little connection between the reasons given and the rule, feeling that there were more sensible ways to deal with the problems her parents identified than rigid adherence to an arbitrary rule. Together the family worked out a more flexible agreement which clearly communicated the expectations of each. Notably, each family member during discussions expressed surprise at the viewpoints of the others, and it was clear that the motivations for previous actions had never been discussed among the family members.

Responses to Loss

Loss or impending loss of a significant other in adolescence threatens the young person's identity, idealism, self-esteem, and self-expression. Losses commonly include the death of a significant other, disruption of friendships, and threatened or actual family disruption. Any of these generates anxiety that is usually discharged in activity. Because death is a particular threat to the adolescent's own identity, it is likely that a teenager in need of counseling will not have taken advantage of previous opportunities to talk about fears and feelings associated with the death of a significant other.

Other losses can also be difficult for the young person to talk about because they are not distinctly identifiable. Such is the case when parents have ongoing but covert marital conflict. According to Despert[9] this kind of "emotional divorce" may be more disturbing to the couple's children than the event of legal divorce.

> The onset of symptoms of anorexia nervosa in a young teenage girl followed the mother's hospitalization for a manic episode. Family therapy with the parents revealed secret events in their lives which had threatened the continuance of the marriage prior to the mother's hospitalization.

Adolescents who have difficulty adjusting to their parents' divorce present with a variety of behaviors. They may not outwardly appear depressed, but their anxiety over the loss or secondary to the parental conflict is commonly manifested in nervous activity such as inability to sit still, rapid speech, and talkativeness. More withdrawn adolescents may have somatic complaints.

In addition to their need to work through their own feelings, these adolescents may be caught in the midst of conflict between the parents. Such a position creates enormous guilt, because the adolescents feel responsible for the parents. The teenager also may become a pawn for indirect expression of parental conflict, as when parents set contradictory expectations of and limits on the young person. In counseling, these adolescents need help to distinguish what they want from what their mothers want and their fathers want. When it appears that a great deal of a parent's conversation with the adolescent is centered on the other parent, it is important to verbalize this observation to the teenager and to recognize how difficult it must be to be caught in the middle. I have found that this approach brings relief, because it removes the burden of guilt and responsibility from the young person. In addition, these adolescents need help in finding constructive methods to relieve tension.

> Dianne, whose parents had divorced and whose father lived away from the home, expressed intense frustration about her difficulty in communicating with him. After a session of role-playing, she was more able to be assertive and constructive in telling him her feelings. When he continued his pattern of behavior, she initiated daily jogging as a way of discharging her anger, and she noticed that arguments with her siblings diminished. She became able after a time to recognize how much she resented her mother's confiding in her and began to seek out activities that would allow her to establish a more separate identity.

When this same adolescent first came for therapy, her mother complained of the daughter's overweight and poor academic performance. The adolescent stated that her own goal was to feel better about herself and to be able to assert herself. At the conclusion of therapy she had lost 15 pounds and was doing better in school, although neither of these areas had been directly addressed in therapy.

THE PRACTICE SETTING AND ITS OPERATION

Community Mental Health Principles

Whenever a person is treated within the community in which he or she resides, certain community-oriented principles should be followed in order to maximize ego strength and adaptibility. In the special case of adolescents, adherence to these principles is no less important.

Principle 1   The client, as a customer-consumer, initiates contact with the service provider. The initial contact centers around a process of negotiation, which begins with identification of needs *as perceived by the client*.

> A young woman reported to me that she had gone to a community mental health center to seek help and had verbalized prolonged depression as her presenting problem. The recommendation of the therapist there had been that she join a group for overweight people. As a result of the mismatch between her identification of the problem and the center's recommendation, she had terminated treatment there.

The initial negotiation must take place in a very careful, systematic manner. Premature speculation about the problem and approaches to be taken will leave the adolescent with feelings of helplessness, hopelessness, and alienation. The therapist must be careful that the treatment plan offered is clearly open to discussion, includes alternatives, and is not more a reflection of the therapist's own value system than an accurate assessment of the client's needs.

Principle 2   The client is an integral part of various social systems.
Adolescents seldom come unaccompanied to their first contact with the treatment center. They are likely to come at the urging of family, teachers, or legal authorities. It is an unfortunate outcome of adolescents' legal, social, and financial status that they do not feel free to initiate contacts with helping agencies.

It is important to notice which social system (school, family, court, peer network, etc.) sends the adolescent to treatment and who comes along to the initial session. Teenagers may be accompanied by members of the social system with which they have the most conflict, or they may, although less frequently, be accompanied by persons from the system that offers them the most support. The proportion of the session dominated by accompanying persons is a meaningful clue, as are the amount of scapegoating of the adolescent and the behavior of the accompanying person during the teenager's time in private with the therapist. A parent who remains in the waiting area during the appointment time communicates a supportive attitude that is absent in the case of a parent who leaves and does not return to pick the adolescent up until well after the appointment is over.

Principle 3   A multidimensional approach to assessment and intervention is necessary for maximizing the success of therapy.

This multidimensional approach requires assessment of the biological, psychological, *and* social systems and the development of interventions appropriate to each. Interdisciplinary collaboration and continuity of care are essential parts of such an approach.

> A young adolescent came for an initial interview upon the recommendation of a psychiatrist conducting marital therapy with her parents. The psychiatrist stated that the mother was concerned about the daughter but that he thought she was developing normally. The initial nursing interview and assessment revealed an emaciated client who had lost 23 pounds in the past two months. Referral to a pediatrician for intensive laboratory testing was the first step in further assessment and intervention.

The Physical Facility

Ideally the adolescent center should be just that—a center for adolescents. The stigma and subsequent damage of psychiatric labels can thus be avoided. It is unfortunate that most counseling centers are designed and operated within the context of illness-oriented settings.

While the atmosphere should not be monotonous or dreary, neither should it be sensorily overstimulating, a mistake that is often made in planning environments for adolescents. Seating in the waiting room should allow choices of seats either near or distant from others. The availability of refreshments helps minimize adolescents' anxiety and serves as a vehicle for relating to peers. When refreshments are available, they should be nutritious.

Different types of counseling require different types of settings. At least two separate areas should be available: a living-room area with a sofa and side chairs for individual and family therapy, and another room with individual chairs for group therapy. It is desirable also to have group activity areas as well as a place that is suitable for a variety of instructional methodologies. A comprehensive center that is not easily accessible to all may find it feasible to develop an outreach program that includes home visits.

Staffing and Staff-Client Interactions

The staffing of counseling centers varies from the intradisciplinary team frequently found in private practice settings to the interdisciplinary team more often seen in the public sector. While an interdisciplinary team is more likely to be multidimensional in approach, the danger of fragmentation of services exists. On the other hand, the intradisciplinary team, although maintaining continuity of therapist contact with the client, is more inclined to evolve a narrow perspective.

The importance of the adolescent's first contact with the setting cannot be overemphasized. In most settings the first contact is with a receptionist. The attitude of the receptionist does much to color the adolescent's fears and expectations regarding the counselor. In my own private practice, being without a receptionist has been an advantage. The adolescent's first contact is with me. The absence of a receptionist in the waiting area seems to create a warmer, freer atmosphere for adolescents and their families. If the instructions to the client and family about the location and use of the waiting area are clear, a more confidential, unrestrained setting can be provided for family interaction prior to the appointment.

It has been my experience that the telephone is an important vehicle for communicating with adolescents. While telephones have been used traditionally by counselors to follow up on missed appointments, their use can be more versatile. Adolescents should be given the therapist's professional card and encouraged to rearrange their own appointments as necessary or to contact the therapist when they feel in need of additional sessions. This practice encourages constructive and adaptive help-seeking behaviors as opposed to destructive, disorganized acting-out. Each adolescent should also be contacted by phone at least twice within the month following the conclusion of therapy, both to evaluate current functioning and to facilitate the teenager's direct contact with the therapist when future assistance is needed. Appointments, when they are for an individual rather than a group, should be arranged directly with the client to facilitate independence and recognize the young person's identity as separate from rather than an extension of the parents.

In order to facilitate adolescents' commitment to the therapeutic relationship, it is important to involve them in some way in the payment for the sessions. I have found it useful to take one of two approaches. If the parents insist on paying for the sessions themselves and live separately from the client and/or refuse to participate in family therapy, I present the adolescent with a copy of the bill at monthly intervals to facilitate his or her awareness of financial matters and to stimulate a sense of responsibility. I negotiate with those adolescents who have their own financial resources (either earnings or an allowance) to pay a portion of the fees, and I bill them separately from their parents. In families seen for family therapy, the adolescent's paying part of the cost minimizes the parents' tendency to scapegoat the teenager and makes all family members equal participants in the therapeutic encounter.

Records

While careful, comprehensive records should be kept for each appointment, it is my belief that they should include as much *objective* information as possible in order to avoid the pitfalls of labeling. Private practitioners are probably at special risk to allow their records to become relatively subjective, because the records are seldom seen by anyone else. The primary danger is that one may become insensitive to one's own bias and then communicate this bias to other systems (school, court, health professionals, etc.) the client is involved with. It is important to keep in mind Rosenthal's[10] work on self-fulfilling prophecy. Bias can be diminished by the processes of supervision and consultation, which should include the review of written records.

Liaison Contacts

Liaison contacts within and between professions should be established for three purposes: case-finding, gathering supplementary information about clients, and intervention (referral). Unfortunately, they are usually used only for referral. Liaison contacts should not be carried out surreptitiously. The adolescent should know from the outset that, in the effort to help, the therapist will get in touch with any resources that might be useful. Specific information about who is to be contacted and for what purpose should be shared with the client in advance. It is sometimes appropriate, when referrals are made, for the counselor to offer to accompany the adolescent to the new setting. Such an approach, besides reducing the client's stress, also enhances continuity of care.

Ethical and Legal Considerations

When adolescents are engaged in therapy without their parents, the issue of confidentiality is complicated by their legal and developmental dependence on parents. The therapist must decide, by investigating the state laws and court decisions, to what extent he or she is legally obliged to inform parents about the treatment. Ethical practice ordinarily demands that parents of minors be informed of the treatment goals and general approaches to be taken. In some cases, however, adolescents seek treatment without telling their parents because of fear of physical harm. Indications of abuse should be reported by the counselor to the appropriate authorities for investigation. Many nurses erroneously believe that only young children are abused. The adolescent most in need of help may be the most difficult to reach because of parental opposition. During one summer I received weekly phone calls from a teenager who wanted to talk about his home situation. He refused to give his full name and was fearful that his stepfather and mother would discover his conversations with me. Counseling programs in schools (see Chapter 15) are one solution to this type of problem.

A second ethical issue is that of the psychiatric label. Labels, especially the official "diagnostic" ones, should be avoided in adolescence because of the damage they do to the development of self-esteem and because labels further disable the client in the eyes of significant others. Labeling is a deterrent to the development of hope and a sense of idealism. Identifying problematic behaviors, such as, "This client is having difficulty with _____," is far preferable to labels, which say in essence, "This client is a _____." When a diagnostic label must be used, for example to enable a client to qualify for third-party reimbursement, a nonspecific one such as "adolescent adjustment reaction" is a workable compromise.

Counseling ethics must include scrupulous care to avoid imposing the therapist's bias on the client. Bias is referred to professionally by a number of terms, including stereotyping, countertransference, and being judgmental. All professionals engaging in interpersonal encounters with persons in need of help must evaluate the ease with which they are able to disguise personal motives beneath professional linguistics.

> I recall a conversation I once had with another therapist about a referral I was considering making to him. The client in question was a former student of mine who had indicated an interest in seeing me professionally, a practice I do not engage in because I believe it is impossible to be objective and to make the transition from the role of teacher to therapist except at the expense of the client. This colleague disagreed with my reasoning and went on to say that he did not hesitate to treat his former students and that he believed the clients could learn a great deal from the role modeling of a person they admired. I suspect that the therapist's own need for admiration may have been a larger factor in the continuance of the relationship with the students than his ostensibly professional motives indicated.

When family therapy is undertaken, the therapist is at risk for several distortions. Specifically, the therapist may (1) tend to see the adolescent as a victim, (2) perceive the family as a victim, or (3) compete with the parents for the parental role. Failure of the therapist to try to involve the family in treatment is sometimes indicative of these countertransference problems.

Selection of Treatment Approaches

The choice of therapeutic method for adolescents is based on several considerations. Those young people who have difficulties at home but whose peer relations and ego strength are good benefit most from family therapy. If the family refuses to participate, these adolescents are helped by a brief course of supportive treatment. Prolonged therapy is inadvisable because it diminishes the teenagers' self-esteem and encourages family scapegoating. An adolescent with poor ego strength and problems with capacity for thought, affect, perception, or reality-testing should be seen in individual therapy. Such a client will be fearful of peer group settings unless they are oriented around activities. Teenagers with situational crises such as illness, divorce, or physical trauma benefit from a group setting. Generally speaking, the adolescents who are helped by group therapy that is not activity-oriented are those of normal or higher intelligence and middle or higher socioeconomic status.

Age is an important consideration in treatment selection. Younger adolescents do not have the facility for verbalization that older teenagers have. Younger clients therefore do better in therapy with an activity orientation. They are also more comfortable in a group comprised of persons of their own sex. Older adolescents profit from mixed groups, which allow them to progress toward the young adulthood developmental stage of intimacy by further solidifying their self-identity through the reflected appraisals of persons of the other sex. Older adolescents also can benefit from co-therapy with both a male and a female group therapist, provided that both counselors share the same philosophy and are comfortable in the professional colleague relationship.

Group therapy is a valuable mode for assessing an adolescent's peer support system. Both to facilitate the therapist's assessment of the client's existing peer support and to help strengthen the peer relationships, the adolescent can be asked to select and bring to the therapy sessions members of his or her peer group.

Whether or not family therapy is to be used, many major advantages accrue if it is possible to have family members present for the initial assessment interviews with the adolescent. In addition to providing the therapist with interactional data not otherwise available, the joint interview focuses on conflicts among all family members and encourages the family toward a therapeutic alliance with the "patient." Parents as well as the adolescent may benefit from the therapist's contacts with the parents. Seeing the client and parents together is valuable because it diminishes the suspicions and distortions that may otherwise arise in the adolescent's mind if the parents are seen alone for the initial interview to talk about their "problem child." Contacts between the counselor and the client's parents should always be in a joint adolescent-parents-therapist session to assure all parties that the therapist is not colluding with the parents in the pathological process of scapegoating the adolescent.

Deciding whether family therapy is the treatment of choice can only be done after a careful assessment of the family. However, problematic acting-out behavior is invariably a symptom of difficulties between the parental pair, and the families of adolescents who act out should be encouraged to engage in family treatment. Even if parents refuse to participate, the adolescent can be assisted and the family interactional patterns can be modified by the therapist's work with the client.

A vital component of the therapeutic process, regardless of the particular approach selected, is the counselor's awareness and facilitation of the adolescent's strengths. The identified strengths can be used to great advantage to work on areas of weakness. It is a mistake to focus solely on problems and weaknesses. In the initial interview, the young person should be asked to identify his or her strong points and accomplishments, and so should the parents. Adolescents have great capacity to grow and change. Recognition of their healthy aspects fosters that capacity, diminishes their fear of being psychiatrically labeled, and facilitates movement toward mastery of adolescent developmental tasks and difficulties.

REFERENCES

1   E. H. Erikson, *Identity: Youth and Crisis*. New York: W. W. Norton, 1968.
2   J. Piaget, *The Language and Thought of the Child*. New York: Meridian Books, 1957.
3   H. S. Sullivan, *The Interpersonal Theory of Psychiatry*. New York: W. W. Norton, 1953.
4   Piaget, op. cit.
5   Sullivan, op. cit.
6   L. Whisnant and L. Zegans, "A Study of Attitudes toward Menarche in White Middle-Class American Adolescent Girls," *American Journal of Psychiatry*, **132**:809–814, 1975.
7   M. R. Whalen, "Amorphous Communication in a Family with Teenagers," in S. Smoyak (ed.), *ThePsychiatric Nurse as a Family Therapist*. New York: John Wiley & Sons, 1975.
8   G. Schneiderman and H. Evans, "An Approach to Families of Acting-Out Adolescents—A Case Study," *Adolescence*, **40**:495–498, Winter 1975.
9   J. L. Despert, *Children of Divorce*. Garden City, N.Y.: Doubleday, 1962.
10 R. Rosenthal and L. Jacobsen, "Teachers' Expectations: Determinants of Pupils' IQ Gains," *Psychological Reports*, **19**:115–118, 1966.

BIBLIOGRAPHY

Brandes, N. and M. Gardner: *Group Therapy for the Adolescent*. New York: Jason Aronson, 1973.
Burgess, A. W. and A. Lazare: *Community Mental Health: Target Populations*. Englewood Cliffs, N.J.: Prentice-Hall, 1976.
Caplan, G. and S. Lebovici: *Adolescence: Psychological Perspectives*. New York: Basic Books, 1969.

Frank, I. and R. K. Frank: "The Management of Adolescent Crisis in Family Practice," *Adolescence*, **37**:25–28, Spring 1975.

Group for the Advancement of Psychiatry: *Normal Adolescence*. New York: Charles Scribner's Sons, 1968.

Howell, J. G. (ed.): *Modern Perspectives in Adolescent Psychiatry*. New York: Brunner/Mazel, 1971.

Jensen, G.: "Adolescent Sexuality," in B. J. Saddock, H. I. Kaplan, and A. M. Freedman (eds.), *The Sexual Experience*. Baltimore: Williams and Wilkins, 1976.

Plachecki, L. J.: "The Adolescent as a Family Scapegoat," In S. Smoyak (ed.), *The Psychiatric Nurse as a Family Therapist*. New York: John Wiley & Sons, 1975.

Rachman, Arnold: *Identity Group Psychotherapy with Adolescents*. Springfield, Ill.: Charles C Thomas, 1975.

Rice, F. P. : *The Adolescent*. Boston: Allyn and Bacon, 1975.

Sorosky, A.: "The Psychological Effects of Divorce on Adolescents," *Adolescence*, **45**:123–136, Spring 1977.

Sugar, M. (ed.): *The Adolescent in Group and Family Therapy*. New York: Brunner/Mazel, 1975.

Chapter 19

Working with Adolescents in a Women's Health Clinic

Elizabeth Randall-David

As an alternative to traditional health care institutions, women's health care clinics have sprung up all over the country in the last decade. Beginning in 1971, when Carol Downer viewed her own cervix and shared this experience with other women in a National Organization for Women meeting in California, the women's self-help movement has established itself as both an alternative and a challenge to the existing medical establishment. The women's health movement emphasizes that women are basically healthy organisms. Many of women's experiences, which are typically seen as pathological by the present medical system with its emphasis on disease processes, are viewed as normal developmental processes by the women's health movement. Thus, menstruation, childbearing, and menopause, to mention just a few, are seen anew, from a perspective of health.

Some of these differences in viewpoint can be accounted for by the fact that the women originally involved in the women's health movement were laywomen not influenced by a medical-system education (either nursing or medicine) with its basis in pathology. On the contrary, these early groups, who formed to learn more about their own bodies, started from the assumption that the best way to begin gathering information was to share their *experiences* as women. This sharing of experiences took the form of verbal interchange, as well as gathering together to view one another's cervixes (hitherto unseen by any laywoman) and exchanging feelings about their bodies and body processes. Beginning with this experiential approach to women's health, the women soon expanded into study groups, delving into medical journals and other available resources to glean whatever information they could. The next step was to organize all of these experiences and information into a form that could be shared with all women—women in large cities where the women's liberation movement had already made a great impact, and women in small, rural towns where the tenets of the women's movement were virtually unknown.

There were really three forms of communication undertaken to accomplish this goal. First, women in California chose to organize their experiences and information in the form of a slide show presentation, followed by a demonstration of how each woman could learn more about her own body through speculum visualization of the cervix and vaginal self-inspection. These women made themselves available to women's groups throughout the country, traveling from community to community with their slide show and demonstration as a means for gathering local women together to share their own experiences and form local ongoing self-help groups. Second, women in the Boston area chose to disseminate the information and experiences they had gathered in the form of a paperback book, *Our Bodies, Ourselves*. This book, often cited as the bible of the women's health movement, deals with varied subjects of interest to women ranging from general topics, such as nutrition and exercise, to topics specific to women's health, such as birth control, childbearing, menstruation, and menopause. The widespread distribution of this book has greatly increased the accessibility of this kind of information to women of varied ages, backgrounds, and educational training. Written in terms that the layperson can understand, *Our Bodies, Ourselves* has done much to demystify the health care experience and instill in women the desire to know more about their bodies as a necessary step in controlling their destinies.

The third approach utilized for distribution and application of women's health care experiences and information was the establishment of women's health clinics. Women in communities throughout the country established women-operated health centers which, at first, concentrated on education, counseling, and referrals, but which later expanded into provision of medical and nursing services as well. Disillusioned with traditional medical facilities, which they not only felt did not serve women adequately but also believed to be actually detrimental to their self-respect, dignity, and health, groups of women banded together to create alternative structures which would provide high-quality health care in a warm and supportive atmosphere. Often these groups met resistance and hostility from the local medical establishment, which attempted to curtail their activities through public health restrictions, city or county ordinances, nonsupport of medical personnel in nearby hospitals, lowering of physicians' fees to be competitive, arresting health care workers for practicing medicine without a license, and so forth. Rather than being discouraged in their attempts to offer a different type of health care, many of the women have become more radicalized from these often nonsupportive, sometimes hostile interchanges.

Although certain problems were found to be specific to a particular community, there were many situations that women-operated clinics had in common. Several organizations, newspapers, and journals have been initiated to facilitate closer communication among women health care workers so that exchange of ideas and ways to combat common problems can be mutually shared. National women's health conferences further facilitate sharing of information and energies among women from different settings and locations. Though some clinics have had a short-lived existence, most of the clinics, once established, have gained such overwhelming support from community women that they have stabilized themselves as essential health care, educational, and political facilities.

In May 1974, a clinic owned and operated by women was established in Gainesville, a university town in north central Florida. The founding philosophy of this clinic was similar to that of other feminist clinics: The objective was to provide high-quality, low-cost gynecological services in an atmosphere which encourages all women—staff and patients alike—to share their information and experiences so that the health care experience is as meaningful and comprehensive as possible. When information is shared and all procedures and treatments are fully explained in lay terminology, health care becomes comprehensible and is demystified. No longer do patients see lab values or diagnoses as mysterious pronouncements that only a doctor or other health professional with extensive training can understand.

In the past, women have been discouraged from participating in their own health care: We have given over this responsibility to our doctors (who eagerly took it) and remained ignorant of our bodies and our emotions. With increased knowledge and encouragement to assume responsibility for their own lives, women are becoming active participants in their own health care. We are learning what questions to ask so that we will have enough information to make informed, intelligent choices about our own bodies.

As was mentioned previously, the emphasis within the women's health care movement is on health rather than disease. Since women are responsible for the health care of their children as well as for themselves, they are the largest group of health care consumers in this country. Quite often, they seek care when they are healthy (e.g., for contraception, abortion, childbirth, yearly Pap smears, etc.) in addition to those times when they need treatment for illness. Thus, they are excellent candidates for preventative health care teaching. For example, all women can be taught how to do a breast self-exam so that they may examine their own breasts monthly for any unusual thickening or lumps. Since most breast masses are discovered by women themselves rather than by physicians or nurse practitioners, the breast self-exam is an important tool for all women to have. Likewise, women are taught about the importance of an annual (or, in some cases, semiannual) Pap smear, a diagnostic screening tool for cervical cancer.

There are many other things that a woman can do to actually prevent pathology. Two of the most common reasons that women seek gynecological care are vaginal and urinary tract infections. However, there is a whole list of measures that can be followed in order to prevent or lessen the occurrence of these infections. The emphasis in women's health care, then, is on each woman's taking responsibility for her own body so that she can remain as healthy as possible. Once she is educated with regard to signs and symptoms to look for, she can seek prompt medical care if a problem should occur.

CHARACTERISTICS OF THE SETTING AND STAFF

The setting in which women's health services are offered is crucial, perhaps especially for adolescents, who are inexperienced in dealing with the health care complex. It should convey openness and acceptance of women of all ages, backgrounds, and life-styles. Often, these messages are conveyed through nonverbal cues, such as comfortable furniture, pleasant music, well-cared-for plants, and posters. What the staff wears can be quite meaningful. Casual, informal clothing imparts a very different tone than starchy white uniforms. Colorful patient gowns are designed to be more comfortable and supportive of ego strength than the white paper ones found in most clinics. Rather than exposing the entire back of the patient as she sits in the room awaiting the examiner, these gowns are designed with a slit down the front which allows the examiner easy access for breast, heart, and lung examination while keeping the woman maximally covered for warmth and privacy.

Speculums and stethoscopes are warmed before use, easily correcting another uncomfortable situation that women have experienced. Potholders are placed over the examining table stirrups so that the woman's feet do

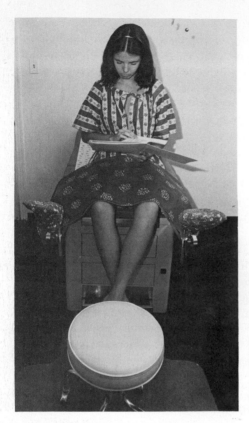

Patients are encouraged to read their clinic charts and ask any questions about their health or their health care. This policy is but one part of the effort to demystify health services, enable patients to assume responsibility for themselves, and provide them with practical experience and information that will help them be active participants in their own health care both in this clinic and in more traditional settings. (*Copyright © 1980 by Anne Campbell.*)

not rest on cold, hard metal when she assumes the lithotomy position. Each room has a mobile above the examining table, giving the patient something to focus on if her attention needs to be diverted from a painful procedure (e.g., IUD insertion or first trimester abortion procedures). A child care room is provided, with a crib and toys for children of all ages. Too often women's needs as mothers are overlooked in the offices of the very professionals who specialize in the birthing of babies (obstetricians and gynecologists). Clinic hours are flexible and varied so that women who work, go to school, have difficulties with baby-sitting arrangements, and so forth, can have a variety of day and evening hours to choose from.

Everyone at the clinic is addressed and spoken of by first name. Doctors, nurses, and patients are introduced to each other by first name in an attempt to reduce the authoritarian, elitist relationship between doctor and patient found in other health care institutions. (When doctors are referred to as "doctor" and the patient is called by her first name, an unequal situation is instantly created which makes it difficult for the patient, perhaps especially if she is young, to feel comfortable in the role of active participant. Instead, she is encouraged to passively accept what the authority has to say about *her* body). Since the health care team is comprised of doctors, nurses, paraprofessionals, counselors, and patients, each person's input is not only valid but necessary. At our clinic, all members of the team are mutually respected for their contributions.

Since the team approach is an integral part of our clinic's health care delivery, the doctor-nurse relationship is very different from that found in most other settings. Doctors are interviewed and hired by the women who work in and own the clinic. Therefore, only those doctors whose philosophies of patient care in general, and, more specifically, whose attitudes toward women are consonant with our own, are employed by the clinic. Doctors are given feedback on an ongoing basis about their technical skills as well as their interpersonal style. While this is never done in front of patients, if a patient is dissatisfied with the doctor's care, either because of his or her style (brusque, patronizing, etc.) or because of his or her technique (rough, didn't fully explain what he or she was doing, etc.), she is encouraged to let the physician know. This can be done by filling out a written evaluation sheet that is provided each patient or by talking with the physician. Either method represents an abrupt departure from the traditionally passive, accepting patient role, and this seems necessary if we are to have responsible, active patients. The feedback sheets, which pertain to all aspects of the woman's experience at the clinic, are carefully reviewed and changes are made accordingly. In this way, each patient has input into the type and quality of care that other women receive at the clinic.

Nurses for the clinic are selected not only on the basis of clinical skills (counseling or obstetric-gynecologic nursing) but also for their awareness of women's issues and perspectives. Since imparting the philosophy of the women's health movement is an integral part of our undertaking, an awareness of these tenets and their implications for treatment is an essential requisite for employment. Since many nurses have received their training in a more traditional context, often the first step of orientation and training is consciousness raising with regard to oppression within the nursing profession. With this reeducation and radicalization, nurses are better able to understand how patients have suffered from sexist, racist, and elitist attitudes in established medical care facilities. All staff members function not only as clinicians but also as patient advocates. As the advocate for her patient, each nurse has the responsibility for seeing that all the patient's questions are answered, that all procedures and findings are explained to her in terms that she can understand, and that she knows about and can assert her rights as a patient within the health care context. It is particularly useful for the nurse or counselor to help the woman see how she can generalize from her experience at the clinic to health care in more traditional settings. In summary, nurses function as educators, clinicians, counselors, and patient advocates within the women's health clinic setting.

SERVICES FOR ADOLESCENTS

The demographic makeup of our patient population is as varied as the community in which we exist. Since this book addresses itself to the nursing of adolescents, the following pages describe only those services that pertain to women in this age group, along with an explanation of how the health care philosophy described above is translated into clinical practicalities.

The Menstruation Workshop

This workshop, designed for mothers and their daughters between 10 and 15, is held monthly in a 2-hour session. Its goal is to bring mothers and daughters closer together on this aspect of sexuality in a positive, educational, nonthreatening atmosphere. The clients' attitudes, myths, and taboos surrounding menstruation are explored in an attempt by the nurses to add a cross-cultural perspective to our own knowledge and belief system. The workshop emphasizes menstruation as a normal developmental process rather than an illness, as expressions such as "the curse," "being hit," "on the rag," "falling off the roof," etc., would indicate. Once the history of cultural attitudes toward menstruation is presented and accurate information about anatomy and physiology is imparted, the participants have a much better idea why a celebration at the onset of menses is more appropriate than the too-common responses of embarrassment or shame.

The larger group is then broken down into two smaller ones: The mothers go into a separate room with one of the clinic staff and talk about attitudes toward their own sexuality as well as their feelings about their daughters' maturing and possibly becoming sexually active in the near future. The daughters stay in the original workshop room (a large carpeted room, where everyone sprawls on the floor or sits on bright, stuffed pillows) and discuss with a staff member their own attitudes about starting their periods, developing breasts and hips, changing relationships with peers and parents, school activities, etc. The daughters are amazingly open, articulate, and in touch with their feelings. The staff member is there to facilitate discussion and answer any questions (particularly those related to physiological processes), but most of the discussion is among the young women themselves. The feedback received about the workshop indicates that both mothers and daughters learn a lot and enjoy the experience.

The Well-Woman Gynecological Clinic

The well-woman gynecological clinic operates 3 days or evenings each week and serves a large number of adolescents as well as older women. It is staffed by four nurses, one doctor, and a front office person. The full range of services provided by the gynecological clinic includes Pap smears, physical exams, pelvic exams, venereal disease screening, diagnosis and treatment, breast exams, vaginal infection diagnosis and treatment, sickle cell screening, birth control counseling and services (i.e., birth control pill prescription, IUD insertion, diaphragm fittings).

Referrals are made to the local medical center or to private physicians if pathology is discovered that needs ongoing care the clinic is not equipped to handle. In this way, only "well woman" care is regularly provided at the clinic.

Interviewing and Teaching at the Well-Woman Gynecological Clinic
Quite often, a young woman is afraid when she goes to a doctor or clinic for a gynecological examination, particularly if it is her first such examination. Regardless of her reason for needing the examination, she approaches it with all sorts of fears and fantasies about what the experience will be like. Fear of the unknown is far worse than the reality of the situation, so one of our first actions in working with any new patient is to reduce anxiety by carefully explaining everything that will happen while the woman is at the clinic. Techniques for doing this will be described later.

Second, a young woman may be embarrassed about the upcoming pelvic and breast exam. In our culture, with its ever-changing attitudes toward sexuality, it is difficult for adolescents as well as adults to know what to expect attitudinally from the examiner. Thus, the clinic staff must create an atmosphere that is nonjudgmental and receptive so that a young woman feels comfortable discussing her feelings and behaviors.

A third reason for an adolescent's concern might be fear that others will find out not only that she has been to the clinic but also what services she received while there. An important point to establish early in the contact with any new patient is that all information is strictly confidential. No patient information will be released in writing or by telephone unless the patient herself has given the clinic written permission to do so.

A fourth fear may be that the examination will be painful. The nurse teaches relaxation techniques that can help reduce the discomfort of the speculum and bimanual exam. This teaching process will be discussed more thoroughly later in this chapter.

Each new patient has a 45-minute individual interview with a nurse who takes a health history, does necessary lab work, and gives pertinent information and appropriate counseling. The purpose of the history is twofold: It elicits necessary information for diagnosis and treatment, and it is used as a tool for health care teaching. The history form is not handed to the woman to fill out. Each question is asked by the nurse, and the rationale for the question is explained. In this way, the nurse can teach the patient about prevention of urinary tract infections, for example, if the patient mentions that she has had several occurrences of this problem in the past year. Or, perhaps, in asking the questions on family history of diabetes, the nurse can point out the familial tendencies associated with this condition and explain why such a history would contraindicate indiscriminate use of oral contraceptives.

The nurse is sensitive to the needs of the individual patient. A young woman who is sexually active will have different needs from the patient who was brought to the clinic by her mother because she has a vaginal infection. Each patient is interviewed alone first. If the young woman would like to include a significant other in the process, this can be arranged during the latter part of the interview.

Most of the adolescent women utilizing the clinic services are already sexually active. Thus, birth control counseling is an important part of the initial interview. The nurse first explains all methods of contraception, including their advantages, disadvantages, side effects, and contraindications. On the basis of the health history, certain methods of contraception may be contraindicated for a particular patient. The reasoning for this is explained carefully to the young woman so that she fully understands this recommendation. We have accomplished nothing if she merely goes to another clinic and convinces someone else to give her this same method.

A second important consideration in helping a young woman decide on a method of birth control is her life-style and social situation. Too often these factors are overlooked as relevant variables in contraception selection. However, insertion of a diaphragm, for example, may not prove practical if intercourse is occurring in the back seat of a car; likewise, prying parents or siblings make concealment of birth control pills too difficult for some adolescents. These factors are as important in *use* effectiveness as any others and should be fully explored.

Likewise, it is important to assess motivation and level of responsibility. How likely is this particular patient to use contraception at the time of intercourse, as is required for methods such as the diaphragm or foam and condoms, or each day in anticipation of intercourse, as in the case of the oral contraceptives? Each woman is strongly encouraged to make her own decision based on all the information shared with her. Ultimately, it is *her* life and *she* needs to take responsibility for it. If the young woman has a stable sexual partner, she might find it helpful to have him sit in on the birth control counseling with her. Use of foam and

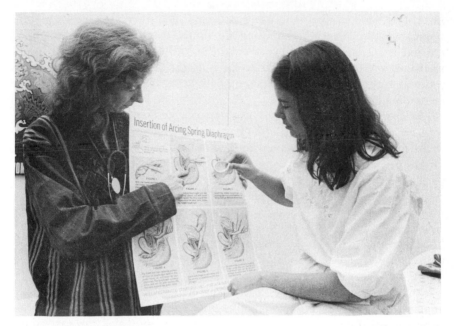

All sexually active women must have access to sound, nonpunitive contraceptive services. They need to know what options are available and which ones may be contraindicated for them and why; and they need to be helped to make their own selection of a method that suits their own needs and circumstances. (*Copyright © 1980 by Anne Campbell.*)

condoms or a diaphragm requires a cooperative partner, so the participation of the involved male is greatly encouraged in the selection phase of the conception control process.

Legally, in the state of Florida, birth control information and services may be provided to sexually active women under the age of 18 years without parental consent. However, many of the public health departments do require written parental permission before providing these services. Since birth control information and services are difficult for adolescents to obtain elsewhere in our community and in surrounding rural towns, it is especially important for our clinic to be as accessible as possible to teenagers. Future plans include opening a *free* teen clinic so that financial concerns can be eliminated. Expanding clinic hours to include more after-school hours will also increase the accessibility of this service. Reaching out into the school systems, so more young people know about our services, will help meet the needs of this previously inadequately served group.

In addition to birth control information, the sexually active adolescent needs knowledge in the prevention, diagnosis, and treatment of venereal disease. With the incidence of these diseases sharply increasing in recent years, this need has become more pressing than ever. The nurse needs to be especially sensitive in handling this subject matter in a nonjudgmental and positive manner. Adolescents can be quite affected, favorably or otherwise, by the vocabulary or tone of voice used. Handout literature is given for reference, and patients are encouraged to have regular checkups.

Following the interview and teaching, each patient is taken to the lab, where a dipstick urinalysis, hematocrit, and vital signs are taken. As in all procedures at the clinic, the rationale for each test, the explanation of normal values, and reasons for any abnormalities are discussed fully with each patient. The woman is then shown how to do a breast self-exam, again with rationale and full explanation of signs and symptoms of possible problems. Each woman practices on a plastic breast model which has four simulated lumps so that she knows what she is looking for during her own self-exam. A handout explaining the technique is given for reinforcement and reference.

The Gynecologic Examination The actual clinical aspect of the woman's visit to the well-woman gynecological clinic may be conducted by the nurse, the doctor, or both. The nurse accompanies the patient to the examining room, gives her instructions on how to put on the patient gown with the slit in the front, and leaves the room. When the woman is ready, the nurse reenters the room and explains what will be done. The patient is shown the instruments that will be used and how they work, i.e., how the speculum is inserted and then opened to permit observation of the cervix. The nurse then does a breast exam, reinforcing previous teaching by demonstration and further explanation of what is normal for that particular woman. When asking the patient to assume the lithotomy position, the nurse reminds her that the exam will be much more comfortable if she relaxes her perineal and abdominal muscles.

The nurse explains techniques of relaxation and breathing to help the woman. Gently, unhurriedly, and with a matter-of-fact approach, the nurse proceeds with the exam, being careful to explain everything that will be done *before* doing it. This increases the trust level and prepares the patient for the next step of the exam. With young patients, it is especially important to determine the correct size speculum to use and whether indeed a speculum is appropriate in that particular exam. Depending on the purpose of the exam and the status of the patient's introitus, a Pap smear or bimanual exam may or may not be needed. Similarly, a gonorrhea culture and/or samples of vaginal secretions will be obtained at this time, if indicated. If the young woman desires oral contraception, the physician does a general physical exam after the nurse has finished with the gynecological exam.

The patient is asked to sit up on the table before the doctor is brought in, so that introductions can be made in a position respectful of the woman's dignity and supportive of her ego strength. The practice of introducing or talking to the patient while she is in the lithotomy position is dehumanizing and disrespectful! Likewise, patients are not "draped" at the clinic because, too often, this creates a mechanical as well as psychological barrier. In this situation the examiner's face is hidden from the woman, so it is difficult for her to ask questions or converse. A draped patient makes it easy for the examiner to relate to one part of the body without regarding the patient as a whole person. Thus, we provide "lap" covers to lay across the lower abdomen if the woman desires that kind of privacy, but we make sure the patient and examiner can maintain eye contact throughout the exam.

The nurse's role shifts from clinician to patient advocate when the physician joins them. The nurse makes sure the woman understands what the doctor is doing and sees to it that all of her questions are answered. If any medication is prescribed, the nurse explains instructions for its use, any side effects that might occur, and any follow-up that may be necessary, such as a reculture after medication for venereal disease is finished. The nurse provides closure at the end of the exam and encourages the woman to call the clinic on the 24-hour hotline if any questions or problems arise.

The Pregnancy Testing Clinic

Many adolescents utilize our pregnancy testing clinic because it is easily accessible (available 4 days per week) and relatively cheap ($3 compared to $7 to $13 in private physicians' offices) and the test results are obtained in only a few minutes. These variables are particularly important for adolescent patients, although women of all ages have expressed appreciation for these same considerations. Pregnancy tests are done on a walk-in basis, though most people have called in advance to obtain instructions for obtaining a valid urine specimen. The woman accompanies her staff member to the lab, where the test is explained to her. The patient herself helps perform the test, thereby further becoming an active participant in her own health care. Having the patient actually see the results and how they were obtained helps to demystify the experience. Too many people still have notions of rabbits dying in the back room!

The staff member explores the woman's feelings about the test results with her. If she has a negative test, birth control counseling may be appropriate. The various types of birth control and where these may be obtained are discussed with the woman. The emphasis is on prevention rather than on how to deal with a problem once it exists. Referrals for contraceptive services are made to public health departments, private doctors, or our own gynecological clinic, depending on where the woman lives, her financial status, and other variables.

If the pregnancy test result is positive, all the alternatives are explored with the patient. If she desires to continue the pregnancy, she is given information regarding the need for good prenatal care, exercise, and nutrition, and she is referred to a private physician or the medical center for continued care. However, young women, especially, are often quite upset to discover that they are pregnant. Immediate counseling is needed to help the woman clarify her feelings and discover what realistic alternatives exist. If the woman chooses to terminate her pregnancy, the first trimester abortion procedure is explained to her and she is referred to our abortion clinic. (Abortion counseling will be discussed at greater length in the next section.) Whatever the test result, women learn a lot from participation in the experience.

The Abortion Clinic

The abortion clinic operates 2 days each week and serves 40 women per week. All staff working at the clinic must feel comfortable with the idea of abortion and every woman's right to choose to terminate an unwanted pregnancy by this method. Special sensitivities and skills are needed to work effectively with the adolescent who seeks a first trimester abortion. Even within the adolescent group of patients, there are very different needs and problems. As in any crisis counseling, the basic goal is to turn what most people see as a traumatic situation into a growth experience. This can be accomplished in a variety of ways. Good counseling helps the woman apply what is learned through the abortion experience to future situations.

The first step in effective abortion counseling is establishing good rapport with the young woman. The counselor-nurse should use language the patient can relate to and understand. Often nonverbal communication, such as the way a counselor sits, facial expressions, tone of voice, or tolerance of silences, conveys to the adolescent how much she can trust and confide in this person. It is usually easiest to start out with some open-ended question that is nonthreatening and proceed from there. The following areas need to be included in abortion counseling:

1   Exploring the patient's feelings about the pregnancy
2   Discussing alternatives for dealing with the pregnancy
3   Learning who significant others are and how they view the pregnancy (if they know about it)
4   Discussing the steps of the abortion procedure and what the patient can expect to feel during each part of the procedure
5   Dealing with her anxieties (commonly they are about pain, future sterility, and violation of confidentiality)
6   Exploring her contraceptive history and future possibilities for birth control
7   Emphasizing the need to follow aftercare instructions diligently and return for postoperative checkup

The following discussion deals with each of these points in turn.

Many adolescent women have very ambivalent feelings about their pregnancy. On the one hand, it is an open confirmation that the young woman is sexually active (except in cases of rape and incest, which will not be dealt with in this chapter). Depending on how accepted sexual activity is in the particular family or community from which the patient comes, this issue may need considerable exploration in counseling. Certainly it is important that the woman not be left with a negative concept about herself as a sexual being as a result of the pregnancy and its termination.

On the other hand, many adolescents have a very romantic notion of what it means to be pregnant and have a child; a young woman may see it as a welcome confirmation that she indeed is a "woman" and can conceive. Others see it as a declaration of independence from their parents. Still others fantasize about a cute little baby (baby doll?) that they can love and play with and that will "belong" to them. One of the purposes of the counseling is to get the adolescent to do some reality testing. What is the young woman's relationship with the father of the child? Can he be counted on for emotional and/or financial support? How could the woman manage if she were to continue the pregnancy and assume the responsibility for the child? These are very relevant questions that quite often have not been thought through by the adolescent in any realistic fashion.

Since the clinic's philosophy emphasizes each woman's taking responsibility for her own life, it is important that the young woman herself make the decision about how to handle her unplanned pregnancy. Nevertheless, it is important for the counselor to know whether the significant others in the patient's life know about the pregnancy and what their feelings are. Sometimes it is her mother or boyfriend who has decided she should have an abortion rather than the woman herself. The clinic offers to facilitate communication between the patient and whomever she would like to work out her decision with. Often the young woman has not told her parents about her pregnancy. Whether or not she decides to inform her parents is the woman's own decision.

The following is the abortion consent form used for women under 18 at the clinic. It is used in addition to our regular abortion consent form to emphasize our philosophies regarding teenage women's rights and responsibilities:

According to the U.S. Supreme Court decision (Planned Parenthood of Central Missouri vs. Danforth, July, 1976) women under the age of 18 years no longer need parental or guardian consent in order to have a first trimester abortion. This legislation ensures the rights of all women, regardless of age or marital status, to choose whether or not to continue an unwanted pregnancy.

Our philosophy at the Gainesville Women's Health Center strongly reaffirms this constitutional right. At the same time, we are also aware that the decision to have an abortion is sometimes a difficult one requiring much thought and consideration. Quite often, it is hard for young women to share their feelings in this situation with their parents. Sometimes the desire not to hurt their parents or be punished or rejected by them causes young women to want to terminate the pregnancy without their parents' knowledge. Ideally, we would like to act as facilitators to increased communication between parents and their daughters. We offer our counseling services to anyone who would like to work with us in bridging this communication gap.

We also recognize that it is the policy of emergency rooms in local hospitals not to treat persons under the age of 18 without written parental consent. Therefore, were a complication to occur at our clinic that required hospital treatment, your parent or guardian would be informed of your condition since his/her signature is necessary before treatment could begin. It is important to consider whether one would want her parents to be informed in this manner of her decision to have an abortion.

Ultimately, the decision to have a first trimester abortion with or without parental/guardian consent or knowledge rests with the individual woman. Having considered all of the points listed above, I assume the responsibility for making the decision to have this abortion without informing my parents/guardian. I understand that if further treatment at another facility is necessary my parents will be informed and their signature required before treatment can begin.

Once the woman has decided to terminate her pregnancy, she needs to know what is involved in having a first trimester abortion. This information is usually shared in a group setting with other women who will be having the same procedure. The nurse or other counselor explains step by step what the process includes and what the normal range of feelings is during each step in the process. Most women are anxious when they first enter the group room but feel considerably relieved when they learn what to expect. Again, fear of the unknown is far worse than the reality. In the area of abortion, which is still surrounded by much emotionalism and by pejorative attitudes, there are all sorts of myths and misinformation which need to be rectified by the clinic staff. Some of the common concerns expressed by women of all ages are: (1) Will it hurt? Patients are reassured to find out that the abortion procedure creates feelings much like menstrual cramps. (2) Will I be sterile after this? Staff members emphasize that it is not a normal occurrence for women to become sterile after an abortion. However, sterility can occur in a small number of people if they get a postabortion infection for which they do not get prompt, adequate treatment. It is emphasized at this point that all patients should carefully follow the aftercare instructions that nurses give them in the recovery room so they can avoid an infection. The need to return to the clinic in two to three weeks for a postoperative checkup is also emphasized.

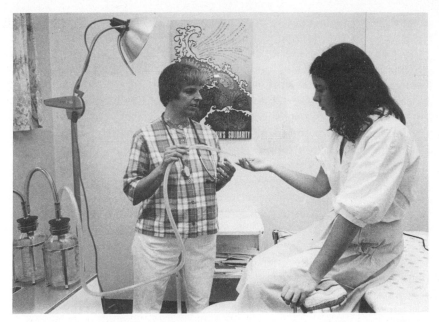

Young women who are contemplating or have decided on abortion need to be fully informed about the procedure and about what an abortion patient experiences. Abortion counseling includes exploring the young woman's reactions to her pregnancy, discussing alternatives to abortion, dealing with her anxieties and other problems about pregnancy and/or abortion, helping her select an effective method of birth control for use after this pregnancy, and (if she elects abortion) teaching to ensure that she will care for herself properly afterward and return for her checkup. (*Copyright © 1980 by Anne Campbell*.)

Of course, one of the most important aspects of abortion counseling is helping the woman prevent the recurrence of unwanted pregnancy. If birth control is needed, the woman and the nurse review the patient's past experience with the use of contraceptives and discuss the methods that might be appropriate for the future. Most (80 percent) of the adolescents seeking abortion services at the clinic have not previously used a reliable method of birth control. For many, conception control information and/or services are not readily available. Still others have mistakenly labored under the notion that "it can't happen to me." Others have engaged in "contraceptive risk taking," a phenomenon not unlike other risks that people take, such as not wearing seat belts, smoking cigarettes, etc. As was discussed earlier, each woman is encouraged to choose a method of birth control and to use her medical history and life-style as important variables in her decision making. This choice is often a difficult one, especially when the adolescent is very young (e.g., 12 years old) and on that basis alone ineligible for the oral contraceptives. Usually foam and condoms are chosen by this age group. It is hoped that all women needing contraception will have chosen a method by the time they return for their postoperative checkup two to three weeks after the abortion.

After the woman has received both group and individual counseling, she has routine lab tests done. These include a repeat pregnancy test, dipstick urinalysis, hematocrit, hemoglobin, blood grouping and typing, and a syphilis test. The lab technologist explains the rationale for each test, the expected normal values, and possible reasons for any deviations from normal. If, for instance, the woman has a low hematocrit, dietary counseling and an iron supplement are offered.

The next day, the woman returns to the clinic for her abortion procedure appointment. She is greeted by the counselor who talked with her the day before. The counselor discusses any feelings or anxieties the woman may have and then prepares her for the abortion itself. Quite often, the first thing the counselor demonstrates to the woman is the actual amount of suction used during the vacuum aspiration procedure. This helps allay fears that the suction will damage the body. After a breast exam, ausculation of heart and lungs, and pelvic exam to determine length of gestation, the physician proceeds to terminate the pregnancy by vacuum aspiration.

The role of the counselor during this time is to help the patient focus her energies and keep her breathing slow and even. Having developed a rapport with the patient from the counseling session the day before, the counselor is able to engage her in conversation that will reduce anxiety during the procedure. By using techniques similar to those employed in the Lamaze method of childbirth, the counselor helps the patient interrupt the pain pathway from point of origin to point of perception. It is also important to help the woman breathe slowly and evenly so she does not hyperventilate or hold her breath during the uncomfortable parts of the procedure. The nurse assists the doctor by checking the woman's medical history and relaying any necessary information to him or her. The nurse works with the counselor to help the patient stay focused and calm during the procedure. The primary responsibility is to the health status of the patient throughout.

The entire abortion procedure by vacuum aspiration lasts an average of 10 minutes. During this time, the woman may experience some cramping similar to the cramps she has during her menstrual period. Though no drugs are routinely given preoperatively, if the woman displays high anxiety, occasionally some Valium p.o. is given to help her relax. The only medication given during the procedure is 10 cc lidocaine paracervically.

After the abortion has been completed, ergotrate or pitocin is given IM to help the uterus contract. The woman then walks to the recovery room, where her vital signs are taken every 15 minutes for 1 hour. After observing her bleeding pattern and emotional state, the recovery room nurse goes over the aftercare instructions with each woman, does follow-up birth control counseling, and dispenses oral contraceptives, to be started that evening if the woman has chosen that method of birth control. Before being discharged, each patient is encouraged to call the clinic on the 24-hour hotline if she has any unusual symptoms, has any questions, or wants to talk to a counselor. A postoperative checkup is scheduled for two to three weeks after the procedure. The nurses conduct these exams in order to assess the normalcy of the postoperative period through patient reporting and pelvic exam. If there is any question about postoperative problems, the doctor is consulted and a plan of action instituted. Approximately 75 percent of patients keep their postoperative appointments.

As was mentioned before, the adolescent has special needs during the abortion procedure. Sometimes, a mother will request that she be present in the room during the abortion for support. The patient is asked whether this is desirable to her. If so, the mother or significant other may be present after spending some time with the counselor. It is important that the counselor be sensitive to the needs of the parents, though the primary responsibility is to the young woman who is the patient.

Future Plans

Future plans for programs of interest to adolescent women include childbirth education and parenting classes; a walk-in free teen clinic for birth control, vaginal infections, and venereal disease; and sexuality groups specifically geared for adolescents. If these services are provided in a nonjudgmental atmosphere by staff that are sensitive to the needs of the adolescent, with input from a consumer board of adolescents themselves, they could provide a much-needed service in our community. It is hoped that through these services we can continue to impart our feminist philosophy of health care to as many young people as possible. We hope they will then push for changes in other parts of the health care system that will improve it for other health care consumers.

BIBLIOGRAPHY

Boston Women's Health Collective: *Our Bodies, Ourselves*. Boston: Simon and Shuster, 1976.

Cherniak, Donna, and Allan Feingold: *Birth Control Handbook*. Montreal Health Press, 1975.

———— and ————: *VD Handbook*. Montreal Health Press, 1975.

Ehrenreich, Barbara, and Dierdre English: *Witches, Midwives, and Nurses: A History of Woman Healers*, 2d ed. Old Westbury, N.Y.: The Feminist Press, 1973.

Frankfort, Ellen: *Vaginal Politics*. New York: Bantam Press, 1972.

Hern, Warren, and Bonnie Andrikopoulos (eds.): *Abortion in the Seventies*. New York: National Abortion Federation, 1977.

Luker, Kristin: *Taking Chances: Abortion and the Decision Not to Contracept*. Berkeley: University of California Press, 1975.

Health Care in a
Juvenile Detention Center

Elizabeth Fitzpatrick

Juvenile offenders have been called the "throwaway children."[1] At other times they are referred to as bad, maladjusted, incorrigible, or undesirable. They are males and females from age 10 through 17, and they come from a variety of economic backgrounds and ethnic origins. The thing they have in common is that they have all been brought before a juvenile court or apprehended by the police. They compose a large population with enormous and, to a large extent, unmet health care needs.

OVERVIEW OF THE POPULATION

The 1970 White House Conference on Children stated that, since 1963, juvenile delinquency had been increasing at a faster rate than the juvenile population.[2] In addition, urban delinquency rates are more than triple the rural rates.[3] During 1965, 300,000 children were detained in more than 250 special detention homes across the country. Another 100,000 were in local jails or police lock-ups.[4] According to current national statistics, one out of six teenagers will at some time enter a juvenile detention center.[5] One author reports that one million juvenile offenders are apprehended in the United States each year.[6]

Youngsters from ages 10 through 17 account for only 16 percent of our national population but constitute 45 percent of all persons arrested for serious crimes.[7] Locally, similar statistics reveal that the juvenile population in Colorado makes up 18 percent of the total population yet commits more than 50 percent of the serious crimes. Colorado statistics for 1975 showed that approximately 59,000 youths were taken into custody and close to 30 percent were placed in a detention center.[8] Nationally, a staggering number of adolescents are detained in institutions and, therefore, without access to normal avenues of health care.

Behavior that violates delinquency statutes is not only commonplace but also widely diverse. Children and adolescents come to juvenile detention centers for many reasons. They are classified as children in need of supervision (CHINS), deliquents, and/or dependent and neglected children. Usually, they are all housed together by age and sex regardless of their legal offense. Offenses can be child-only infringements, such as running away, truancy, being beyond control of parent, or curfew violation. Other juveniles are detained for much more serious offenses, such as felonies, assault, drug abuse, theft, burglary, homicide, rape, or any other crime for which adults can also be arrested. Today child-only offenses account for more than half the case loads of the juvenile courts.[9] Children can also be detained for their own protection because of child abuse, sexual abuse, or any other condition that may threaten their well-being.

HEALTH NEEDS AND THE SERVICES AVAILABLE IN DETENTION CENTERS

The supposition that health problems are uncommon during adolescence is rapidly becoming recognized as a misconception. Detention center residents emphatically illustrate the fact that not all youths are in good health. Detainees are a high-risk sample. Many are from deprived backgrounds. Others have been "on the run" for extended periods of time, living away from home and supervision. Their health care is episodic and fragmented, if not nonexistent. Few can remember the last time they were examined for health reasons, routine or otherwise. A great many of the adolescents who come to detention centers bring preexisting emotional, dental, and medical problems. Because of overcrowding and minimal exercise and fresh air, all incarcerated youth become prime targets for communicable disease. In a New York City detention center, of more than 20,000 youthful detainees examined by the staff of Montefiore Hospital over a 3-year period, 45 percent were found to have medical problems.[10] A sample of these problems is listed below.

Infectious—1,107
Toxic—1,287
Metabolic—134
Traumatic—193
Neoplastic—35
Congenital—121
Allergic—30
Psychiatric—61
Miscellaneous—271[11]

Another 14,976 ill detainees were managed on an ambulatory basis. In 1974, a 6-month study of 132 youths in a Denver detention center revealed that 86 percent had one or more significant health problems, i.e., some disorder that would require follow-up after the young person's transfer to some long-term institution.[12]

Fewer than half of the detention centers in the nation give routine physical examinations. More than 25 percent give no admission examination at all. Eighteen percent of the juvenile detention facilities can make no professional medical services available at any time.[13] Rarely does a detention center have a full-time medical staff or an affiliation with a hospital.

ESTABLISHING HEALTH CARE PROGRAMS

It is becoming increasingly evident that the number of adolescents in detention, and the insufficiency of their health care, cannot be overlooked. Recently, more and more attention has been focused on the juvenile delinquent and his or her problems, including health care. Many segments of our population are concerned. In 1973, the American Academy of Pediatrics Committee on Youth established health standards for juvenile court residential facilities.[14] These standards have been endorsed by the National Council of Juvenile Court Judges.

The Nurse's Participation in Health Delivery

As adjustments are made to implement the standards, it is evident that nursing will play a major role and have significant impact in delivering health care to this select group of adolescents. The nurse will work in close association with many other professionals but will, in all likelihood, be the daily health care provider. She or he will be an important member of a team that will decide on treatment and care of the incarcerated adolescent. Other members of the team will include pediatrician, psy-

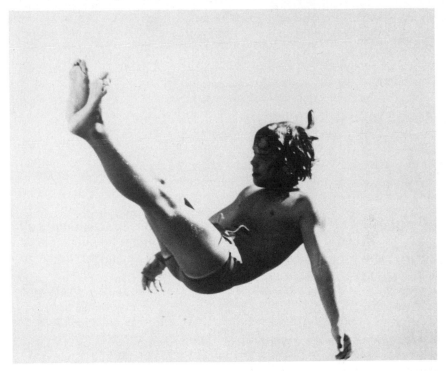

Contrary to commonly held opinion, a great many adolescents are not in the best of health. Juvenile detainees in particular usually have histories of erratic life-styles and poor health practices, and a great many enter detention with mental or physical health problems. Incarceration itself creates additional health risks. (*Copyright © 1980 by Anne Campbell.*)

chiatrist or psychologist, police representative, juvenile intake officer, welfare representative, school representative, parent, detention counselor, court officer, the child's attorney, and the child. Each will have something unique to contribute to the future of the juvenile detainee.

A detention center health program established in Denver has served as a model for other local centers in the state. Although health programs for Colorado youth in detention are not ideal, the state is working toward meeting all the standards recommended by the American Academy of Pediatrics. The center's daily population ranges between 50 and 125, increasing during the school year. The following material, based largely upon experience with the Denver setting, is a compilation of the writer's recommendations about the organization and functions of a health service for detained adolescents.

The health service should operate autonomously from the detention functions of the institution. The health care providers, while certainly cognizant of the security and custodial purposes of the detention center, should not be responsible for them. Where nurses or other health workers must also represent the security "establishment," their relationship to the adolescent detainee becomes colored by the young person's attitudes toward persons with that kind of authority, and their approachability and effectiveness as health care providers is diminished.

Our clinic's physical layout included two examining rooms, an interview area, a records and storage room, a waiting and rest area, and an isolation room. This arrangement permitted complete privacy and maintained the human rights and dignity of the patient. These considerations are of course basic ethical issues which obtain in all health care delivery settings; in addition, they are particularly important components of working with incarcerated teenagers in such a way as to optimize adolescents' participation and cooperation in their own health care programs. Many times, young people in detention are hostile, depressed, and uncooperative. They are upset and anxious about their situation. Away from home, confined, and stripped of personal belongings, the youngster struggles to maintain identity and self-respect. Health care providers must be constantly aware of the emotional status of the patient and how it might affect their role in delivering health care.

In most states, the court has the legal authority to approve health care for the detainees. In addition, appropriate permission should be sought from parents, when possible, and always from the child. Ordinarily, the young person is concerned about his or her health and, if approached with respect and honesty, will be cooperative. Often a few nurse-patient meetings will take place before confidence and trust are obtained, and only then can procedures be performed. The practitioner should be direct, respectful, and nonjudgmental. Using these approaches, an environment of mutual respect will be established and satisfactory rapport should ensue.

Our facility was staffed by two full-time school nurse practitioners and a part-time consulting pediatrician. An affiliation with the University of Colorado Medical Center Adolescent Fellowship program provided consultation by their adolescent fellows. This coverage did not staff a 24-hour, 7-day-week health service. Because of this, complete cooperation from community health care agencies and the police department was necessary. The police department provided patient transportation out of the center whenever necessary. The health agencies in the community were used not only during the hours when health care was unavailable in the detention center but also for broader services than our facility could provide. These included outpatient and bed patient care, diagnostic facilities, specialist consultation, pharmacy, and dental care. Community agencies were also used to ensure continuity of health care when a resident was transferred from the detention center back into the community. Following release, appropriate health records were sent to the new source of health care.

In our facility, the nurse practitioner was the primary care provider. She worked in cooperation with the consulting pediatrician to establish policies, procedures, and standards consistent with those recommended by the American Academy of Pediatrics. The attainment of those standards should be a goal of all juvenile detention centers. As stated in those standards:

> Every institution which confines juveniles should have a health program designed to protect and promote the physical and mental well-being of residents, to discover those in need of short-term or long-term medical and dental treatment, and to contribute to their rehabilitation by appropriate diagnosis and treatment and provision of continuity of care following release.[15]

The role of the nurse as the primary health care provider in maintaining these standards is complex. Often the nurse is the only primary health contact for a detainee who has had no other source of health care. The influence the nurse has on that youngster's future attitude toward his or her health care will be lasting. Comprehensive well-child care should be offered and delivered, including health assessments. The health assessments include a complete health history as well as a thorough physical examination. The social and behavioral history are very important: In addition to serving the usual purposes, the entire assessment is considered by the courts in planning the adolescent's overall rehabilitation program. The nurse needs to be equipped and authorized to update immunizations and must have laboratory facilities or technician backup for routine tests such as urinalysis, CBC, venereal disease testing, pregnancy testing, and tuberculosis screening.

Those children who are ill or injured must be assessed to determine the acuteness and severity of their disorder and to decide what referrals should be made. The nurse institutes and supervises rehabilitative measures for individuals with long-term illnesses or disabilities. It is not unusual to have an adolescent who is a known diabetic or epileptic in detention. Frequently, it is difficult and quite challenging to care for, for example, diabetics who refuse to eat, take insulin, check their urine, and so forth. The nurse must be able to provide skillful management of both physical and emotional emergencies and must have access to psychiatric help in the event of suicide threats and other acute emotional problems. Nurses need to be able to identify, and respond appropriately to, signs of drug abuse and dependence and must be able to offer care to those young people who have been abused physically and sexually.

Referral is an important aspect of nursing practice in the relatively isolated practice setting of a detention center. The nurse must be able to identify deviation from healthy physical or behavioral functioning and

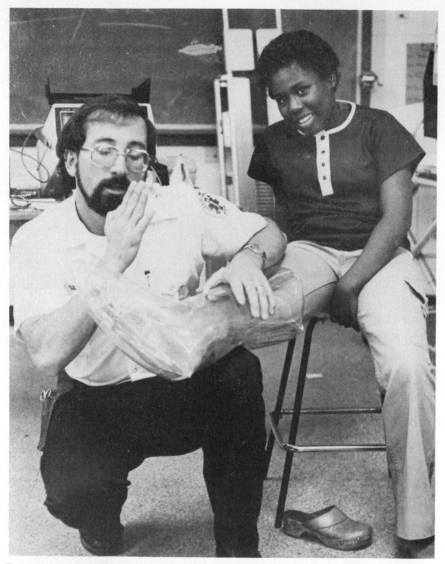

Teenagers in detention are good candidates for health teaching programs. (*Copyright* ©
1980 by Anne Campbell.)

make appropriate referrals. Collaboration with other health professionals
is necessary, and provision for the young person's total health should be
the goal. The nurse should also provide contact with community agencies
to ensure continuity of care for those youths leaving detention.

The detention setting is, in some ways, ideal as a facilitator of the
teaching aspect of nursing. The nurse in this situation, having a "captive

audience," can provide counseling, teaching, and anticipatory guidance in such areas as venereal disease, conception control, pregnancy, abortion, medical self-help programs, and the importance of health supervision.

Another very important nursing function is collecting relevant data. Health records should be maintained on all detainees kept overnight. Access to records should be restricted to the patient and those persons involved with providing for the *health* needs of the adolescent. These records should be transferred with patients to their new source of health care. Care must be exercised to maintain ethical standards in the keeping and sharing of records, as in all aspects of treatment of the adolescent. Most states do have laws that uphold the rights of minors. Two major Supreme Court decisions—the Gault decision in 1967 and the 1966 Miranda decision—ensure children's and adolescents' constitutional rights. They prevent loss of liberty and guarantee the right to counsel and protection. These decisions have caused a virtual overhaul of procedural methods of the juvenile courts of the United States,[16] and their eventual impact upon health care in court residential facilities may be great.

The following account of a typical day in our institution demonstrates some of the challenges and complexities of health care provision in a juvenile detention center. An admitting officer "books" the adolescent. Part of the booking procedure is to ask the youth pertinent questions regarding his or her health status. This information is transferred to the nurse's office. Each morning and evening the nurse reviews these papers and is notified of all admissions and releases in the center. Since many juveniles are detained only a few hours and others are kept for several months, the extent of their health care depends upon two considerations: any obvious need for immediate attention, and the duration of incarceration.

After this information is reviewed, the nurse usually visits each unit and administers prescribed medications. Following this a sick call is held in the clinic. Each unit has a specific time during which its residents are seen in the clinic, and the adolescents know what those times are. Youngsters come to the clinic if they are ill or injured, need some specific treatment, have a health concern they need to discuss, are new admissions, or just want to talk. Follow-ups of previous visits are also conducted during sick call. Subsequently, referrals to the physician or to a community agency are arranged, and newly admitted individuals who are to be detained more than 48 hours are given a complete health assessment.

The nurse's workday involves many additional activities. The nurse is sometimes called upon to testify in court regarding a juvenile's health status and attends staff meetings at which many court-related personnel discuss future placement alternatives for a particular youth. These meetings deal with all aspects of the young person's condition, situation, and prospects, and the nurse has a major role at such conferences.

Many problems come up daily that need the attention of the nurse and may involve collaboration with the entire staff. Examples from my experience follow.

- An adolescent boy comes in "high" and, while not needing hospitalization, does need close nursing observation.
- A boy whose jaw is wired shut because of a fracture is not permitted by the counselor to keep his wire cutters in his room: "It is a weapon."
- A girl is admitted to the juvenile detention center while being treated for venereal disease. Her antibiotics have been confiscated by the police, who mistook them for dangerous drugs. The drugs, after being analyzed and identified, were destroyed rather than returned to the girl. She must be restarted on costly antibiotics.
- A girl who is a known epileptic has been on the run for several weeks and has not been taking her prescribed anticonvulsant. She has had several seizures in the interim.
- A girl who has been picked up for assault and is obviously pregnant has yet to receive any prenatal care.
- A boy who is quite despondent has threatened suicide. The counselors brush him off as a "fake."

The following longer case extracts may serve to demonstrate the complicated social backgrounds of adolescents who come to detention settings. The physical and psychological health problems that arise from those backgrounds often are also complicated.

William was a 15-year-old black male who came to my attention when admitted to the detention center for a six-month stay. His offenses included car theft, truancy, being beyond control of his parent, and inhaling toxic vapors. He was the youngest of three brothers all known by the court. He lived at home with his mother and brothers. Each of the boys had a different father and, at the present time, there was no father in the home. Their mother worked during the day and was not home much in the evening hours. Supervision was minimal. I saw William in the clinic for an admission examination. The history and physical revealed that the vision in his left eye had been greatly diminished since he had been struck on the left side of his head by a brick one year earlier. He had no peripheral vision. The lens of his right eye was clouded, and vision from that eye was poor. William had been seen by a local general practitioner soon after his injury and had been told that his loss of vision was temporary and would correct itself. The boy was very accepting of his injury and was patiently waiting for his vision to return. We sent him to an ophthalmologist who made the diagnosis of detached retina and recommended surgery, although the prognosis was poor due to the length of time that had elapsed between injury and treatment. The surgery was performed and, surprising all, William recovered 75 percent of his vision.

He was released to his home with both medical and probation follow-up. We did not hear from him for over a year except for friendly, "nonofficial" visits. He was released from probation, thought to be well-adjusted. In a tragic postscript, William suddenly collapsed and died. Autopsy revealed no cause of death, but speculation was that he had once again been inhaling toxic vapors and had done so the evening of his death.

Maria was an attractive 17-year-old Latin-American female who looked older than her age. She came to the attention of the court when her boyfriend was picked up on a drug charge. She had been living on her own, quite successfully, for two years. She had a part-time job, but she was arrested when the police discovered that she was "under age." While in detention, she had many physical complaints. Physical examination disclosed that she had a urinary tract infection, gonorrhea, and a strep throat. Appropriate treatment was started and the infections cleared. She was counseled about available health agencies in the community that could assist her with her needs after she was released from detention (teen clinic, Planned Parenthood, etc.). After evaluation by the court, it was decided to emancipate Maria and allow her to live on her own as previously. She was, however, assigned to a social worker to help her with any future problems.

Terry was a 16-year-old obese, unkempt Caucasian female who was acting quite immaturely. She was admitted while the court staff evaluated her for placement in a long-term institution. She had been living with a 38-year-old black man whom she professed to love, but for whom she had been working as a prostitute. Physical examination revealed many bruises and scars from beatings by this man. She also had a venereal disease. Her general hygiene and dental condition were extremely poor. Social history included a fantasy history of multiple pregnancies, miscarriages, and abortions, none of which could be documented. What was apparent was a sexually active teenager who did not use any birth control precautions. She was obviously mentally and psychosocially retarded. Family history revealed a chaotic family life with an apparent incestuous relationship between Terry and her father. There was proof that the father was sexually abusing Terry's younger sister. Her mother was aware of what was going on but did not interfere. It was evident that the entire family needed intervention and rehabilitation that would entail prolonged therapy. Terry was sent to an institution for disturbed adolescents. Her family was referred to an agency that would initiate family therapy. Terry's sister was temporarily removed from the home. Prognosis for the entire family was guarded, since their family dynamics had been disturbed for such an extended time.

CONCLUDING REMARKS

From this brief discussion it is evident that health care of juvenile offenders presents many challenges for the nurse working within the detention center. The youth to be served are troubled youth, most of them products of a long history of suboptimal mental and physical health environments and experiences. They have had trouble in school, at home, and in their communities. Some have not had substantial peer support, and some others have had a kind that compounds their difficulties rather than promoting adjustment and health. Many have lacked growth- and health-promoting guidance from significant adults. The institutional setting within which the nurse practices offers numerous constraints to that practice, because its established purpose, security, frequently conflicts with or takes precedence over health programs for its residents.

The challenge holds many promises, however. Adolescence is a period of fluidity and great susceptibility to influence, and the nurse who works with detained youth can be a singular force for positive change. Experience at the Denver center and elsewhere has shown that an effective health program for incarcerated teenagers plays an essential role in their rehabilitation. As more and more correctional institutions move toward establishing and fully supporting adequate health programs, nurses can find a rich opportunity for improving the services offered to these young people and for helping them move from their difficult pasts toward adulthood.

REFERENCES

1 L. A. Richette, *The Throwaway Children*. New York: Delta Publishing Co., 1969.
2 White House Conference on Children, *Profiles of Children*. Washington, D.C.: U.S. Government Printing Office, 1970.
3 National Council on Crime and Delinquency, *Standard Juvenile Court Act*, 6th ed., New York, 1959.
4 S. Norman, "The Youth Service Bureau," in National Council on Crime and Delinquency, *Standard Juvenile Court Act*, 6th ed., New York, 1959.
5 U.S. Department of Health, Education, and Welfare, Office of Youth Development, *Juvenile Court Statistics for 1973*. Washington, D.C., 1975.
6 D. C. Gibbon, *Delinquent Behavior*. Englewood Cliffs, N.J.: Prentice-Hall, 1970.
7 U.S. Congressional Record, *Bayh Juvenile Justice and Delinquency Prevention Act Extension*, March 17, 1977, Vol. 123, No. 47, 95th Congress, 1st Session.
8 *Juvenile Crime in Colorado, 1975*, Law Enforcement Assistance Administration, Region VIII statistical report compiled by Juvenile Specialist Carl Hamm, 1976.
9 U.S. Congressional Record, op. cit.
10 Montefiore Hospital and Medical Center Program at Juvenile Center, New York City, December 1971.
11 Ibid.
12 Medical Statistical Survey for Youth Services, "A Health Study of 132 Detained Youth," conducted by E. Fitzpatrick, Denver, 1974.

13   Census of Children's Residential Institutions in the United States, Puerto Rico and the Virgin Islands, 1966, conducted by D. M. Pappenfort and D. M. Kilpatrick, Vols. 1 and 7, Social Service Monographs 2d Series, School of Social Service Administration, University of Chicago, 1970.
14   Committee on Youth, American Academy of Pediatrics, "Health Standards for Juvenile Court Residential Facilities," *Pediatrics*, **52**:452– 457, September 1973.
15   Ibid.
16   R. E. Cushman and R. F. Cushman, *Cases in Constitutional Law*, 3d ed. New York: Appleton-Century-Crofts, 1968.

BIBLIOGRAPHY

Baum, Frederic S., and Frederick B. Sussman: *Law of Juvenile Delinquency*, 3d ed. Dobbs Ferry, N.Y.: Oceana Publications, 1968.

Birch, H. C., and J. D. Gussow: *Disadvantaged Children: Health, Nutrition and School Failure*. New York: Harcourt, Brace and World, 1970.

Blount, J. H., W. W. Darrow, and R. E. Johnston: "Venereal Disease in Adolescents," *Pediatric Clinics of North America*, **20**:1021–1033, November 1973.

Breslow, Lewter: "Some Essentials in a National Program for Child Health: A Summary," *Pediatric Clinics of North America*, **16**:909–913, November 1969.

Children in Custody—Advance Report on the Juvenile Detention and Correctional Facility Census of 1972–1973, U.S. Department of Justice, LEAA, National Criminal Justice Information and Statistic Service, Washington, D.C., 1975.

Coffey, Alan R.: *Juvenile Corrections: Treatment and Rehabilitations*. Englewood Cliffs, N.J.: Prentice-Hall, 1975.

Cole, Larry: *Our Children's Keepers: Inside America's Kid Prisons*. New York: Grossman Publishers, 1972.

Conger, John J.: *Adolescence and Youth*. New York: Harper and Row, 1973.

Fine, L. L.: "What's a Normal Adolescent? A Guide to the Assessment of Adolescent Behavior," *Clinical Pediatrics*, **12**:1, January 1973.

Gemignani, Robert J.: *Youth Services System, Diverting Youth from the Juvenile Justice System*, U.S. Department of Health, Education, and Welfare, Youth Development and Delinquency Prevention Administration, Washington, D.C., July-August 1972.

Hubbard, C. W.: *Family Planning Education: Parenthood and Social Disease Control*. St. Louis: C. V. Mosby Co., 1973.

James, Howard: *Children in Trouble*. New York: The Christian Science Publishing Society, 1970.

———: *The Little Victims: How America Treats Its Children*. New York: David McKay Co., 1975.

Kramer, J. P.: "The Adolescent Addict: The Progression of Youth Throughout the Drug Culture," *Clinical Pediatrics*, **11**:382, July 1972.

Litt, S., and M. Cohen: "Prisons, Adolescents and the Right to Quality Medical Care," *American Journal of Public Health*, **64**:894, 1974.

McAnarney, Elizabeth, and McAveney, William J.: "The Adolescent and the Pediatrician: Their Future Together," *Clinical Pediatrics*, **16**(2):169–172, February 1977.

McCandless, B. R.: *Adolescent Behavior and Development*. Hinsdale, Ill.: Dryden Press, 1970.

Mitford, Jessica: *Kind and Unusual Punishment: The Prison Business*. New York: Alfred A. Knopf, 1973.

"A Model Act Providing for Consent of Minors for Health Services," Report of the Committee on Youth, American Academy of Pediatrics, *Pediatrics*, **51**:293, February 1973.

Noshpitz, J. D.: "The Antisocial or Asocial Adolescent," *Clinical Proceedings of Children's Hospital of the District of Columbia*, **27**:138, April 1971.

———: "Drugs and Adolescence," *Clinical Proceeding of Children's Hospital of the District of Columbia*, **27**:138, April 1971.

Pappenfort, Donnell, Dee Morgan Kilpatrick, and Robert W. Roberts: *Child Caring: Social Policy and the Institution*. Chicago: Aldine Publishing Co., 1973.

The Pediatric Clinics of North America, "Symposium on Behavioral Pediatrics," **22**:3, August 1975.

Ross, D. C., and D. C. Ross, Jr.: "Youthful Alienation and Social Mobility, A Re-evaluation of the Whole Social Mobility Ethos Is Urgently Needed," *Clinical Pediatrics*, **12**:22–27, January 1973.

Sternlieb, J. J., and L. Munan: "A Survey of Health Problems, Practices, and Needs of Youth," *Pediatrics*, **49**:177–186, February 1972.

"Teenage Pregnancy and the Problem of Abortion," Report of the Committee on Youth, American Academy of Pediatrics, *Pediatrics*, **49**:303, February 1972.

"Venereal Disease and the Pediatrician," Report of the Committee on Youth, American Academy of Pediatrics, *Pediatrics*, **50**:492, September 1972.

Chapter 21

Nursing of Adolescents in a Psychiatric Inpatient Setting

Phyllis J. Baldwin
Sally A. Julien

The primary task of adolescence is to cope with the onset of puberty and to make the transition from childhood to adulthood. Perhaps the most arduous aspect of this task is dealing with the rapidity of body changes stimulated by internal forces over which the adolescent has little control.

As the biochemical changes of puberty stimulate the development of secondary sex characteristics, the libidinal concerns of childhood resurface. The adolescent becomes preoccupied with dependency need satisfaction: the need for approval, control over aggressive and sexual impulses, and the struggle for autonomy and independence and for a psychosexual identity. While these needs and concerns were previously resolved and mastered in regard to the realities of childhood, they now must be reworked in preparation for adulthood. In the face of such physical and psychic tension, the adolescent ego must provide protection from anxiety, control unacceptable impulses, and act as agent and ally in the realignment of body image and relationships with family, peers, and society.

Where the body was experienced as good and efficient in childhood, adolescents, because of rapid growth and weight redistribution, experience the body as too big, too small, gangly, inept, and unattractive. In the latency phase, the child, unbothered by sexual drives and instincts, developed family and peer relationships that allowed comfortable patterns of dependence and independence. Adolescents must learn to manage a renewed rise in drive tensions from within the self which alters these patterns. Weighing family norms against peer norms, adolescents must balance their responses to both and compete for individual acceptance without suffering alienation. They find themselves in league and in competition with peers as they test their own progress in physical and social maturation. Finally, at puberty young people must come to grips with genital sexuality. To do this adolescents must accept gender identity and transfer object love previously lodged with the mother or father to potential, nonincestuous sources of sexual gratification.

Watching the young person traverse the difficulties of adolescence commands awe and respect. At perhaps no other point in the human life span will the ego structure undergo a more rigorous test of strength and integrity. During this time all defense mechanisms and maneuvers will be utilized to achieve satisfactory adjustments in the transition from child to adult.

The degree of psychic energy available for adolescent task mastery depends on the degree to which developmental conflicts were mastered in earlier phases. If there was an unsatisfactory resolution of these at an earlier period, the adolescent must either abandon the work of adolescence in favor of the preadolescence conflict resolution or attempt mastery at both levels, which is apt to result in overwhelming ego stress.

It is easy to appreciate the difficulties experienced by young people who are propelled into adolescence by the physical maturation process but whose egos are not sufficiently mature to protect and assist them. Such adolescents typically have difficulty controlling aggressive impulses, exhibit signs of anxiety and confusion, rely heavily on reality testing, and show immature responses to other people and the environment. It is such troubled youngsters who are seen in the inpatient adolescent treatment programs throughout the country and for whom the therapeutic services offered there are critical. Whatever resolutions and growth can be achieved will be incorporated into the adult personality. Failure in this regard results in a marred ego which will remain vulnerable to anxiety and stress throughout adulthood.

In view of the critical importance of the successful negotiation of adolescence, the negative impact of emotional failure on the ego structure, and the implications for the person's ability to function as an adult, all knowledge and resources must be mobilized to help the emotionally disturbed adolescent achieve successful resolution of conflicts and devel-

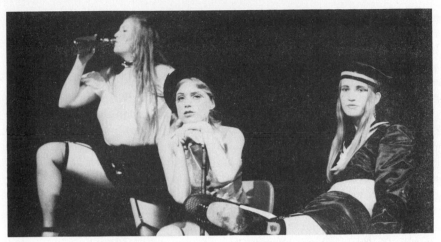

Nurses must understand behavior in order to apply the nursing process effectively. Adolescents' behavior, enigmatic at times, nevertheless conforms to laws of behavioral science. (*Copyright © 1980 by Anne Campbell.*)

opmental tasks. This is so not only because of the intrinsic human dignity of the person, but for ecological and economic reasons as well.

Society is wrestling with multiple social problems: the breakdown of the family, the increase in violent crime, human wastage through alcoholism and drug dependency, unemployment, and ever-increasing welfare rolls. The economic drain on society to support its dependent and deviant members is causing public outcry. At a time when inflation erodes the taxpayers' ability to meet their own health, education, and welfare requirements, the average citizen has little ability to recognize and respond to the needs of the poor and ill. Economic pressures on health professionals to provide cost-effective care have never been greater. These pressures have led not only to increasing governmental insistence on quality care standards and documentation but to the development of alternate forms of care as well.

Community-based mental health counseling, brief hospitalization, and reliance on psychotropic medications to control and inhibit the manifest symptoms of psychiatric illness are being recommended as alternatives to the more traditional and conservative forms of psychiatric treatment. Indeed, state psychiatric hospital beds are steadily being phased out as a result of rising costs and shrinking budget allocations. Patients previously cared for by these agencies for chronic mental health problems are now flooding community mental health centers and other community agencies whose budgets are equally unable to provide adequate service. Although alternate approaches to mental illness, while potentially promising, have failed to produce documentably better care for the psychiatrically ill, the professionals of adolescent inpatient treatment programs must rise to the challenge of demonstrating the efficacy of inpatient services or face budgetary extinction. The latter will result in loss of necessary services to adolescents and their families. To document their services effectively, professionals must demonstrate in process and outcome that the patient's health status has been positively affected by the concentrated inpatient treatment services. Further, it needs to be demonstrated that the progress noted during the period of hospitalization can be sustained within the patient's home and community.

The starting point of such documentation is a precise diagnostic assessment of each patient's health and pathology. With a working hypothesis of the origins and dynamics of an individual's psychiatric problems, the interdisciplinary team has a baseline on which to construct effective treatment strategies. To the degree this can be accomplished, nursing can identify the meaning and purpose of behavior in order to plan and initiate corrective milieu experiences.

The fundamental characteristic of therapeutic care is that its actions are *purposeful*. In all phases of the nursing process, from assessment through planning, intervention, and evaluation, psychiatric nursing care must be based on knowledge. Nursing care that is not based on knowledge will be reactive, purposeless, and custodial.

Psychiatric nurses must be well grounded in the behavioral sciences, particularly normal growth and development and theories of psychopathology. They must view themselves as more than parent surrogates, teachers, or friends; they should view themselves as essentially behavioral scientists. Working from the nursing assessment and diagnostic formulation, psychiatric nurses must initiate purposeful interventions and evaluate patients' behavioral response to the interventions. Interventions that fail to produce the expected adaptational response must be modified.

THE THERAPEUTIC MILIEU

Whether an adolescent inpatient unit is located in a large medical center or near a peaceful country lake, it must have certain characteristics in order to successfully treat disturbed adolescents. The living environment must be safe, comfortable, and suitable for adolescent activities of daily living.

Every effort should be made to ensure that the adolescent's need for privacy and an individualized living space is respected. Although this is more difficult to achieve on a unit with large wards or dormlike rooms, the arrangement of furniture and the use of posters, photos, and art work displays can serve to demarcate personal space, create a sense of privacy, and humanize an otherwise sterile environment. Within reason, adolescents should be encouraged to bring meaningful possessions from home.

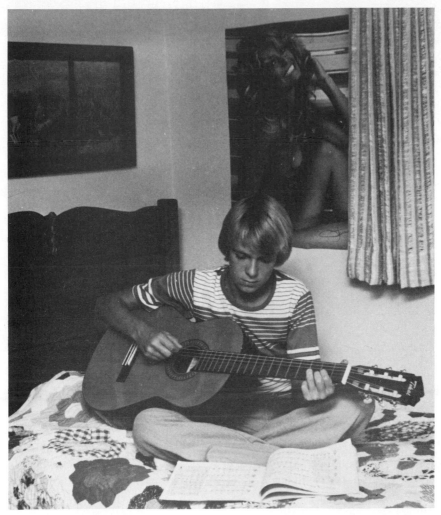

A personalized hospital environment and appropriate responsibility for it can facilitate normality and health. *(Copyright © 1980 by Patricia Yaros.)*

Items such as musical instruments, favorite games, or personal recreational equipment allow the adolescent continuity with home and encourage individual skill development during the period of hospitalization. An adequate supply of recreational resources and equipment should be available to adolescent patients for the appropriate expression of creative and aggressive tensions.

Treatment staff should encourage the appropriate development of the adolescent's sense of responsibility to himself or herself, the other inpatients, and the environment. Expectations must be stressed that the inpatients help to keep their environment as clean and well repaired as is reasonable. The individuals' rooms should be kept clean, beds should be made, and clothing should be laundered and kept in good repair. If some patients are periodically unable to manage these tasks alone, perhaps because of their depression or inability to organize around a task, staff should help them do so. As the adolescent cleans a room with a member of the nursing staff, or together they fix a chair broken during an emotional outburst, the patient learns not only the satisfaction of personal organization and the gratification of work accomplished but also the warmth of doing things together.

Common areas on the unit must also be kept in a livable state. Although the unit may have a housekeeping staff, the patients and staff should be expected to clean up after themselves. Furniture or equipment that is broken must be fixed, as often as possible by the person who caused the breakage, with the help of the staff when necessary. This provides an excellent opportunity for adolescents to take responsibility for their actions and achieve a corrective emotional experience in the management of guilt.

The inpatient adolescent unit must ensure each patient's physical safety. Simultaneously, the goal must be to protect the health and welfare of those patients unable to protect themselves and to set high expectations that adolescent patients assume responsibility for and control over their own behavior. The best method of achieving these goals is by providing adequate numbers of caring staff members who will establish behavioral limits and support the adolescents' adaptational efforts.

The milieu exists to provide the adolescent with a "proving ground" to test strengths and reveal weaknesses in the presence of staff members who recognize the adolescent's need to establish control over his or her life and who will provide support and assistance as needed.

A patient's loss of behavioral control should be viewed as a temporary problem. The therapeutic objective is to help the patient establish active control over his or her affects and impulses as quickly as possible. The use of tranquilizing medication or seclusion from caring adults in the environment will frequently increase the adolescent's sense of isolation and helplessness. Physical holding techniques, on the other hand, can be used effectively to protect and control unacceptable behavior without subjecting the patient to the prolonged effects of medication or the dehumanization of seclusion.

The consistent realistic use of rules and limit-setting helps provide a sense of security within the patient group. This decreases the adolescent's need to test limits and allows the patient's energy to be applied toward accomplishing desired change.

Consistent rules and regulations of living that consider the needs of both patients and staff add to the effectiveness of the unit. Such policies should be based on sound principles of clinical care rather than on the staff's convenience. While rules are essential, too many rules in a treatment setting will produce a regimented atmosphere that is not conducive to the expression of individuality or creativity within the milieu. Such conditions are apt to provoke natural rebellion in adolescents already prone to acting-out behaviors.

The interpersonal atmosphere should be geared to enhancing the strengths and functional abilities of its residents. Not only must the nursing staff be emotionally stable themselves, but they must be able to engage in a therapeutic relationship and to role model successful personal and interactional styles. They must be aware of their own strengths and sensitivities and should have some distance from and insight into their own adolescent experience. Without such distance and insight the staff member can easily overidentify with the adolescent and unwittingly participate in the patient's pathological dynamics.

It is important that the staff be comprised of a balanced proportion of men and women. Adolescents by nature are seeking sexual role models with whom to identify and to emulate. The dress, deportment, habits, and values of the staff members will be critically scrutinized and then rejected or incorporated in relation to the pathological or adaptational significance they present to the adolescent patients.

Activities and school programs are the major ego interests of the adolescent. Creative and coordinated school and activity programs are intrinsic to the inpatient adolescent program. They not only provide academic and social opportunities for the adolescent patient, but also create a predictable daily structure, which is helpful to the adolescent struggling with internal confusion.

Activity and school programs must be viewed as an integral part of the patient's individualized treatment program. To the greatest extent possible, such programs should be tailored to remedy identified social, physical, and academic deficits and to motivate the patient to achieve his or her fullest potential.

Many disturbed adolescents have experienced failure both in learning and in social interactions. Many find the structured, individualized approach of the inpatient school an exhilarating experience. Jerry, a 16-year-old male who had trouble finishing projects or assignments, is an example.

> Jerry feared the results of his work would be less than perfect. Midway through a four-week film class, in which he was the director, it became apparent to him that the quality of acting within the film was not going to win any awards. He became discouraged and began to cut classes, saying that the whole thing was "boring." Jerry's treatment team insisted that he continue his work on the film, and the film instructor began to teach him about editing. To his delight, his mistakes ended up on the cutting room

floor, and the finished product met his expectations. Thus, he learned that mistakes could be corrected and experienced a valuable success.

There should be room in the school curriculum for traditional academic courses, vocational classes, and specialized instruction. Short learning modules of perhaps six or eight weeks on such subjects as photography, ecology, poetry, and creative writing provide an opportunity for the teaching staff to provide an innovative and meaningful curriculum for an individual patient or patient group. Further, the academic and activity programs should not only offer opportunity for individual learning and skill mastery but also respond to the adolescent's need for peer group identity and interaction. Thus, activities that require group cohesion and cooperation for goal achievement should be encouraged in the program curriculum. Camping expeditions, canoeing classes, intramural sports, and school plays are a few examples.

Carefully planned evening and weekend activity programs offer the adolescent opportunities to channel physical and emotional energies into constructive activity, provide personal enrichment, and provide extended opportunity for corrective mastery of personal and interpersonal conflicts. Such programs should reflect the interests and involvement of the patients themselves. When adolescents share responsibility for their activities, they become personally invested in their successful outcomes. If, on the other hand, adults are seen as controlling the activities, the adolescent will respond to the person or adult rather than to the intrinsic appeal of the activity.

The adolescent's inpatient experience should include meaningful contact with the community at large. This decreases the feeling of isolation and abandonment that many adolescents experience during hospitalization. Such activities dispel the stigma of being a "psychiatric patient." As one adolescent so aptly put it, "I feel less like a 'crazy' when I'm at a football game with the group."

Individual patients or patient groups may be encouraged to volunteer their services in community service programs that appeal to the humanitarian and idealistic nature of the adolescent, such as a gerontology center, the humane society, or an ecology center. Patients who are ready to assume limited personal responsibility may be encouraged to attend classes at the YWCA or YMCA. Those ready to assume greater responsibility may be encouraged to attend public school.

THE ADMISSION PROCESS

Patient Selection and Admission Screening

Any treatment program should develop a set of admission criteria to guide its decisions regarding admissions. To do this the treatment program must consider its treatment capabilities, the type of program and services it

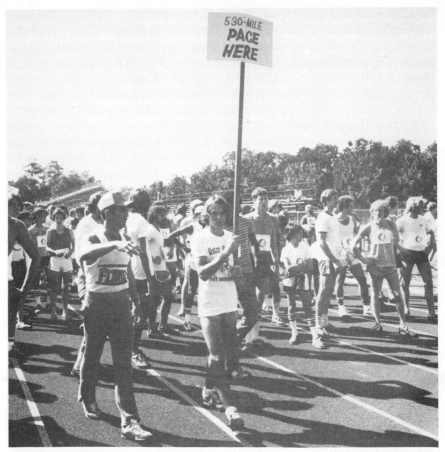

Inpatients should interact with well people in the community to help normalize behavior and diminish self-labeling as psychiatrically ill. (*Copyright © 1980 by Anne Campbell.*)

purports to deliver, and the types of patients who will benefit from its physical and program structure. It should determine the number of patients who can be accommodated for diagnostic evaluation, for short-term therapy, and for long-term treatment.

No treatment program is fully prepared to deal with every type of psychiatric problem. Each program usually has a philosophy of treatment or is structured around the treatment capabilities of its staff. Some units are psychoanalytic in orientation; others use a behavior modification framework; others are oriented toward short-term treatment. Regardless of the philosophy and treatment framework, patients should be selected for admission in accordance with their predicted ability to benefit from the services available.

The availability of adequate clinical personnel is a critical factor to be weighed when considering new admissions. There must be adequate nursing resources to provide intensive care of those patients requiring close supervision, as well as to provide general care and activity options to those patients ready to resume more normalized activities of daily living. To fail in the provision of both types of care is apt to jeopardize the safety of the more disturbed patients and frustrate the healthier population to regress and act out to win the time and attention of the staff.

Thus, the admission team must ask themselves: What level of care does the admission candidate require? Can such care be provided without jeopardizing the care of the patient population currently residing on the unit? To have large numbers of psychotic patients, sociopathic patients, drug abusers, or suicidal patients on the unit at the same time courts adolescent gang formation, wherein one patient's pathology supports that of another and peer reinforcers overpower those of the treatment program. This dynamic jeopardizes the corrective living milieu, robs patients of the motivation to change behavior, and consumes enormous amounts of staff energy in policing the patients and their activities.

Preadmission Home Visit

Patients and families anticipating psychiatric hospitalization experience three sources of anxieties: (1) those normally associated with hospitalization, (2) those related to internal feelings of guilt and failure, and (3) those related to the general myths and fantasies about the nature of psychiatric hospitalization.

The significance any individual attaches to psychiatric hospitalization will to some extent be related to his or her view of the nature of the patient's problem and the degree to which he or she feels responsible for the problem experienced. Parents of inpatient adolescents frequently view hospitalization as a sign of their own impotence and failure to adequately meet the needs of their child. From the adolescent's perspective, hospitalization can represent the ultimate parental punishment for misbehavior.

The anxiety generated by such internal feelings of failure and guilt is apt to be compounded by the rampant myths and fantasies regarding the nature of psychiatric hospitalization and treatment. The public stereotypes created by popular literature and cinema such as *The Three Faces of Eve*, *The Snake Pit*, *Beyond the Looking Glass*, and *I Never Promised You a Rose Garden* evoke degrading, demeaning, and violent images. Sensitive nursing support during the preadmission period can provide a helpful and welcome opportunity for the patient and the family to deal with the realities of pending hospitalization.

A preadmission home visit offers the patient and family early contact with nursing staff and establishes a supportive relationship that will continue during the transition from home to hospital. It is a vehicle by which the patient and family may receive information that will help allay their fears.

The purpose of the nurse's home visit is twofold: (1) to allay the anxiety of the patient and family regarding pending hospitalization and (2) to gather nursing data in preparation for the patient's admission to the treatment program.

Ordinarily, arrangements for the home visit should be made by the nurse who will be the most directly responsible for the patient's care within the treatment milieu. The visit should be planned to occur at a time when the entire family can be present. The nurse who initiates contact with the parents in setting up the preadmission home visit should provide a simple explanation about the nature and purpose of the visit.

In preparing for the preadmission home visit, the nurse should read all available information on the nature and circumstances of the teenager's problem which have led to the decision in favor of hospitalization. The nurse should also gather specific information regarding the admission: date, time, room assignment, and school placement. Finally, a preadmission home visit folder should be compiled containing maps and directions to the home, home phone number, hospital patient information booklet, nursing assessment outline, health history form, pencil and paper, and other necessary items.

As can be expected, the first few minutes of the interview are the most awkward. Parents are typically concerned about the tidiness of the house and that common courtesies are extended to the strangers. Commonly, the parents make family introductions spontaneously; however, the nurse must be cognizant of signs of anxiety. Occasionally parents lose their composure and forget to introduce family members or to direct the interviewers to be seated. If necessary, the nurse should make discreet inquiries, for example, ''Are you Jane's brother?'' or ''Where would you prefer to visit?''

The identified patient will sometimes refuse to participate in the interview and stay in his or her bedroom or in the family room. For this reason we prefer to schedule two staff persons to participate in the home visit: one to conduct the interview with the family and the other to initiate contact with the patient on an individual basis. In such a fashion, the nursing staff are able to demonstrate their interest and concern for both without prejudice. In the treatment of adolescents this is of prime importance, since alliance with the parents is apt to be construed by the patient as an alliance against the adolescent.

One of the best ways for the nurse to break the ice with the entire family is to engage their common interest: What will the hospital be like? Pictures of the unit give concrete reassurance and dispel troublesome fantasies. They also provide a natural springboard for discussion about the daily living routines of the treatment milieu.

The nurse should inform the patient and family about the organizational operation of the unit and the policies that govern the patients participating in the program. The major interest will center on visiting privileges, mail, phone calls, and so on. However, the nurse should also respond to the unasked questions: Who will take care of the adolescent at night? Who will provide care if he or she becomes ill? When and under what circumstances will the parents be informed of illness or injury? How will, for example, orthodontic follow-up be arranged? Will the adolescent ever be placed in isolation or restraint? It is our belief that the use of restraints and isolation should be discussed openly. The patient and family should be told the truth, that out-of-control behavior jeopardizes not only the patient but the safety of other patients and staff as well. Such discussion will provoke anxiety, but this can be offset by further discussion of the criteria for using restraints and isolation, precautions that are taken to protect the patient, the degree of care and supervision provided to patients in restraints and isolation, and the benefits that can accrue from the application of such techniques.

Of equal importance to alleviating anxiety surrounding the hospitalization experience is the nursing assessment component of the home visit interview. Rather than risk inadvertent omission of important nursing data, and in order to systematize the assessment content, we have developed an assessment guide for the nurse to use during the home visit. This can be used as necessary to direct the interview discussion or to jog the memory if the content is not covered spontaneously. The assessment guide can be found in Table 21-1.

Because we expect the nurse to write a formal home visit summary and to use the interview data to design a nursing care plan prior to admission, we encourage the nurse to make notations during the interview. While some nurses feel uncomfortable making such notations in the presence of the patient and family, we encourage them to legitimize this action with the family rather than trust vital information to memory. Usually a simple statement regarding the importance of the information in preparing for the patient's admission will appeal to the patient and family because of its demonstrated interest in the individuality of the patient.

The nursing assessment usually covers the patient's current activities of daily living, the patient's physical health status, and the patient's relationship abilities. During this portion of the interview, care must be taken that the patient be given the opportunity to speak for himself or herself, without jeopardizing the contribution of the parents and siblings.

The nurse must be prepared to guide and direct the interview in such a fashion that neither the patient nor the family are overly protected,

Table 21-1 Preadmission Assessment Guide

I. Activities of Daily Living
A. A.M. Wake-Up
1. What time does patient rise in A.M.?
2. Mood and routine upon waking?
3. To what degree is patient self-sufficient in regard to hygiene and grooming?
4. To what degree is patient responsible for own room and personal belongings?

B. Eating Habits
1. Nature of appetite?
2. Mealtimes in home? (time and social climate)
3. Snacking habits?
4. Attitude toward eating and mealtimes?
5. Food preferences and/or idiosyncracies?
6. Food allergies?
7. Family table rules?
8. Overt signs of repetition, compulsions, or phobias involving food?

C. Hygiene and Grooming
1. Any unique hygiene needs, such as daily hair washing, special shampoos, lotions?
2. Shower vs. bath preference?
3. Bathing frequency?
4. Shaving
    (a) *Boys*: facial (frequency; type of razor)
    (b) *Girls*: axillary and legs (frequency; type of razor)
5. Degree of interest in appearance?
6. Overt manifestations of repetition, compulsions, or phobias involving hygiene?

D. Toilet Patterns
1. Presence of encopresis or enuresis? If so, at what frequency? Under what circumstances? How managed in the home?

E. Bedtime
1. Usual bedtime?
2. Usual activities in preparation for bed? (e.g., reads self to sleep; watches TV)
3. Is patient responsible for going to bed at expected time, or is this a point of contention in family?
4. Sleep patterns? Does patient sleep lightly? Deeply? Episodically? Poorly?
5. Does patient experience nightmares, bad dreams? How frequently?
6. Does patient use a night light or other sleep aids?
7. Does patient use sleeping pills?
8. Does patient sleepwalk?
9. Does patient ever sleep in other than own bed?
10. Does patient share room with a sibling or other family member?
11. Does patient share a bed with a sibling or other family member?

II. Physical Status
A. Speech and Verbal Communication
1. How verbally expressive is patient?
2. Can patient be depended on to articulate wants and needs?
3. Any known speech impediments?
4. Any evidence of immature speech modes, e.g., baby talk?

Table 21-1   Preadmission Assessment Guide (*Continued*)

  B. Hearing
    1. Any known hearing deficits?
    2. Any hearing aids required?
    3. Does patient use selective hearing? How frequently? Cite example.

  C. Vision
    1. Any known visual problems?
    2. Glasses or other visual aids?

  D. Nutritional State
    1. Is patient within normal weight for age and height?
    2. If overweight, have diets been tried in past? What is patient and family perception of this problem?
    3. If underweight or overweight, how concerned are patient and family?
    4. Is patient taking vitamins? Why? What kind?

  E. Elimination
    1. Any persistent difficulty with constipation and/or diarrhea? If so, how is this treated in the home? Medicines, enemas?
    2. Any past history of colitis, urinary tract infections, kidney disease?

  F. Reproduction
    1. Girls—have they begun menses? How regular is menstrual cycle? Does patient experience cramping, excessive flow?
    2. Boys—degree of secondary sex development: voice change, facial hair, axillary hair, wet dreams?
    3. Has patient received basic sex education? From whom? To what degree does patient understand conception, birth?
    4. Is patient sexually active? Is patient knowledgeable about birth control? If sexually active, is patient using birth control methods?
    5. Does patient engage in masturbatory activities? How discreet is patient with these?

  G. Motor Abilities
    1. Any difficulties with coordination and/or balance?
    2. To what degree does patient enjoy gross motor activities?
    3. Any difficulties with fine motor coordination?

  H. Previous Health History
    1. Past childhood illnesses?
    2. Immunization history?
    3. Past medical illness/trauma?
    4. Any recurrent illnesses?
    5. Any known allergies? How treated?
    6. Any health problems patient would like to bring to the doctor's attention during the admission physical?
    7. Name, address, and telephone of attending physician?
    8. Mental status?

III. **Relationship Abilities**
  A. Peer Relationships
    1. Does patient have many friends of the same sex/opposite sex? If so, how frequently does patient see friends?
    2. Favorite games or interests pursued with peers?

   3. What is interactional mode? Shy? Outgoing? Aggressive? Imitative? Isolative?

   4. Any difficulties in peer relationships? If so, cite specifics.

B. Relationship to Self

   1. Is patient responsive to rules of safety and health?

   2. Has patient exhibited suicidal gestures? If so, cite examples.

   3. Does patient drink, smoke, take drugs?

C. Relationship to Adults

   1. What is nature of parent-child relationship? Argumentative? Obstinate? Passive? Silent? Dependent?

   2. Does patient have any significant relationships with other adults? Describe.

   3. What is nature of teacher-child relationship? Does patient have record of truancy, delinquency, or difficulty with the court? Describe.

   4. What are patient's modes of reaction to frustration, disappointment, positive achievement?

   5. What modes of discipline are used by parents? Are they successful in deterring unacceptable behavior?

---

scapegoated, or excluded. Since portions of the nursing assessment can best be answered by the patient, by the parents, or by a combination of both, the interview can be structured to enhance such communication. The patient can be given latitude to answer the questions related to activities of daily living, with the interviewer seeking parental validation. The parents can be acknowledged as the legitimate source of information on the patient's physical health history. Both the patient and family can be relied on to supply information related to the patient's interactional and social skills.

Usually at some point in the interview one of the nursing staff will go with the patient to his or her room. Whether this is initiated by the patient or staff, the adolescent will generally respond in a shy but positive fashion to this gesture of interest. The staff can use this opportunity to discuss in greater detail those things that may and should be brought to the hospital on admission. It is also a unique opportunity to have a more intimate discussion with the patient about worries and concerns that he or she may be reluctant to verbalize in the presence of parents.

Such individual time with the patient also makes possible a similar discussion with the parents. In view of the adolescent's sensitivity to questions of a sexual nature, this may be the only opportune time the nurse can ask questions regarding the patient's physical maturation status without causing embarrassment to the adolescent. In addition, it may be the only time the parents have to speak candidly on discipline matters. It is important that the nurse remain nonjudgmental as he or she inquires about the disciplinary approaches the parents have used in the past and their relative success or failure. Such information is vital to the management plan for the patient within the hospital, and such information will not be forthcoming without the support and sensitivity of the interviewing nurse.

In summary, the entire home visit interview must be structured and guided to increase the comfort and receptivity of the patient and family. To this end, nurses must divorce themselves from their own moral and cultural biases and immerse themselves in those of the patient and family. Nurses must feel free to be guided by the verbal and nonverbal cues of the family, probing gently but firmly for the information necessary to complete a preliminary nursing care plan.

There are times when a preadmission home visit is not feasible. If the patient's admission occurs under emergency circumstances, if the adolescent has already been separated from his or her family, or if the parents refuse to participate in the patient's treatment, a preadmission/admission interview should be substituted for the home visit.

Like the home visit, the preadmission/admission interview should be formally structured both to provide the patient with information about the milieu and the treatment program and to acquire that information vital to the planning of his or her care.

Patient Orientation to the Hospital Milieu

The adolescent's first hours on the inpatient unit should receive careful nursing attention. The patient's initial impressions of the nursing staff as sources of comfort and protection will be positively or negatively affected by the welcome and care he or she receives during these early hours.

Hospitalization not only subjects the adolescent to a strange and frightening environment but also thrusts him or her into a microcosmic society of which he or she is the newest member. Further, the adolescent generally enters into this experience not by choice but by coercion. Thus, the admission itself will generate in the adolescent patient numerous and conflicting affects, such as fear, anger, guilt, shame, and a secret sense of relief.

The nursing staff must be prepared to greet the patient promptly upon his or her arrival on the unit. The first order of business should be to show the patient and family the patient's room and to help unpack and settle personal belongings. Following this, the nursing staff should introduce the newly admitted adolescent to the other patients and staff on the unit. Often more experienced patients are very sensitive to the new patient's apprehension and are eager to show the newly admitted adolescent the various rooms on the unit. Remarks like "It's not half bad around here once you get used to it" are often heard. This peer support often visibly reassures the newly admitted adolescent.

The patient should be briefed on the unit's daily routines shortly after admission. Awareness of bedtime, meal time, and wake-up time gives the adolescent an orientation and structure to relate to. A review of basic unit rules will help the adolescent anticipate and comply with the environmental expectations. Such knowledge may prevent the adolescent from unwittingly violating the unit norms and being reprimanded unnecessarily early in the hospital stay. Often the new patient's anxiety will interfere with his or her ability to retain verbal information. For this reason written lists and explanations of the unit rules and regulations are helpful and can serve as the patient's self-reference guide.

The new adolescent patient should be drawn into the mainstream of unit activity as soon as possible. The patient's participation in activities with other patients will enhance a sense of belonging and minimize the "new kid" identity. The nursing staff should inform the patient of activity options, verbally encourage his or her participation, and actively draw the patient into activities.

Planning and Delivery of Nursing Care

The adolescent patient should be encouraged to take an active role in the planning of his or her individual care. This involves the adolescent's sharing some responsibility with the rest of the treatment team for identifying problems, finding solutions to those problems, and setting realistic treatment goals. Unless adolescents are involved in the planning of their own treatment, a resistance can develop in which all the "well-intentioned" adults in the environment are locked in a struggle to change an adolescent who may not be interested in changing a particular piece of behavior at a given time. On the other hand, growth can be facilitated if the adolescent experiences the treatment team as sharing common goals with him or her and "being on his or her side" in the painful struggle toward adaptation.

Unless a patient's admission is predetermined to be brief for the purpose of situational crisis resolution, a designated time frame should be established by the team for the purpose of observation and assessment. All team members should be accountable for both general observation and the collection of more refined data that will be useful in making a diagnostic formulation. Nurses must deliberately use their time and energy to observe the patient in as wide a variety of activities and circumstances as possible.

Unless a patient is actively psychotic, it can be expected that a brief "honeymoon" period will occur, during which the patient will actively attempt to mask symptoms and deny the existence of emotional problems. This phenomenon can probably be accounted for as the mobilization of defenses against the heightened anxiety precipitated by hospitalization. The patient's honeymoon "flight into health" can be productively used by the nursing staff to identify overt defense mechanisms used by the

patient in the management of anxiety and to assess the adaptational efficiency of those defenses and the apparent ego strengths the patient has
drawn on in the management of anxiety.

As the patient's symptomatology emerges, nurses must be ready to
focus their observational skills on the patient's developmental status and
the nature of the symptomatology. Under what circumstances does acting-
out occur? What is the apparent purpose of the acting-out behavior? How
does the symptomatology correspond with that experienced prior to hospitalization? To what degree is the patient's functional ability affected?
Under what circumstances can the patient modify or control his or her
behavior? To what extent is the patient able to maintain age-appropriate
interests and tasks?

While it is the responsibility of the psychotherapist to develop a
diagnostic formulation, the observational contributions of the psychiatric
nurse will assist the psychotherapist in this task. The information gathered
will serve to support, modify, or contradict the diagnostic hypothesis until
the most accurate formulation can be achieved.

At the end of the diagnostic period, the psychotherapist should articulate to the treatment team the diagnostic formulation, the dynamics
of the patient's pathology, the meaning and purpose behind the symptomatology, and the broad therapeutic goals to be achieved to return the
patient to maximum functional ability. The nurse must use this information
to identify the clinical problems to be addressed in the nursing care plan
and the priority of interventions to be pursued.

Based on the theory that the quantity of psychic energy available to
a person is constant and that conflict "binds" psychic energy and thereby
decreases the amount of energy available for continued growth and mastery of the environment, the nurse should use the diagnostic formulation
to identify the strata of conflicts which bind the energies of the adolescent
and which decrease the adolescent's ability to master adolescent tasks.
The nurse should note where the individual has become fixated or re-
gressed in development, and that is where the thrust of nursing intervention
should be placed. With the resolution of such problems, the individual
will have freed energy to function at a higher level. When the nurse and
the milieu thus contribute to the patient's health and well-being, the nurse
can be said to have facilitated progress. Such progress can be documented
and the clinical interventions revised to address remaining problems until
the patient is able to manage living apart from the hospital setting.

Inpatient facilities frequently command equipment and resources generally unavailable to the average family. These serve as tools in the patient's milieu treatment. They must be used skillfully. Nursing staff should
rarely use activities and interpersonal experiences for the patient's en-

tertainment or diversion. Instead they must be used as opportunities to assist the patient in working out identified problems that interfere with adaptation and health.

For example, if a particular patient has unresolved oral conflicts that affect his ability to trust and interact, movies, arts and crafts, and dances, while otherwise age appropriate and "nice," will contribute little to the resolution of the patient's identified problems. Instead, engaging in cooking, eating, gardening, and nurturing of animals may more appropriately address the patient's identified needs, provide legitimate sources of gratification, provide new opportunities to identify and rework conflicts, and reduce anxiety. Professional knowledge and personal creativity must be focused on the design of interventions to be used in the patient's care.

The success of any given intervention will depend not only on the degree to which it corresponds to the patient's identified needs but also on the nurse's ability to manage the transference phenomenon as it arises in his or her relationship with the patient. *Transference* has been refined as a concept since its identification by Freud in his early work. Essentially it refers to the patient's re-creation of earlier developmental conflicts in the interaction with other significant adults. Usually it is an unconscious mechanism by which the patient engages in reality testing either to reconfirm the conflict as previously experienced or as a new opportunity to master and resolve the conflict.

If the transference phenomenon is to be managed as an opportunity to rework conflict, it is important that the nurse critically examine the affects the patient's behavior engenders in the nurse, scrutinize the behavioral dynamic, and respond not in retaliation but in a careful and reflective fashion. If, for example, the patient must be insulting and derogatory to put interpersonal distance between self and the nurse or to precipitate rejection as it was previously experienced, the nurse must have his or her affects and intellect well in hand or risk reacting with anger to the patient, and in thus reacting to the patient reconfirming the conflict dynamic. If instead the nurse can find acceptable ways of giving the patient interpersonal space, acknowledge the patient's affects, and remain emotionally available to the patient, the nurse is apt to thwart the conflict dynamic and supply the patient with a corrective emotional experience, an experience that the patient can retest, internalize, and build new adaptations on.

Since transference is an unconscious process, the nurse will need the assistance of an objective, supportive clinician who will help examine the patient's behavior and the affects engendered within the nurse. To the extent these are not openly shared by the nurse, his or her responses to the patient will be motivated by unconscious forces and may interfere

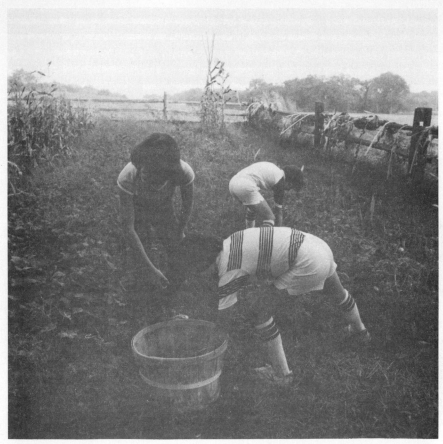

Activity programs are integral parts of inpatient treatment and should be designed to promote the development of interpersonal or personal skills and improved ways of coping with real-life situations. Insofar as possible, activities should be tailored to remedy identified social, physical, and academic deficits of each particular patient. (*Copyright © 1980 by Anne Campbell.*)

with the nurse's ability to make helpful and purposeful responses to the patient. Further, the transference and countertransference will rob the patient of the opportunity to learn new modes of behavior.

PRIMARY NURSING IN THE ADOLESCENT TREATMENT PROGRAM

With the development of humanistic trends in psychology and philosophy, increasing complaints regarding the delivery of health care services, and legislative pressure for documentation of quality care standards, the concept of *primary nursing care* is taking root as a method by which patient care can be coordinated, goal oriented, and monitored for quality.

Primary nursing or caretaking has been defined by Lodgson as "the nursing care provided to the patient by one nurse who plans with the patient the care that the patient and the nurse decide is needed—care that results from the coordination with other disciplines and collaboration with the primary physician."[1]

Pragmatically, this model of patient care makes the primary nurse responsible and accountable for the nursing care regimen including observation, assessment, planning, and execution of the nursing care to be delivered to specified patients. It is premised on a significant and consistent relationship with the patient; the relationship develops from direct patient contact.

Primary nursing offers definite advantages over the team nursing model. The team nursing model is premised on a lack of sufficient numbers of registered nurses to serve the needs of the unit population. The team then is generally composed of one or two RNs charged with the responsibilities of coordinating and supervising the care rendered by a group of lesser-trained personnel. This concept effectively removes the professional nurse from the patient and replaces her with lesser-trained personnel who are given daily patient assignments which match the needs of patients with the skill level of the team member. The patient's care and welfare are lodged with the nursing care team rather than specific persons. "When a patient is the responsibility of a group of people, he is no one's responsibility."[2]

The University of Michigan Adolescent Psychiatric Unit has adopted a primary nursing delivery system. In order to make the best use of nursing personnel and time, all primary nursing staff work permanent evening shifts. Smaller numbers of nursing staff are used to provide nursing coverage on the day and midnight shifts. These patterns are used because (1) school and activity therapy programs staffed by the respective disciplines provide the programmatic structure for patients during the day; (2) unstructured evening hours offer extensive opportunity for significant nursing staff-patient interaction and involvement; and (3) the midnight hours need only sufficient numbers of staff to manage occasional patient care problems. Accordingly, nursing staff patterns were established to provide appropriate nursing coverage for the unit census of 18 patients. These patterns may be found in Table 21-2.

To begin the transition to the primary nursing model, all nursing staff currently assigned to evenings were designated as either primary staff or back-up staff. The primary staff were then given permanent assignments to specific patients, and patient-staff modules were organized. The module configurations may be found in Figure 21-1. The objective of the primary

Table 21-2   Staffing Pattern Used to Ensure Maximum Staff-Patient Contact at the Times the Patients Are Most Available to Unit Staff

Shift	Census	Staff	Staff-patient ratio
Midnight	18	3 × 7 days	1:6
Days	18	3 × 5 days (M–F)	1:6
		6 × 2 days (weekends)	1:3
Evenings	18	8 × 5 days (M–F)	1:2.25
		7 × 2 days (weekends)	1:2.5

care model was to provide each patient with consistent caretakers and to lodge with those caretakers the responsibility for designing and implementing a nursing care plan reflective of the needs of these individual patients. To this end the functions of the primary staff were defined as:

1   Establish an effective therapeutic relationship with designated patients.
2   Formulate in writing and carry out a specific plan of care in consultation with the treatment team and psychotherapist.
3   Serve as a patient role model; structure activities and experiences to facilitate conflict resolution and/or adaptation and growth; provide affection and limit-setting in activities of daily living.
4   Provide teaching and counseling to patients about health care matters.
5   Participate in team conferences and communicate pertinent clinical information.
6   Maintain clinical records on the patient care given and the patient's response to care rendered.
7   Provide written progress summaries as requested.
8   Participate in weekly clinical supervision with the designated supervisor.

The role and responsibility of the back-up staff was to complement the primary staff. The back-up staff was charged with the responsibility of knowing and carrying out all facets of the plans and programs designed by the primary staff in that staff's absence. Back-up personnel's functional duties were defined as:

1   Establish an effective therapeutic relationship with designated patients.
2   Carry out the patient care plan as designed by the primary staff in the primary staff's absence.
3   Serve as a role model, source of affection, and source of limit-setting for patients in activities of daily living.
4   Participate in clinical supervision with designated supervisor.

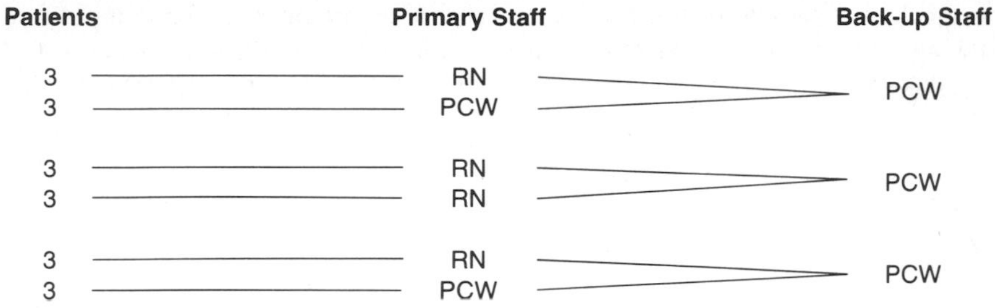

Patients	Primary Staff	Back-up Staff

3 ——————————— RN

3 ——————————— PCW   PCW

3 ——————————— RN

3 ——————————— RN   PCW

3 ——————————— RN

3 ——————————— PCW   PCW

Figure 21-1 Patient-staff groupings established for the evening shift. *Psychiatric care workers* (PCWs) are nonprofessional personnel whose minimal qualifications include high school graduation, effective written and spoken communication skills, and experience in dealing with people in an empathic way that demonstrates their suitability as healthy role models. In our setting many have had college work in such fields as special education, psychology, and social work. Psychiatric care workers are expected to function as patient role models, provide general supervision to ensure patients' safety and welfare, and implement the nursing and medical care plans.

It was envisioned that to make this patient care model work effectively, the primary and back-up staffs needed adequate time to discuss patient care issues and develop a complementary relationship. Moreover, effective clinical supervision needed to be provided in the management of intense patient-staff relationships and in the planning of creative nursing care approaches.

In order to meet the first requirement a staff schedule was structured to give staff the opportunity to work together and receive supervision on a planned weekly basis. An example of the scheduling pattern may be found in Table 21-3.

To meet the second requirement, to provide the nursing staff with expert nursing supervision and ongoing staff development, a clinical nurse specialist was employed. The clinical specialist works a flexitime schedule, which allows him or her to maximize visibility and involvement with the adolescent patients and the nursing staff.

It is the responsibility of the clinical nurse specialist to provide clinical leadership and expertise to the nursing staff involved with the adolescent patients by using his or her knowledge and expertise to promote current nursing practices, to facilitate creative and innovative nursing practice, and to foster the personal and professional growth of the nursing personnel. The clinical nurse specialist exercises these responsibilities by conducting formal and informal clinical supervision sessions, inservice and staff development programs, and unit orientation programs for new employees.

The clinical supervision provided by the clinical nurse specialist places its emphasis on the application and integration of clinical theory with the design, conduct, and evaluation of nursing intervention. Its purpose is to provide nursing service personnel with supportive direction in

Table 21-3   Sample Day-off Scheduling Pattern for Each of the Three Staff Modules Shown in Figure 21-1

	Staff schedule							
	S	S	M	T	W	T	F	S
Primary staff member	E	E	X	E	E	E	E	X
Primary staff member	E	E	E	E	E	E	X	E
Back-up staff member	X	X	E	E	E	X	E	E
Primary staff member	X	X	E	E	E	E	E	E
Primary staff member	E	E	X	E	E	E	E	X
Back-up staff member	E	E	E	X	E	E	X	E
Primary staff member	E	E	E	X	E	E	E	X
Primary staff member	E	E	E	E	E	E	X	X
Back-up staff member	X	X	E	E	X	E	E	E

E = Evening shift; X = Day off.

their clinical work and to monitor the quality of nursing care through the use of critical clinical inquiry.

Through careful organizational planning and proper clinical and administrative support, the primary nursing care model offers considerable promise as a delivery system that promotes optimal therapeutic care for adolescent patients. It facilitates the integration and continuity of care from preadmission to discharge. Finally, it creates a system of nursing care accountability, whereby nursing personnel critique and validate their practice and receive recognition on the basis of their clinical performance.

REFERENCES

1   A. Lodgson, "Why Primary Nursing?" *Nursing Clinics of North America*, 8(2):283–291, June 1973, p. 284.
2   M. Manthey et al., "Primary Nursing: A Return to the Concept of 'My Nurse' and 'My Patient,' " *Nursing Forum*, 9(1):64–83, 1970, pp. 72–73.

BIBLIOGRAPHY

Baker, A. A. (ed.): *Comprehensive Psychiatric Care*. London: Blackwell Scientific Publications, 1976.
Topalis, Mary, and Donna Aguilera: *Psychiatric Nursing* (7th ed.). St. Louis: C. V. Mosby, 1978.

Index